Measurement Procedures in Speech, Hearing, and Language

to
Professor John W. Black

MEASUREMENT PROCEDURES IN SPEECH, HEARING, AND LANGUAGE

Edited by **Sadanand Singh, Ph.D.**
Professor of Hearing and Speech Sciences
Ohio University School of Hearing and Speech Sciences

University Park Press
Baltimore • London • Tokyo

University Park Press
International Publishers in Science and Medicine
Chamber of Commerce Building
Baltimore, Maryland 21202

Copyright 1975 by University Park Press

Typeset in the United States by The Composing Room of Michigan
Printed in the United States by Universal Lithographers, Inc.

Library of Congress Cataloging in Publication Data
Main entry under title:
Measurement procedures in speech, hearing, and language.
    Includes index.
    1. Audiology—Technique. 2. Audiometry. 3. Speech—Physiological
    aspects. 4. Speech disorders in children. I. Singh, Sadanand. [DNLM: 1.
Hearing teats. 2. Language. 3. Speech. WV272 S617m]
RF294.M4   617.8'9'028   75-5791
ISBN 0-8391-0753-6

Contents

Contributors

Joseph G. Agnello, Ph.D.
Professor of Speech and Hearing
  Sciences
University of Cincinnati
Cincinnati, Ohio

Carl W. Asp, Ph.D.
Professor and Director
Aural Habilitation and Rehabilitation
Department of Audiology and
  Speech Pathology
University of Tennessee
Knoxville, Tennessee

John W. Black, Ph.D.
Professor of Speech
Ohio State University
Columbus, Ohio

Arthur J. Compton, Ph.D.
Research Speech and Language
  Pathologist
San Francisco Hearing and Speech
  Center
San Francisco, California

Malcolm H. Hast, Ph.D.
Professor and Director of Research
Department of Otolaryngology and
  Maxillofacial Surgery
The Medical School
Northwestern University
Evanston, Illinois

Robert B. Mahaffey, Ph.D.
Associate Professor

The Institute of Speech and Hearing
  Sciences
The University of North Carolina at
  Chapel Hill
Chapel Hill, North Carolina

Donald M. Morehead, Ph.D.
Associate Professor
Department of Child Development
California State University, Hayward
Hayward, California

Charles W. Nixon, Ph.D.
Chief, Biological Acoustics
Aerospace Medical Research
  Laboratory
Wright-Patterson Air Force Base
Dayton, Ohio

John J. O'Neill, Ph.D.
Professor and Head
Department of Speech and Hearing
  Science
University of Illinois
Champaign, Illinois

Herbert J. Oyer, Ph.D.
Professor, Audiology and Speech
  Sciences
Dean, College of Communication
  Arts
Michigan State University
East Lansing, Michigan

Robert Peters, Ph.D.
Professor and Director

Institute of Speech and Hearing
  Sciences
The University of North Carolina at
  Chapel Hill
Chapel Hill, North Carolina

Russell L. Sergeant, Ph.D.
Associate Professor
Communication Sciences Program
School of Health Science
Hunter College of the City University
  of New York
New York, New York

Jon K. Shallop, Ph.D.
Professor of Hearing and Speech
  Sciences
Ohio University
Athens, Ohio

Sadanand Singh, Ph.D. (Hindi), Ph.D.
  (Speech)
Professor of Hearing and Speech
  Sciences
Ohio University
Athens, Ohio

Yukio Takefuta, Ph.D.
Associate Professor
Chiba University
College of Education
Department of English
Chiba-ken 280, Japan;
Consultant, Ohio Department of
  Health
Columbus, Ohio

Oscar I. Tosi, Ph.D.
Professor and Director
Speech and Hearing Research
  Laboratory
Michigan State University
East Lansing, Michigan

Preface

The growth and maturation of a science depends on the extent of internal discipline exerted by the scientist in the field. The extent of the validity of a science is determined by the quality of measurement procedures perfected. Viewing a number of areas of hearing and speech it becomes clear that the last four decades of the acquisition of such a discipline have entitled the study of hearing and speech behaviors to be labeled a "science." This volume therefore represents an effort to describe some important methodological advances and their recent consequences in our field of study.

Fifteen chapters on the selected aspects of measurement procedures are included in this book. All authors had dual professional commitments in undertaking their assignments. First, they jointly felt the void of a text which would examine the quality of selected measurement procedures for the use of students and professionals in speech, hearing, and language sciences. The maturation of these areas of study demands an account of the prevalent measurement procedures employed at the data collection, analysis, interpretation, and implication stages. Second, they wished to dedicate this work to Professor John Wilson Black of the Ohio State University, who has participated in the perfection of the measurement procedures in hearing, speech, and language throughout the last four decades. He has ceaselessly conducted experiments, trained students, and influenced professional decisions in speech, hearing, and language. All contributors to this volume have studied under Professor Black.

The fifteen chapters have been organized in three sections: Language, Perception–Audition, and Production–Acoustics. Two chapters deal with language, eight chapters with perception and audition, and five chapters with production and acoustics.

The selection of the chapters within each section, as well as the intended readership of this book, is broadly based. However, I am acutely aware of the lack of an inclusion of certain areas, e.g., vocal tract and respiration measurements. These exclusions were primarily attributable to the fact that this topic has been dealt with elsewhere. The materials presented in this book are generally intended for advanced undergraduate and graduate students and for the practicing professionals in speech, hearing, and language sciences.

The authors are individually responsible for their chapters. No effort has been made by the editor to reconcile the differences of views or to resolve differences in terminological usage. Most of these differences have been viewed as an integral part of one's methodological and theoretical stands.

A deep sense of appreciation is expressed to Professor Black, who wrote the Introduction for this book. While he has expressed unequivocal support for this collection, he had no knowledge that this book was being organized in his honor. I also express my thanks to Professor Arthur J. Bronstein, who gave encouragements at the very onset of this project; to Ron Allison and Bette Zilles, who helped prepare the indices; and to several of our graduate students, who assisted in comparing references with the original sources. The Baker Fund Award of Ohio University to the editor partially supported this work.

Sadanand Singh, Ph.D.

Introduction:
Sidelights on Measurements

John W. Black, Ph.D.
Professor of Speech
Ohio State University

CONTENTS

DEVELOPMENT OF PSYCHOPHYSICS

Leipzig

Techniques for measuring hearing and speech originated in the developments of psychophysics and the psychological laboratory, which date from the 19th century. An important center of research was at Leipzig. In 1817, Fechner and Weber independently went to Leipzig (Boring, 1929). Weber was an assistant in the faculty of medicine and became a professor of comparative anatomy. He later became a professor of physiology and worked with various senses, particularly touch. He hinted in generalizations about ratios, as if they were increments of the stimulus that affected sensation in a special way, and then extended his work on touch to vision and to the hearing of tones. However, he formulated no law.

Fechner, who did not know Weber, is described by Boring as a versatile man who first acquired modest fame as a professor of physics but who, in later life, was a philosopher, characterized as a humanist, satirist, poet, and aestheticist. Although his present fame rests with psychophysics, this reputation was forced upon him through the importance of a "lesser" publication, *The Elements of Psychophysics* (1860). He discovered Weber's ratios independently, and upon discovering Weber's work he designated as Weber's law the constant ratio between "just noticeable differences" and the value of the stimulus.

1

Fechner, a philosopher-physicist, and Weber, an anatomist-physiologist, did not view as their first interest the measurement of sensations or any development from this measurement. Yet they were the very founders of measurement techniques.

Leipzig continued to pioneer the field of measurement procedures. In 1875, Wundt came from Heidelberg and Zurich to a chair of philosophy at Leipzig. He was a physiologist who had become a psychologist, and he headed Leipzig's psychological laboratory. One of his students was E. W. Scripture, from the United States. Scripture's experiences can be found in Murchison's *A History of Psychology in Autobiography* (Scripture, 1936), a gold mine of information about the influence of the laboratory at Leipzig. He wrote:

> Entering Wundt's Psychological Laboratory in Leipzig in 1888 I learned to listen to little ivory balls striking a board and to say whether I perceived a difference between two sounds or not. I also learned to press a button when the bell rang. As a result of such pursuits I grasped the fact that psychic measurements could be made. This understanding developed into a belief that can be best expressed in the words of Lord Kelvin: 'When you . . . can express what you are speaking about in numbers, you know something about it; but when you cannot express it in numbers, your knowledge is of a meagre and unsatisfactory kind; it may be the beginning of knowledge, but you have scarcely in your thoughts advanced to the stage of science. (Thompson: *Popular Lectures and Addresses*. London, 1889, 1, 73.)'
>
> The logical conclusion is: *only statements based on measurements are reliable*. The corollary is: statements without measurements are not worth listening to. The belief is strengthened by the fact that wherever measurements are introduced most previous statements are shown to consist of illusions and delusions or to be quite meaningless.
>
> . . . I have finally got far enough to grasp the idea that the universe consists solely of numbers arrived at by measurement.

I extend my reliance on Scripture's autobiography with an account of a specific instance.

> At the meetings of classical societies continual clashes occurred between a professor of Greek at Harvard and another at Yale concerning the nature of Greek verse. One asserted that it must have been quantitative (that is, consisting of long and short syllables) "just as in English." The other asserted that it must necessarily have consisted of differences in stress, "just as in English." Each appealed to the audiences for opinions on English verse as they heard it. Some of them heard it one way, some heard it the other way; others gave the matter up as undecided. The Yale professor appealed to me to do something with apparatus. I thereupon traced off the curve of speech from a gramophone record of the nursery rime "Cock Robin." The results were unexpected. The characteristics of English speech that produced the rhythm were found to be five, namely, change in speed (long and short), change in intensity (stress), change in pitch, change in quality, and change in precision of enunciation. The only persons in the controversy who were right were those who had said they did not know.
>
> The most astounding result was that the curves contradicted every one of the prevailing notions concerning metrics. The metrists assume

that English verse is based on four typical forms, the iambus, the trochee, the anapest, and the dactyl. These are only four out of more than fifty forms and how they got them all wrong owing to ignorance of classical verse are matters of no importance. Important is the way in which they have deluded people and maltreated the poets. For example, blank verse is the verse that Shakespeare wrote. The metrist, however, says that blank verse is "iambic pentameter." This is a form that never existed and never could exist in any language. He draws up a scheme into which he tries to fit Shakespeare's lines. As only a small portion of the lines can be forced into the scheme he proceeds to give Shakespeare "licenses" for innumerable deviations.

This topic is continued through three pages in the autobiography. Scripture's students are aware that the analysis of "Cock Robin" was carried into *The Elements of Experimental Phonetics* as well as *The Study of Speech Curves* (Scripture, 1904, 1906).

The Leipzig Influence

Scripture, of course, was not the only student to be influenced by Wundt. At Leipzig began the training of the first generation of psychologists in Germany, from America, and from other parts of the world. Besides Scripture, other foreign students from the United States who went to Leipzig to study with Wundt included Stanley Hall, Cattell, Frank Angell, Titchener, Witmer, Warren, Stratton, Judd—all experimental psychologists seeking measurements. The impact of this group on hearing and speech is readily apparent. One line of influence is through Scripture to Carl Emil Seashore to Lee Travis, Joseph Tiffin, Milton Metfessel, Don Lewis, and Grant Fairbanks, among others— from Wundt to his students, their students, and their students' students. Scripture's student Seashore (1930) described his experiences.

I entered Yale the day the psychology laboratory was opened and on Ladd's advice entered the laboratory course. Four of us graduate students registered in the laboratory the first day. There were about 60 graduate students at Yale that year. We were quite exclusive, close to the professors. We wore silk hats and Prince Albert coats to class.

The course was too rudimentary and too devoid of book learning to suit me. I resented Scripture's frequent reference to the futility of getting psychology from books, especially his speaking lightly of Ladd, from whom I felt I was getting things far more valuable than this laboratory stuff. I did not see then what laboratory experiments were about. We spent a long time on experiments that seemed nearer to telegraphy than psychology.

Toward the end of the year, an incident happened which proved to be a sharp turning point. Although still busy absorbing Ladd's system, I began to feel the need of independent work on a problem; so one day I went to Professor Ladd and told him I would be interested in doing some work on the subject of inhibitions. "That is a pretty interesting subject," he replied, "you will find a full account of it in my large book, p. 143 ff." We had not reached that point in the class, so I looked it up, and indeed it was a very interesting account and for a while proved a solution for my embryonic impulse for investigation. But the original idea that I could do something with that subject came back, so I went across the street to Scripture and expressed the same desire. He listened intently and then slapped me on the shoulder, a very unusual thing for him to do, and said, "Try it." That "Try it," as opposed to reference to authority, gave me a fresh start, and from that moment I date my scientific birth as a psychologist . . . I became willing to try the experimental method. I failed in finding a good approach to the proposed subject; but I got my hands into the laboratory and soon found tangible problems of interest, although I was still untrained and did not have my bearings.

In the laboratory I skirmished extensively before settling down to a problem for research. My first article to be published was a report on the measurement of speed of adaptations in accommodation of the eye for far and near points. So far as I know, the validity of those data has never been questioned. My next problem was the measurement of hallucinations and illusions. I produced hallucinations in the various senses by objective suggestion and compared the intensity of these with the intensity of the true sensation. Out of these grew the topic for my dissertation which dealt primarily with normal illusions of weight. Although the term may have been used before, that investigation gave status to and new interpretations of the term "normal" illusions.

The department was cleaned out . . . It took psychology and philosophy a long time to rehabilitate themselves at Yale. Scripture was swept out with Ladd, although they had practically nothing in common . . . The President should have recognized in Scripture the new approach to mental science, of which Scripture was champion. Instead he threw the baby out with the bath. Scripture came to Yale with good training and a splendid grasp of the approaches to the "new psychology." He was temperamental and enthusiastic. With students he was both patient and critical. If he had enjoyed the freedom that came to Cattell and Munsterberg and Titchener, he would have played a notable role in the founding of American psychology as these men did . . . I am the only one of his pupils in that earliest period who survived the ordeal and remained clearly in the field of experimental psychology.

While at Yale, Seashore had "drunk deep of the Pierian Spring" of Leipzig. A postscript to this story can be found in *The Elements of Experimental Phonetics* (Scripture, 1904), in which Scripture described several pieces of the custom-built equipment at the Yale laboratory, and of which he noted:

This line of work aroused much interest at the time; my pupil, assistant, and friend, Seashore, with his group in Iowa has continued it in his brilliant investigation of speech and vocal music. I have never been able to understand why experimental psychology never attempted to use the methods of experimental phonetics for investigating the most complete form of expression that the mind posesses.

Berry (1965) lists several pieces of "Seashore equipment" as having originated with Scripture, including the Tonoscope and the Iowa Pitch-audiometer. She also includes the Iowa Piano Camera, but Tiffin notes that this was his development in the Seashore laboratory (Tiffin, personal communication).

As firsthand evidence of his interest in speech Seashore writes (1930):

It has been very gratifying to find through laboratory experiments that the scientific principles which underlie the psychology of speech are in the large part the same as those underlying the psychology of music and that the instruments and techniques for research in speech are largely the same as those employed in the psychology of music. I have perhaps made two distinctive contributions which enable this University [Iowa] to offer the doctorate in speech with self-respect. The first is that a student who is to qualify in this field is not to be taught primarily by a "Professor of Speech," but, beyond the more or less elementary work on the artistic side, by specialists in the underlying fields; that is, he is to study anatomy with an anatomist, acoustics with a physicist, phonetics with a phonetician, psychology with a psychologist, and speech pathology with a psychiatrist. He may then conduct his research within any of these fields of scientific approach, the most frequent being that of psychology by the techniques ordinarily employed in the psychology of music. For this reason, we have developed the plan of staff members with joint appointment in the Departments of Speech and Psychology.

In the second place we have been able to transfer to research in speech most of the techniques developed in the psychology of music. For this reason we have been able to make progress in the psychology of speech many times as fast as the corresponding results were obtained in music.

A third feature consists in the organization of remedial work. The voice is an index to character and is also a salient element of character itself. From infancy upward the neglect of voice-training represents one of the largest gaps in our educational system. The program which I have assisted in evolving and promoting consists of the development of scientific aids to the early development of speech in the home and in the pre-school and kindergarten. It provides a service for the twelve grades in our high school and in the freshman class of the University. In this service, children and students are analyzed annually to determine the presence of speech impediments of any kind, and a remedial service is provided and enforced as outlined in the program for the Institute of Mental Hygiene. This service has enormous possibilities for the building of character through the development of effective and pleasing voice as well as by the removal of impediments. While I take some credit for having originated this movement, its success is due entirely to the very hearty following of the project in the Department of Speech.

There is a most tempting field for research in the psychology of speech, both normal and pathological, and the development of the instruments and techniques in this Department has given great impetus to investigation.

Evidently, interest in the subject of metrics, investigated by Scripture in his "Cock Robin" analysis, was passed on to Seashore. Whether or not the topic was among the ones investigated in the Wundt laboratory is unknown; but the range of topics there must have been considerable, simply judging by the varied interests of the scholars who were trained by Wundt.

One of Seashore's students, Wilbur Schramm, now known for his work in mass communication, made an extensive study of the oral reading of English poetry. He used the oscillograph, a high speed output-level recorder, and a strobophotographic camera. This work, done under the direction of Seashore, led to the monograph, *Approaches to a Science of English Verse* (1935) with 12 chapter headings: the need, the approach, the syllable, the accent, stress, melody: characteristics, melody: sources, rhythm, rhyme, the metrical foot, artistic deviation from regularity, and verse.

I prize a letter from my former colleague, the late John Crowe Ransom, to whom I lent Schramm's monograph and who obviously held a different view.

> Schramm's book on meters doesn't accomplish very much, though it is perfectly sound. For example, he shows by his machine recorder that readers do not give exactly the same time to the different feet of the poetic line; he charts their variations and says that it is a gross error to assume the foot means a uniform time interval; but concludes presently that what the foot really is, is an idealized "standard" which is not ever consistently realized but is approximated. That is precisely what everyone who has studied metrics should have known in the first place. Again a great deal of measurements has been got through with the most vigorous method possible, and it turns out love's labor lost.

Conclusions

Although Wundt headed a movement that had international implications in the development of laboratories of measurement, his, however, was not the only laboratory. I have read recently in a source which I cannot now locate a rather surprising statement that Binet, before joining with Simon, was as productive as Wundt, and I note in the autobiography of Edouard Claparede, "During this stay in Paris I became an intimate friend of Binet who used to be at home every Thursday in his laboratory." Lester (1974) notes that the Laboratory of Experimental Psychology in Paris "is the psychological research facility with the longest continuity in France. Binet was the second director; when he moved off in the direction of applied work with Simon, he was replaced by Pieron. The fourth director is now active." Claparede, incidentally, wrote of his short stay in Leipzig. "I had also put down my name for a 'praktikum' of psychology . . . Unluckily I was the fifth on the list and Wundt had taken it into his head that only four students should attend this course."

Tuning forks and the sound cage seemed to provide the only answer for most questions about measurements of audition. Both were required if one was to pursue Steven's *Handbook of Experimental Psychology* (1951). Both are obvious in photographs of Scripture's laboratory. Both were in use along with vacuum tube devices in Seashore's laboratory in the 1920's. Seashore aided the pioneering ventures of Reger and the collaborative investigations of Reger, in otolaryngology, and Lewis, in psychology. Audiology as we know it drew heavily on the contributions of auditionists and came to fruition during and in the wake of World War II.

The subject of measurement techniques in hearing and speech has been handled in a variety of ways. Stevens has treated measurement in a broad and concise manner in the first chapter of his *Handbook of Experimental Psychology* (1951; personal correspondence). Other authors have made extensive treatments of the topic in a relatively untechnical manner, such as Guilford in his *Psychometric Methods* (1936), and in a more technical vein, such as Lewis in *Quantitative Methods in Psychology* (1960) and an introductory chapter, "A little calculus," in Peters and Van Voorhis' *Statistical Procedures and Their Mathematical Bases* (1940). The scope of some treatments is more limited, as in Hirsh's *The Measurement of Hearing* (1952). Such contributions are available, as crutches for many of us, and do not need to be abstracted here.

The work of these and other authors evolved from the earlier work done in psychophysics and in the psychological laboratory, and these have been recent developments. The late Dr. Pierce, who headed the faculty where I taught for 14 years and who was for 40 years president of a small Ohio college, foresaw the importance of psychophysics and the psychological laboratory. He spoke in 1897 to the Ohio College Association on the topic "Has psychophysics a place in the college curriculum?" As a college president, and long before the introduction of the elective system in the college curriculum, he said:

> The growth of the laboratory method in the teaching of psychology has been one of the most striking and rapid movements in modern education ... The laboratory for the study of mental science is now an essential part of a German university, and every year witnesses a growth in the additions to the number of psychological experiment-rooms in American universities ... The equipment required for a psychological laboratory is very simple, and provisions for such experiments can generally be conveniently made in connection with the physics laboratory, and the method once adopted students can be given, at very slight cost, the opportunity to study the phenomenon of consciousness, objectively and experimentally (Pierce, 1897).

DETERMINATION OF MEASURES

I turn now to a second topic, the determination of measures. The measure is a digit. It is obtained in circumstances such that each estimate, as it is obtained, is a true estimate of the outcome of the procedure. This means that the measure is repeatable and is not selected from available estimates. The measure is meaningful under the conditions in which it was obtained, and should be so described. Interpretations of the meaning of the measure are only inferences and extrapolations made by the experimenter or a "reader;" they do not cast doubt on the legitimacy of the measure as such. This paragraph is only an extension of two common words, reliability and validity. The idea is inherent that the measures only reflect the planning and procedures of the experimenter.

Measurements in speech and hearing are made from supraliminal stimuli and from stimuli that range from sub- to supraliminal. Furthermore, the stimuli have: 1) discernible physical properties, as did the "little ivory balls striking a board" to which Scripture learned to listen, or 2) no physical properties, at least in the immediate situation, as in the instance of rating or ranking the "handicaps" introduced by different speech and hearing disorders. Although this is an implied dichotomy, it probably ranges through many degrees. The same method for obtaining a measure may be used throughout the range; therefore, I shall not make a distinction between "psychophysical" and "psychometric" judgments.

Equal Appearing Intervals

I begin with supraliminal stimuli. A large proportion of measures in hearing and speech are derived from a procedure of "equal appearing intervals." A subject is given a range of digits and a definition of the extreme values, which is *high* and which is *low*. Scripture might have rated the thuds that resulted from a ball hitting a board by designating 1 to represent a slightly audible sound, and 9 to represent a seemingly maximal sound. Thorndike (1915), in an important illustration of the scaling of handwriting, defined zero merit arbitrarily as: "That handwriting recognizable as such, but not legible at all and possessing no beauty." He defined 18 (top) as the quality of the samples of writing in the copybook. He also took steps to support the assumption that his scale was linear, that 10 represented a merit greater than 8 by the same amount that 8 represented a merit greater than 6. Typical samples were selected for various scale intervals and were used to "train" further judges and, from Thorndike's work, teachers of the elementary schools of New York City.

Thurstone (1952) paid little heed to Thorndike's scaling:

Cattell seems to be the first to have extended the psychophysical methods to stimuli other than simple sensory values. He applied the psychophysical procedures with some variations to the measurement of estimated degrees of eminence of scientific men. Here, for the first time, the methods were used on stimuli which do not have any simple stimulus magnitude. When the methods are used on lifted weights, line lengths, and brightnesses, the experiments yield two scales. One is a scale of physical stimulus magnitude such as the actual weight in grams, the length of the lines in centimeters, or the photometrically determined brightness of the gray papers. It is known in psychophysics as the R-scale. The second scale is the psychological continuum, which is known as the S-scale. Its unit is the equally often noticed stimulus difference. Fechner's law describes the logarithmic relation between these two scales. Weber's law describes the average error of perception as a constant fraction of the physical stimulus magnitude. When Cattell extended the use of these methods to social stimuli he constructed, in effect, a psychological scale, the unit of measurement for which was the equally often noticed difference or some approximation to it.

Thurstone himself was interested in measuring attitudes. His contributions are sufficiently important to warrant a digression.

Thurstone began his education as a student of engineering. He wandered into a psychology course, and relates (Thurstone, 1952):

> I used to wonder what the elementary course could be like if the course that I was taking was called 'advanced'. I soon became accustomed to the fact that prerequisites did not mean anything and that there was no real sequence of courses in psychology even though they were listed by number and title to give an appearance of a sequence where one course was supposed to build upon another.

I continue to draw upon his autobiography:

> Now we turn to psychophysics which is psychological measurement proper. It is another line of development that was started soon after our arrival at the University of Chicago. When I started to teach psychological measurement in 1924, it was natural that I should encourage the students to learn something about psychophysical methods. The standard reference was, of course, the two big volumes on quantitative psychology by Titchener. The determination of a limen was the basic problem in old-fashioned psychophysics. In order to be scholarly in this field, one was supposed to know about the old debates on how to compute the limen for lifted weights to two decimal places with a standard stimulus of one hundred grams. One could hardly worry about anything more trivial. Who cares for the exact determination of anybody's limen for lifted weights? In teaching this subject I felt that we must do something about this absurdity by introducing more interesting stimuli. Instead of lifted weights we used a list of offenses presented in pairs with the instruction that they should be judged as to their relative seriousness. The subject checked one of each pair of offenses to indicate which he thought was the more serious. Instead of selecting one of the offenses as a standard, we asked the subjects to compare every stimulus with every other stimulus. It was now apparent that the classical method of constant stimuli is a special case of the more complete psychophysical method of paired comparison. We followed this same procedure with a list of nationalities that were also presented in pairs. For each pair of nationalities the subject was asked to check the one which he would prefer to associate with. I did not realize at the time that it was going to be necessary to rewrite the fundamental theory of psychophysics in order to cope with data of this type.

Out of this background arose Thurstone's willingness to use "psychophysical toys" in measurements in social psychophysics. He developed a number of attitude scales on subjects such as the treatment of criminals, patriotism, Sunday observance of the church, war, the Negro, prohibition, the unions, communism, the social position of women, immigration, birth control, the Chinese, the Germans, the law, censorship, evolution, capital punishment, the economic position of women, and others.

A study illustrating the range of topics enumerated in the foregoing paragraph was the work of Thurstone and Chave in *The Measurement of Attitude* (1929). This was a matter of measuring the attitudes of people about the church. One hundred thirty statements were made. They were placed in 11 piles by each of 300 judges, with the low end of an 11-point scale indicating the opinion that the judge viewed the statement favorable toward the church and with the upper end indicating that it was unfavorable. Subsequently, the selected "reliable" statements were presented to large numbers of judges of different ages, faiths, and of both sexes. The selected items represented a small ambiguity among the 130 criterion judges. The items also represented a range of median values on the 11-point scale.

As a result of Thurstone's work with social values, such as is illustrated by his attitude scale with regard to the church, he developed his "law of comparative judgment." In doing so, he formalized the definitions of certain terms: "discriminal process," "discriminal dispersion," the "modal discriminal process," "discriminal deviation," and the "discriminal difference" (Thurstone, 1927).

The discriminal process is simply the decision making that attends the selection of an answer. This decision varies from time to time with the same person. The variation leads to discriminal dispersion. However, there is one process that occurs more frequently than the others, and of course, this is the modal discriminal process. All of these can be determined for a subject's responses on the 11-point scale. Accounting for the dispersion, the difference between two modal discriminal processes, perhaps 7 and 8, respectively, leads to the discriminal difference. These concepts would have been useful in the development of psychophysical theory and with experiences with "ivory balls;" instead they became the undergirding for the application of equal appearing intervals to "nonphysical events."

The emphasis here on Thurstone is because Thurstone and Chave (1929) is the only reference given by Lewis and Sherman (1951) in the extension of the method of equal appearing intervals to hearing and speech. Their work, reported as "Measuring the severity of stuttering," completed before 1940 and first presented orally in 1950, set a pattern for researchers too numerous to acknowledge. The work itself has been replicated as well as extended to articulation, nasality, cleft palate speech, language development, and backward-played speech, among others. In the course of Sherman's many follow-up studies, she found that, at least in the instance of scaling cleft palate speech, the mean and median values of the dispersion of the judges are equally serviceable (Sherman, 1970). Thurstone and his followers had used the median value.

Magnitude Estimation

The reader may wish to draw a sharp line between equal appearing intervals and ratio scales. Weber and Fechner started working with constant ratios.

Thorndike, Thurstone, and Lewis and Sherman might have given their judges another set of instructions. Thorndike could have said: "18 is the writing of the work book; writing that is one half as good will receive a 9," and so on. Thurstone and Chave could have done the same with attitudes toward the church; and Lewis and Sherman could have done this with regard to the severity of stuttering. The terms discriminal process, discriminal dispersion, and the others would be equally applicable. The outcomes also might be highly similar. Sherman and Silverman (1968) reported no correlation below 0.92 with the results obtained with three methods of judgment of the "intricacy of children's language usage."

Irrespective of the point of view of the preceding paragraph, ratio scales have assumed particular importance through the work of Stevens. He permitted subjects to use any scale of digits that was convenient for them, individually, as long as the subject used "double," "one half," etc. The experimenter transformed each of the values of a subject into a proportion of the total for that subject. Through this procedure, Stevens developed a number of functions that represented subjects' responses to sound, light, tactile vibration, and a host of other stimuli. He extended this to include cross modality responses, accepting, for example, the length of a line in lieu of a digit. Singh and I individually have extended this procedure in an attempt to measure the relative similarity-dissimilarity of English consonants (Black, 1969, 1970; Singh, Woods, and Becker, 1972).

I had another interesting experience with Stevens and ratio scales. Experimental subjects heard a white noise sustained for 2 sec and were asked to match the intensity of the sound while saying /a/. They were then asked to produce the vowel one half as loud as the one they heard. They heard the sound again and were asked to reproduce the vowel twice as loud as they heard it. In a personal communication in 1955, Stevens wrote:

> I was delighted to receive "the control of the sound pressure level of voice." In part two you describe an experiment on the bisection of loudness intervals employing a noise with a spectrum that slopes 60 per octave. I did a lot of work on the bisection problem a couple of years ago, which I hope someday to publish. Actually some of the data have appeared in the enclosed paper, "On the averaging of data." Some more of my results appear in the last section of "The measurement of loudness." I am getting this paper ready for publication and in it I would like to call attention to your results since they agree rather well with what the loudness function would predict. Your results for bisection and for extending the range upward are consistent with my data obtained with the ascending order of listening.
>
> When you try to extend the range downward you seem to run into certain troubles. I am not surprised that your subjects found this a more difficult task. In setting this task we also run into the peculiar fact that unless we are careful we end up by setting a task that is logically impossible. What I mean is that a reduction of about 10 dB produces a sound that is half as loud as the first sound. If this is true then a reduction of more than 10 dB would make it impossible to find a third sound that was as far below the second as the second was below the first. For

example 100 dB gives a loudness of 60 sones and 88 dB gives a loudness of 27 sones, but no stimulus will give a loudness that is as far below 27 as 27 is below 60. Of course, so long as the fact is not too obviously impossible most subjects will go ahead and make a setting because their subjective criteria are at best tenuous and unstable.

Other Methods

There are other methods for achieving the purpose served by the foregoing procedures, equal appearing intervals and magnitude estimation, whether or not the end is applied.

Thurstone attributes the introduction of the method of triads to Richardson. This is commonly referred to as the ABX method and was used by Singh, Woods, and Becker (1972). The subject is presented with three stimuli and asked to indicate which two are the more similar or, as usually employed, is asked whether the third is more like the first or second. This is a convenient device for scaling stimuli.

Another technique for scaling is provided in paired comparisons, described above by Thurstone, and in attributed scope, which encompasses "the constant method" of classical psychophysics. Possibly this was first used in regard to measurements in speech and hearing by Lewis and Tiffin (1934). They scaled six voices in terms of general effectiveness, pitch, loudness, and quality and then attempted to find physical correlates for each set of subjective judgments. Through largely replicating this study I found the tediousness of the method and the necessity for limiting an application to a few stimuli (Black, 1942).

In the foregoing discussion of magnitude estimation, the situation was mentioned in which persons were asked to produce a sound of the same loudness as the sound they heard. This procedure in situations that emphasize articulation and perhaps voice quality is routine in speech therapy. One person says to another, in effect: "Make the sound as I make it." It is also a manner of teaching taken for granted by teachers of foreign languages. Here is the "method of production." In the dull context of "ivory balls" it led to "draw a line of the same length as this line." In that circumstance the disparity between the stimulus and the response was easily measured. This gave rise to a dispersion of disparities, and the consequent handling of the data is often treated as the origin of the statistics that relate to measures of central tendency, of dispersion, and significant differences. Measurements of discrepancies between the stimulus and the response, however, are rarely made in the speech therapy situation. This "failure" on our part strongly calls for measurement and quantification in a context of "accountability" and in settings in which Wundt's descendants cannot restrict enrollments to four.

Another dominant source of measurements in hearing relates to the identification of supraliminal stimuli. This naming of what is heard is an application of the method of absolute judgment, a method that was developed in experiments with vision. All tests that rely on verbal materials and that are used in audiology are applications of absolute judgment. In this instance, the subject is naming the word that he hears. There are other applications, many of them less applied than intelligibility tests. Extensive work has been conducted at the Haskins Laboratories (New Haven, Conn.) with synthetic speech. The phonemes that are identified by listeners change with altered transients that precede the synthetic formants of vowels. They also change with differences in the duration of the approach to a consonant. I made another application of absolute judgment by asking students of phonetics to transcribe backward-played syllables, although the stimuli were not described as such (Black, 1973). Some phonemes retained their identity when played backwards; others did not. The discrepancies here "become digits" when placed in a confusion matrix. In all instances, however, there was marked agreement among the listeners about the "phoneme" they heard.

All of the foregoing discussion has treated supraliminal instances. For example, if one is determining the shortest detectable pause he must be presented suprathreshold stimuli that include pauses that are subliminal with respect to the object of the experiment. Also, in measurements of hearing, there is always the need to determine absolute threshold, that is, to determine the sensitivity of an ear to sound. A conventional procedure for this is pure tone audiometry. Tones are presented subliminally and at successively higher intensities until they are reported present. This, of course, is the "method of minimal change" or the "method of limits." It is applied at each of several selected frequencies. The applied purposes of the audiologist suggest or impose shortcuts in the procedures: 5-dB increments, the introduction of bracketing, and the like. Even so, the report of the audiologist implies that the subject was unable to detect an acoustic signal below a stipulated level.

The behavior of the subject who is being tested by an audiologist provides a great deal of data that until recently have been ignored. The introduction of signal detection theory has made four types of responses meaningful: responses when a signal is present, responses when a signal is absent, no response when a signal is present, and no response when a signal is absent. These four behaviors lend themselves to comparative evaluation.

The audiologist is also interested in supraliminal stimuli. He shares with the student of speech an interest in the identification of spoken verbal material. The audiologist uses nonsense syllables, one-syllable words, two-syllable words, sentences, and whatever verbal material may be standardized to assess speech reception thresholds and to quantify the ability of a subject to understand verbal material 1) in quiet and 2) in noise.

The student of speech may use the same assortment of stimuli as the audiologist does to measure the *intelligibility* of a speaker, that is, the capability of a speaker to utter speech signals in a manner such that they are understandable. Engineers, likewise, have a stake in this process, for they use the measures as indices of the relative effectiveness of transmitting or receiving equipment. Indeed, the whole process of testing with verbal material was developed in the context of the relative efficiency of telephone systems.

Conclusions

The procedures that have been described above are only examples of the ones that may yield meaningful measures in speech and hearing. The researcher will select from ones that have been used or, importantly, from ones that he develops for a particular procedure, ones that are expedient for the task at hand. The fact that he is modifying an old psychophysical instrument or making a new one may not occur to him until he is well along in his work. Then it may become clear that the procedure he has developed is a distant relative of "ivory balls" in Leipzig, and is, in addition, as possibly relevant to today's social matters as Thurstone hoped his stimuli were.

REFERENCES

Berry, M. F. 1965. Historical vignettes of leadership in speech and hearing. I. Speech pathology. ASHA 7.

Black, J. W. 1942. A study of voice merit. Q. J. Speech 28: 67–74.

Black, J. W. 1969. Relative perceptual similarity of sixty initial consonants. Ohio State University Research Foundation.

Black, J. W. 1970. Interconsonantal distances. In A. J. Bronstein, C. L. Shaver, and C. Stevens (eds.), Essays in Honor of Claude M. Wise, pp. 74–96. Standard Printing, Hannibal, Mo.

Black, J. W. 1973. The "phonemic" content of backward-reproduced speech. J. Speech Hear. Res. 16: 165–174.

Boring, E. G. 1929. A History of Experimental Psychology. Century, New York. 699 p.

Guilford, J. P. 1936. Psychometric Methods. 2nd Ed. McGraw-Hill, New York. 566 p.

Hirsh, I. J. 1952. The Measurement of Hearing. McGraw-Hill, New York. 364 p.

Lester, J. T. 1974. Psychology in France. European Scientific Notes. Office of Naval Research, London.

Lewis, D. 1960. Quantitative Methods in Psychology. McGraw-Hill, New York. 558 p.

Lewis, D., and D. Sherman. 1951. Measuring the severity of stuttering. J. Speech Hear. Disord. 16: 320–326.

Lewis, D., and J. Tiffin. 1934. A psychophysical study of individual differences in speaking ability. Arch. Speech 1: 43–60.

Peters, C. C., and W. R. Van Voorhis. 1940. Statistical Procedures and Their Mathematical Bases. McGraw-Hill, New York. 516 p.

Pierce, W. F. 1897. Has psychophysics a place in the college curriculum? Speech given to the Ohio College Association.

Schramm, W. L. 1935. Approaches to a Science of English Verse. University of Iowa Studies, Iowa City.

Scripture, E. W. 1904. The Elements of Experimental Phonetics. Charles Scribner's Sons, New York. 623 p.

Scripture, E. W. 1906. Researches in Experimental Phonetics. The Study of Speech Curves. The Carnegie Institute of Washington, Washington, D.C. 204 p.

Scripture, E. W. 1936. *In* G. Murchison (ed.), History of Psychology in Autobiography, pp. 231–261. Vol. 3. Clark University Press, Worcester, Mass.

Seashore, C. E. 1930. *In* C. Murchison (ed.), History of Psychology in Autobiography, pp. 225–297. Vol. 1. Clark University Press, Worcester, Mass.

Sherman, D. 1970. Usefulness of the mean in psychological scaling of cleft palate speech. Cleft Palate J. 7: 622–629.

Sherman, D., and F. H. Silverman. 1968. Three psychological scaling methods applied to language development. J. Speech Hear. Res. 11: 837–841.

Singh, S., D. R. Woods, and G. M. Becker. 1972. Perceptual structures of 22 prevocalic English consonants. J. Acoust. Soc. Amer. 52: 1698–1713.

Stevens, S. S. (ed.). 1951. Handbook of Experimental Psychology, pp. 1–49. John Wiley & Sons, New York.

Stevens, S. S. 1970. Notes for a life story. Recollections assembled for History of Psychology in Autobiography, pp. 1–34. Harvard Psychoacoustics Labs, Cambridge, Mass.

Thorndike, E. L. 1915. Handwriting. Teachers College, Columbia University, New York. 41 p.

Thurstone, L. L. 1927. A law of comparative judgment. Psychol. Review. 34: 273–286.

Thurstone, L. L. 1952. *In* E. G. Boring, H. S. Langfeld, H. Werner, and R. M. Yerks (eds.), History of Psychology in Autobiography, pp. 295–321. Vol. 4. Clark University Press, Worcester, Mass.

Thurstone, L. L., and E. J. Chave. 1929. The Measurement of Attitude. The University of Chicago Press, Chicago. 96 p.

LANGUAGE

The Study of Linguistically Deficient Children

Donald M. Morehead, Ph.D.
Associate Professor
Department of Child Development
California State University, Hayward

CONTENTS

INTRODUCTION

Linguistically deficient children represent an extremely heterogeneous population difficult to categorize into clearly defined subgroups. This diverse population is described here as those children who fail to comprehend and/or produce a first language consistent with their mental age. This working definition has the advantage of separating bilingual and bicultural children from the populations of linguistically deficient children (Ginsberg, 1972). In addition, it excludes retarded children who do not show a linguistic level of development that is inconsistent with their mental age.

Until the late 1950's, the primary concern in both normal and deficient child research was the study of overt and observable aspects of production and perception. However, this early work also showed considerable interest in formal measures of linguistic complexity. Several measures such as the mean-length-of-response and type-token ratio were used extensively (McCarthy, 1954; Powers, 1957; Templin, 1957). It was not until the appearance of Jakobson, Fant, and Halle's (1952) classic work on distinctive feature theory that the shift to studying more abstract and less observable aspects of the phonological system in particular and of language in general began.

When Chomsky's transformational theory was published in 1957, the movement away from the study of overt performance to that of abstract

19

description now included syntax, and in some basic ways, semantics. Chomsky (1957) also clarified many of the basic descriptions related to perception and production by emphasizing the more general distinction between competence and performance. In 1968, two important works appeared. The first, by Chomsky and Halle, advanced a transformational theory of phonology, and the second, by Fillmore, proposed that semantics, rather than syntax, might be central to the study of language. This second proposal has had significant effects on the recent directions in the study of child language (Bloom, 1970; Bowerman, 1973; Brown, 1973; E. Clark, 1973a; H. Clark, 1973b; Schlesinger, 1971; Slobin, 1973).

More recently, considerable attention has been directed in both linguistics and psychology to the importance of early cognitive development as a general prefiguration to language development as well as to those functions which may act as specific precursors to language (Bloom, 1973; Brown, 1973; Greenfield, Smith, and Laufer, in press; Morehead and Morehead, 1974; MacNamara, 1972; Sinclair, 1971, 1973). Finally, there have been a number of recent attempts to characterize the relationship between the acquisition of certain linguistic forms and their cognitive level of development (Sinclair, 1969) and also the relationship between the strategies used by children in acquisition and integration of linguistic structures (Bever, 1970; Bloom, Lightbown, and Hood, 1974; Clark and Garnica, 1974; Cromer, 1974a; Ervin-Tripp, 1973; Greenfield, Nelson, and Saltzman, 1972; Slobin, 1973; Sinclair, 1973). Studies attempting to describe the underlying knowledge and strategies used in the acquisition and integration of language demonstrate the tremendous shift from consideration of surface aspects to those aspects which may be basic to all mental behavior, including language.

The study of language-deficient children has paralleled that of normal children with an almost singular focus on syntax and morphology. This chapter begins with a review of that research, including the relevant studies with normal children. Except for several studies on the relationship of language dysfunction and general mental development (de Ajuriaguerra, 1966; Inhelder, 1966), little attention has been given to linguistically deficient children in other areas of language development. For this reason, recent studies of comprehension and imitation and of semantic and cognitive development that offer specific direction for research with linguistically deficient children are also discussed. Finally, an attempt is made to abstract and discuss the methodological issues that seem most relevant to the study of linguistically deficient children.

SYNTAX

In the early 1960's, three important longitudinal studies on early language acquisition were reported (Braine, 1963; Brown and Bellugi, 1964; Miller and

Ervin, 1964). In these studies spontaneous speech samples were collected, generally in the child's home, and transcribed for syntactic rather than phonetic or semantic detail. The utterances were largely two words, and all three studies used two-word classes ("pivot and open," "modifier and noun," "operator and nonoperator") to derive highly similar rules describing the child's linguistic structures. The analysis of the samples was largely distributional; that is, the primary concern was how words were grouped into classes through co-occurrence. Little attention was directed toward the function of these classes in expressing the child's grammatical relations or semantic intentions. Thus, the analysis was confined primarily to the surface rather than the underlying structures that define grammatical relations and semantic meanings of the child's utterances. The pivot grammar characterization of early language became the mainstay in child language, so much so that it was not until Bloom (1970) and Schlesinger (1971) introduced semantic intention that the analysis changed.

At the same time, Menyuk (1963) reported the early results from a large cross sectional study of children between 3 and 7 years old. In this study, she focused on change in sentence structure as a condition of increasing chronological age and on adult grammatical acceptability to determine those structures restricted to the children's usage. She generally assumed a categorical position in the early analysis of her data; that is, each structure was considered to be composed of one or several categories derived from specific rules. She found that young children (3.0–3.8 years) generally omit a category, that kindergarten children (5.6 years) generally substitute within members of a category, and that first grade children (6.5 years) generally use a category redundantly.

From this cross sectional study (summarized in Menyuk, 1969), she made the first comparison of normal and deficient children using a transformational model to construct grammars describing each child's corpus or language sample. Menyuk (1964) recorded language samples for 10 deficient children with no apparent deficits other than language, and compared them with those of 10 normal children selected from the larger study. Rather extensive situational sampling under three different conditions was used: 1) responses to a standardized projective test, 2) conversation with the experimenter, and 3) conversation with three peers while playing "family." The groups were matched on standard criteria of age, IQ, and socioeconomic status. The age range of the children was from 3 to 6 years. The verbal IQ of all the subjects was well above normal, and they were from middle class families. Fewer than 100 sentences were collected for each group.

When the linguistically deficient children were compared with normal children, Menyuk (1964) found that they most often omitted categories in both their spontaneous samples and in their repetition or imitation of sentences. Few statistically significant findings were reported on the use of transformations or restricted forms (forms in which categories were omitted, substituted, redundant, or restricted by, for example, failure to make "wh" conversions) by the two groups, although there was a trend toward difference in the structures used by the two groups. A high rate of omissions was found for the deficient group, suggesting that they were functioning in a way similar to the young preschool children tested earlier by Menyuk (1963). Brown (1973) also found a high omission rate in obligatory as well as optional contexts for very young children.

The comparison of a normal 2-year-old with a deficient 3-year-old was included to determine if the trend of difference found in the comparison of the two groups could be supported or whether the deficient children were simply functioning at a lower linguistic level. The normal child's language sample was collected longitudinally while the deficient child's sample was collected during short sampling periods. In addition, no systematic attempt was made to match the two children on specific criteria. The findings of this comparison showed a discrepancy in the forms used similar to that found in the larger group comparison.

Another early investigation of deficient language was reported by Lee (1966). She developed four "levels" of developmental sentence types, using data summarized by McNeill (1966) from the early work of Brown and Bellugi (1964), Braine (1963), Miller and Ervin (1964) and, in addition, included data from Weir (1962). Using these sentence types, she compared language samples of a 3-year-old normal child and a 4.6-year-old deficient child. The normal child's utterances were reported to be more closely aligned to the sentence types characterizing each of the four levels, with fewer omissions of some sentence types than those of the deficient child. Moreover, the deficient child also produced a few idiosyncratic forms that were not predicted by the sentence types used in the comparison. Unfortunately, the sampling situations used for the two children were grossly different, including the apparent necessity for the deficient child to be "prodded with questions to elicit speech at all" (Lee, 1966, p. 322). Furthermore, the data base for the developmental sentence types was dependent on surface comparison of spontaneous sentence types constructed from children's utterances other than those used in the comparison.

Two recent studies, Lackner (1968) and Morehead and Ingram (1973), incorporated significant changes in the methods used to study language-deficient children. In a study of five retarded children, Lackner (1968) collected 1,000 utterances of spontaneous speech for each child interacting with the experimenter and other children during three time periods when the children were most talkative. The major portion of the sample was recorded in the early morning, before their afternoon naps, and before retiring in the evening. It was not reported whether or not contextual information was obtained for the language samples. For each language sample the mean sentence length (in words) was used to order the five children who ranged in mental age from 2.3 years to 8.10 years. Complete phrase structure grammars were written for each corpus, and the occurrence of specific transformations was noted. Moreover, six different sentence types representing increasing levels of complexity were chosen, and their frequencies of occurrence were tabulated for each sample. The sentence types were simple declarative, interrogative, negative, passive, negative passive, and negative passive interrogative. In addition, comprehension and imitation tasks were used to modify the grammars written from the production data. Thus, the grammars not only revealed the degree of well formedness, in so far as each was considered as a subset of the adult grammar, but they also reflected the child's ability to comprehend and imitate novel sentences. By using this method, Lackner (1968) was attempting to follow Chomsky's (1965) requirement that grammars must account for creativity as well as grammaticality.

Lackner (1968) used five normal children as controls to establish the chronological age correspondence of each of the five retarded children's grammars. Using the sentence comprehension and imitation tasks, he constructed from the retarded children's grammars sentences more complex than or deviant from those that the child spontaneously used, and he presented them both to the five retarded and to the five normal children. From the performance of both groups he determined which chronological age best suited each retarded child's grammar.

The results of Lackner's (1968) study show that there is a close similarity between the mean sentence length of a normal child and that of a retarded child whose mental age is comparable to that of a normal child. More complex sentence types appeared as mental age increased, and the phrase structure grammars became more differentiated with fewer omissions and redundancies of major linguistic categories, such as noun phrase, verb phrase, and preposition. The number of transformations used in spontaneous speech and understood in the comprehension task also increased with age. Moreover, both the normal and the retarded children could understand and imitate any sentence generated from the grammars assigned to their respective linguistic levels. If the sentences exceeded the children's grammatical level, then both the normal and the retarded children modified the sentences on the imitation task in such a way that the sentences were made to conform to their levels of grammatical complexity. An important finding in this study is that the grammars written for the retarded children were capable of specifying the comprehensive and imitative performance of the normal children assigned to their level. Furthermore, no qualitative difference was found in the behavior of the two groups on the comprehension and imitation tasks. These results show that the two groups follow a similar developmental sequence with the retarded children demonstrating delay or arrest rather than difference in development. Some additional support for Lackner's (1968) major findings comes from a less exhaustive study reported by Graham and Graham (1971), who also found that retarded children used syntactic structures very similar to those used by a normal control group.

Morehead and Ingram (1973) reported a study comparing 15 normal and 15 linguistically deficient children. The normal group was selected to represent the mental age period of 18–36 months, a period of intense learning of basic syntax for normal children. Children in the two groups were matched according to linguistic level as determined by mean morpheme per utterance. In addition, three subjects from each group closely approximated the mean morpheme per utterance for each of the five linguistic levels previously determined by Brown (1973). The chronological age range for the normal group was 17–37 months, while the age range of the deficient group was 42–114 months. The language-deficient group was restricted to children whose only detectable problem was failure to acquire language at a normal rate.

The language samples were collected under three conditions: 1) spontaneous interaction with the experimenter or parent, 2) structured play, and 3) elicitation using a children's picture book. An observer recorded what was said to the child, the child's utterance, and an interpretation of the utterance. This contextual information was used to determine the semantic intention of the child, allowing a more exact determination of the grammatical relations in each utterance, and to divide each sample into spontaneous versus response utterances. All single words were eliminated from each sample, leaving about 100 relational utterances for each subject at the two lower levels and about 200 relational utterances for each subject at the three upper levels of linguistic development. The mean number of utterances for the normal group was 175, and the mean number of utterances for the deficient group was 148. Because of the relatively small samples, only forms occurring two or more times were included in the analysis.

Rosenbaum's (1967) adaptation of Chomsky's (1965) transformational grammar was used to write base grammars for each language sample, since it incorporates some changes in earlier methods of linguistic analysis. Initially, separate grammars were written for both spontaneous and response utterances to control for unknown performance variables, primarily in the deficient group, and for differential effects that might have existed in collecting the samples. Few differences in the two types of utterances were found, and the utterances were then pooled for comparison.

Five aspects of linguistic development were compared across the five linguistic levels: 1) phrase structure rules, 2) transformations, 3) construction types, 4) inflectional morphology, and 5) minor lexical categories. Phrase structure and transformational analysis allowed a qualitative comparison of the basic organization of the children's linguistic systems. A number of quantitative measures were also developed to assess the relative occurrence of transformations, the number of transformations per utterance, the diversity of construction types, the occurrence of inflections, and minor lexical categories.

The phrase structure grammars as well as the proportion of utterances reflecting phrase structure relations were highly similar in both groups. Forty different transformations were identified and assigned absolute ranks based on their percentage of occurrence. When the transformations were compared as a group, they were found to be nearly identical; individual comparison showed four of the transformations occurring with significantly greater frequency in the normal group and two showing significantly greater frequency in the deficient group. Of the 20 transformations that occurred with low frequency, the normal children produced these transformations, taken together, significantly more often. Since the infrequent transformations occurred 5% or less of the time with the frequent transformations occurring 40–50% of the time, this comparison based on percentage of occurrence provides a method for ascertaining which transformations may be more difficult. For example, the normal children used, although not significantly, twice as many infrequently occurring transformations at the three upper linguistic levels as did the deficient children. This comparison also may be used to assess those infrequently used transformations which contribute to linguistic diversity since the infrequently occurring transformations did not always overlap at a particular linguistic level for the two groups. This measure was also an attempt to quantify this aspect of productive capacity.

Transformations were also grouped into four major categories: 1) sentence transformations, 2) noun transformations, 3) verb transformations, and 4) question transformations. Significant differences were found between each of the five linguistic levels for both groups. However, significant group differences were only found for question transformations, indicating that deficient children do not often use the question form as a means of obtaining new information. There is little reason to believe that this transformation is in some sense more difficult than more frequently used transformations. Both the number and types of transformations increased with advancing linguistic level for both groups. Finally, the mean number of transformations per utterance was compared for both groups. Again, the number of transformations used in a given utterance significantly increased with linguistic level while no significant group differences were found.

Each utterance was classified by determining the number of major lexical categories (e.g., noun, verb) within each construction type or grammatical relation (e.g., noun-verb, verb-noun). Two measures were then derived from the different construction types identified for the two groups. The first measure was derived by dividing the mean number of lexical categories per construction type by the total number of different constructions occurring in a sample, giving a percentage score for each construction type. The mean number of lexical categories was included in the measure to control for the fact that constructions such as "boy hit ball" and "the boy hit ball" had been pooled for this analysis (see Brown, 1973, pp. 184–186, for a discussion of multimorpheme utterance scoring). Clear differences between the two groups were obtained on this measure across the five levels of linguistic development.

A second measure—the percentage of occurrence of each construction type in the total language samples of both groups—was used to determine if different construction type development corresponded with advancing chronological age. A comparison of diverse construction type development with age showed a high correlation for the normal children and a low correlation for the deficient children. The significant group differences found for diverse construction type development indicate that deficient children do not use as many different construction types as do normal children at a comparable linguistic level. As Brown (1973) points out, adding a word to a particular construction type often does more than simply increase its length; it can also change its entire form. For example, in a noun-verb-noun construction such as "boy hit ball," the child can add an article without changing the form of the sentence (e.g., "the boy hit ball"), while the addition of a locative changes the form to noun-verb-noun-locative (e.g., "boy hit ball here"). Apparently, deficient children add a word to a construction but in ways that less often vary the form of that construction. Finally, this finding is further supported by the fact that infrequent use of some transformations will also affect the number of different constructions generated from a basic set of linguistic components and their relations.

Word-morpheme ratios were computed for each group to determine the occurrence of inflections such as plural, past tense, and possessive. Utterances either had no inflections, one inflection, or two inflections (e.g., two words/two morphemes; two words/three morphemes; five words/seven morphemes). Linguistic level effects were significant for both groups with no significant group differences. Pronouns, demonstratives, "wh" forms, prepositions, and modals were also compared to determine the level and order at which these minor lexical categories appeared for the two groups. With the exception of the deficient group's having more pronouns at the third level, only minor differences were found in the level or order of appearance of these minor lexical items.

In contrast to the earlier work reported by Menyuk (1964) and Lee (1966), the studies by Lackner (1968) and Morehead and Ingram (1973) clearly show that when linguistically deficient children are matched to normal children by linguistic criteria, they do not demonstrate linguistic systems that are qualitatively different. These results underscore the necessity for matching deficient and normal children on criteria other than chronological age or IQ. For example, in the Morehead and Ingram (1973) study, there was a marked delay in the onset and acquisition time of syntax for the deficient group. On the average, these children appeared to take three times as long as the normal children to initiate and acquire linguistic systems comparable to Brown's (1973) fifth linguistic level. Despite this considerable delay, the major difference between the two groups was quantitative rather than qualitative, with the deficient children failing to use their systems in as diverse a way to produce highly varied utterances.

Until recently, Bloomfield's (1933) notion that all nonoral communicative systems were imperfect derivations of spoken language was widely accepted. Stokoe (1972) has made an eloquent argument for viewing American sign language or the language of the deaf as a fully integrated linguistic system. As a result, three recent studies of young deaf children of deaf parents have shown that these children develop early language in a way very similar to that of young normal children. More specifically, Moores (1974) has reported preliminary results indicating that young deaf children sign their first word at a younger age than normal or blind children, supporting the view that early word acquisition is partially dependent on visual imitation (Piaget, 1962). Moreover, Bellugi and Klima (1972) and Schlesinger and Meadow (1972) have found considerable evidence in the general assessment of communication in young deaf children that their grammatical relations and corresponding semantic intentions develop with similar form and complexity to those of young normal children.

Studies of syntactic development in both normal and deficient children have relied almost exclusively on the analysis of spontaneous language samples. This method avoids the artificiality of controlled experimentation and is easily used with young children. Considerable change in the methods used to study spontaneous language samples has occurred since the early studies with normal children were reported. However, the use of spontaneous language samples still presents unique problems for the study of both normal and deficient children. In the studies reviewed here, particularly those using deficient populations, the important methodological issues seem to be: 1) language sampling, 2) the matching of normal and deficient populations, and 3) the method of linguistic and statistical analysis.

Researchers have long recognized that context and sample size can effect the content and complexity of the utterances as well as the reliability of the sample (McCarthy, 1954; Templin, 1957). Recently, Bloom (1970), Brown (1973), Bowerman (1973), and Schlesinger (1971) have provided convincing evidence that in order to determine the grammatical relations of children's utterances, it is necessary to know the semantic intentions of the child. To do this, extensive contextual information must be collected for each utterance in a sample. In addition, language samples, even those used in cross sectional research, should use controlled time sampling techniques developed in longitudinal studies (Bloom, 1970; Bowerman, 1973; Brown, 1973). Moreover, Snow (1972) and Shatz and Gelman (1973) have demonstrated that children's spontaneous utterances vary significantly depending on the context of the verbal interactions. For example, adults modify their language patterns depending on the age of the child to whom they are speaking and 4-year-old children speak quite differently to 2-year-old children than to adults. These studies suggest that situational sampling may be inadequate even if varied conditions are used and that samples should be collected in a broad inter-personal milieu of natural discourse. In the studies of deficient language, Menyuk (1964), Lackner (1968), and Morehead and Ingram (1973) attempted to control for situational variance while Lee (1966) did not (Bloom, 1967).

As mentioned earlier, the size of the language sample has also been shown to be critical to detailed analysis, particularly analysis using frequency counts (Bloom, 1970; Brown, 1973). Although 50 utterances have generally been assumed to be an adequate sample for the calculation of rather gross measures such as mean length of utterance (MLU) in normal children (Shriner, 1967), at least 100 utterances per time sampling period are necessary for reliable calculation of MLU with linguistically deficient children (Tyack, 1973). Moreover, there is ample evidence which now suggests that much larger samples ranging from 700–1,500 utterances are required for any attempt at detailed linguistic analysis (Bloom, 1970; Brown, 1973). Of the four studies of deficient language discussed previously, only Lackner (1968) collected an adequate sample for detailed linguistic analysis.

The conventions used to determine which utterances are to be included for analysis also can affect the results obtained from the comparison of samples from different populations. Since the dependent variable is usually full control of the structures to be analyzed, several investigators have used a criterion which somewhat arbitrarily requires that a given structure appear five times or more to be included in the sample used for analysis (Bloom, 1970; deVilliers and deVilliers, 1973). In the Morehead and Ingram (1973) study, the criterion was two or more occurrences because of the relatively small sample sizes. In addition, some researchers in syntax have chosen to include single words (Brown, 1973) while others have not (Morehead and Ingram, 1973)–a decision determined by the individual goals of the researcher. Finally, correction factors, such as equating for different total sample size in group comparison, are important computational considerations.

Once the contextual conditions, size, and conventions of the samples have been determined, it is necessary to group the samples, particularly in comparison studies of normal and deficient populations, according to some criterion. In the past, samples have generally been matched according to chronological age, IQ, and socioeconomic level (Menyuk, 1964). Although no strict criterion exists for matching samples, it is now generally assumed that linguistic level and mental age are the most appropriate criteria. The use of either of these criteria depends on the populations being studied and the goals of the individual researcher. For example, in studies using retarded subjects, mental age may be as useful as linguistic level, while studies using language-deficient children and also controlling for mental age may use only linguistic level.

Mental age generally has been determined by standardized testing procedures. This method has become a point of controversy, and many researchers now are using tasks derived from cognitive-developmental theories such as that of Piaget (1970). In the past, an approximation of linguistic age or level was usually determined by standardized tests such as the Peabody Picture Vocabulary Test (Dunn, 1965). Recently, MLU has once again emerged as a reliable index of linguistic development until sentences reach four to five words or the child is approximately 3–4 years of age. MLU is reliable during this period because almost everything a child does in organizing an early linguistic system increases length (Bloom, 1970; Bowerman, 1973; Brown, 1973; McCarthy, 1954; Menyuk, 1969).

Brown (1973) has developed useful guidelines for calculating MLU and upper bound, a measure of the longest sentence in a sample. These guidelines are listed in Table 1. From MLU and upper bound, Brown (1973) has established five levels of linguistic development. These levels and their corresponding MLU's, upper bounds, and approximate chronological ages are given in Table 2.

Several changes can be made in using MLU, particularly with language-deficient children, to increase its reliability as a measure of linguistic maturity. First, all structures in a given sample which appear fewer than five times should be eliminated. Second, the *median* length of utterance is less sensitive than the *mean* to the variance found at either of the two extremes of a language sample. Finally, the *mean* lower and upper bounds, rather than the longest or shortest utterance, provide further evidence regarding sentence length distribution in the sample. For example, in a 100-utterance sample taken from a language-deficient child, the 10 shortest sentences, the 10 longest sentences, and the remaining 80 sentences may have a distribution pattern different from that of a comparable normal language sample even though the MLU in each case is very similar. These controls are important in the study of language-deficient children because of the potential variance in performance of the same child within and across time sampling periods.

Two approaches now dominate analysis in child language studies and reflect the current status of linguistic theory. The first approach uses a modified transformational method (Bloom, 1970; Brown, 1973). The second approach adheres more closely to recent developments in semantic theory (Bowerman, 1973; Slobin, 1973). Brown (1973) provides an excellent discussion of both approaches, and in addition, gives a detailed account of the acquisition order of general linguistic structures and their meanings developing between 18 and 30 months of age. I return to the question of linguistic analysis in the section on semantics and cognition.

The linguistic analysis of deaf language seriously needs extensive investigation and requires separate discussion. For example, for apparent reasons, language sampling should include audiovisual data collection, a method that is

Table 1. Brown's (1973) guidelines for calculating mean length of utterance and upper bound

---

1. Start with the second page of the transcription unless that page involves a recitation of some kind. In this latter case, start with the first recitation-free stretch. Count the first 100 utterances satisfying the following rules.

2. Only fully transcribed utterances are used; use none with blanks. Portions of utterances, entered in parentheses to indicate doubtful transcription, are used.

3. Include all exact utterance repetitions (marked with a plus sign in records). Stuttering is marked as repeated efforts at a single word; count the word once in the most complete form produced. In the few cases where a word is produced for emphasis or the like (no, no, no) count each occurrence.

4. Do not count fillers such as "mm" or "oh," but do count "no," "yeah," and "hi."

5. All compound words (two or more free morphemes), proper names, and ritualized reduplications count as single words (for example: birthday, rackety-boom, choo-choo, quack-quack, night-night, pocket-book, see saw). The justification is that there is no evidence that the constituent morphemes function as such for these children.

6. Count as one morpheme all irregular pasts of the verb (got, did, went, saw). Justification is that there is no evidence that the child relates these to present forms.

7. Count as one morpheme all diminutives (doggie, mommy) because these children at least do not seem to use the suffix productively. Diminutives are the standard forms used by the child.

8. Count as separate morphemes all auxiliaries (is, have, will, can, must, would), and also all catenatives (gonna, wanna, hafta). The latter counted as single morphemes rather than as "going to" or "want to" because evidence is that they function so for the children. Count as separate morphemes all inflections, for example, possessive /s/, plural /s/, third person singular /s/, regular past /d/, progressive /in/.

9. The range count follows the above rules but is always calculated for the total transcription rather than for 100 utterances.

---

now being urged for the study of normal children as well. Formal linguistic analysis of American sign language provided by Stokoe (1972) and suggestions for segmenting signs described in Schlesinger and Meadow (1972) now allow more extensive analysis of deaf language samples. Moreover, since the preliminary evidence suggests a developmental sequence similar to that of normal children, much of the work on presyntactic development (Bloom, 1973; E. Clark, 1973a; Greenfield, Smith, and Laufer, in press; Morehead and Morehead, 1974) and on early postsyntactic development (summarized in Brown, 1973) can now be used for research and training in early deaf language research.

The development of clear operational definitions for extracting criterion measures from any linguistic data base often violates the assumptions that

Table 2. Brown's (1973) five linguistic levels and their corresponding mean utterance length, upper bound, and approximate mean chronological age

Linguistic level	Mean morpheme per utterance	Upper bound	Approximate mean chronological age (months)
I	1.75	5	24.0–26.0
II	2.25	7	28.0–30.0
III	2.75	9	31.0–33.0
IV	3.50	11	36.0–38.0
V	4.00	13	41.0–43.0

must be met for many standard statistical tests. Many studies have used frequency and proportion data because these measures allow the researcher to capture the diversity with which a given formative may be used in different contexts. Diverse use of a given form probably indicates more complete grammatical understanding and interpretation of that form and, as such, is an important performance variable to measure. In addition, the use of proportion or percentage can demonstrate increments in the occurrence of specific construction types independent of increases in the total number of construction types across time sampling periods. Studies by Bloom (1970), Bowerman (1973), and Brown (1973) have demonstrated that frequency and proportion data can be extremely informative. An alternative to the use of frequency and proportion data for occurring linguistic structures is the presentation of data in terms of the number of subjects using a specific structure (Menyuk, 1964, 1969). This alternative to the use of frequency data is preferred by many researchers.

In both longitudinal and cross sectional studies, researchers have often generalized their findings based on the analysis or testing of a small set of linguistic structures to overall language functioning. H. Clark (1973a) has recently pointed to the inherent fallacies of such an approach and has presented detailed methodological considerations related to the selection of testing materials and certain limitations on the kinds of statistical analysis available to language research.

MORPHOLOGY

Almost without exception, frequency and variety of utterance types and their degree of occurrence have been used as major acquisition criteria for studying the development of syntax in both normal and deficient children. As Brown (1973) points out, any sample of spontaneous production is likely to be affected by both the child's underlying competence and his communicative intentions at the time the sample is collected. The study of morphology gets around this problem somewhat since morphemes have obligatory contexts in which the child uses these forms with greater consistency as they become part of his integrated linguistic system.

Brown (1973) has provided a detailed description of the acquisition of 14 grammatical morphemes in three young normal children, including a word structure grammar and possible semantic meanings which characterize these morphemes. Recently, deVilliers and deVilliers (1973) in a cross sectional study collected spontaneous speech samples averaging 360 utterances for 21 children between the ages of 16 and 40 months and then analyzed these samples for the same 14 grammatical morphemes studied by Brown (1973). Brown (1973) found evidence in his longitudinal study that both MLU and chronological age were reasonable predictors of morpheme acquisition. More-over, he found that the order of acquisition was nearly invariant for the three children. Because of the smaller sample size in the deVilliers and deVilliers (1973) study, they could not use Brown's (1973) acquisition criterion of 90% presence of each morpheme in three successive time samplings. MLU could be used to order three successive children and retain the 90% criterion used by Brown (1973). However, the variance in the MLU's of the children in the deVilliers and deVilliers (1973) study was too great to use successive MLU order. As a result, the morphemes were first ranked according to the lowest MLU sample in which each morpheme first occurred in 90% or more of obligatory contexts. A second procedure based on Brown's (1973) finding of near invariance in the acquisition order of morphemes was to rank the mean percentage that each morpheme appeared across all the children. In addition, they used the criterion of five or more occurrences in obligatory contexts for a given morpheme.

The 14 morphemes identified by Brown (1973) and used in the deVilliers and deVilliers (1973) study are: 1) present progressive, 2 and 3) prepositions "in" and "on," 4) plural, 5) past irregular, 6) possessive, 7) uncontractible copula, 8) articles, 9) past regular, 10) third person regular, 11) third person irregular, 12) uncontractible auxiliary, 13) contractible copula, and 14) con-tractible auxiliary. There was a high correlation found between the acquisi-tion order of the 14 morphemes in Brown's (1973) longitudinal data and the cross sectional data of deVilliers and deVilliers (1973). Moreover, high corre-lations with Brown's (1973) findings occurred when either the modified 90% in obligatory contexts criterion or the ranked mean percentages criterion was used. As mentioned earlier, Brown (1973) anticipated that both MLU and chronological age might be important predictors for the usage of particular morphemes. However, the deVilliers (1973) found a clear advantage of MLU over chronological age as a reliable predictor.

Methods for studying morphology in linguistically deficient children have been adapted from Berko's (1958) early work. Using an elicitation technique that supplied the obligatory contexts, she studied the times at which the plural, progressive, past tense, possessive, and third person singular inflections and their allomorphs appeared in preschool and first grade children's responses. Lovell and Bradbury (1967) used Berko's (1958) method and results with normal children and compared them with a large group of retarded children with a mean IQ of 70. The results indicated that performance of mildly retarded children, measured according to the number of subjects producing the correct morpheme or allomorph, was poorer than that of Berko's (1958) first grade children. Since the retarded children were between 14 and 15 years of age, Lovell and Bradbury (1967) concluded that these children were unable to generalize to new lexical items in contexts that required the use of particular inflections. In a follow-up study, Bradbury and Lunzer (1972) found that retarded children could learn inflectional rules but were less successful than normal children on a transfer task requiring the use of those rules.

A more complete study using Berko's (1958) methods and normal controls was reported by Newfield and Schlanger (1968). They compared 30 retarded children with a mean chronological age of 10.4 years and a mean mental age of 6.2 years with 30 normal children having a mean chronological age of 6.10 years. Since no intelligence scores were available for the normal group, the Peabody Picture Vocabulary Test was administered to both groups, showing approximately a 2-year difference in favor of the normal group. The results showed that the order of morpheme acquisition was nearly identical for both groups across both nonsense and real word items although the retarded children learned these forms at a slower rate.

Cooper (1967) constructed a 48-item morphology test in a study comparing 140 congenitally deaf children with 176 hearing children. Chronological age ranged from 7 to near 20 years for both groups, and only an approximate match of the two groups according to age was possible. Given the advanced age of the normal subjects, it is not surprising that their performance on the test was superior to that of the deaf population. The interesting finding here is that the percentage passing score for items ranked according to difficulty was very similar for the two groups.

Recently, morphological research with deficient children has followed the shift in research with normal children from elicitation techniques to studies using cross sectional data derived from language samples. One of the more important features of the deVilliers' (1973) study is that it demonstrates that cross sectional data are extremely useful in providing independent support for major findings derived from the more laborious and time-consuming longitudinal analysis. This particular research strategy can be very effective in using the large amount of linguistic data available on normal children to study specific and relevant questions regarding language development in deficient children.

Johnston and Schery (in press) have used just such an approach to study the development of grammatical morphemes in language-deficient children. They selected 287 children from 3 to 16 years of age who were part of a special program in a large metropolitan school system. Although the group was extremely heterogeneous, all the children were of normal intelligence and judged to have a deficit primarily in language. A sample of 100 utterances for each child was elicited during play sessions with a language therapist. The linguistic level of each child was determined by the mean number of words per utterance. Because of the relatively small samples and contextual sampling restrictions, only eight of Brown's (1973) grammatical morphemes could be analyzed for both rate and order of acquisition.

The relationship between linguistic level and performance on the grammatical morphemes was used to determine the rate of acquisition. Two measures were used: 1) the percentage of children at each linguistic level who used a given morpheme at least once, and 2) the percentage of children who used a given morpheme 80% of the time. They found that both usage and occurrence of the eight morphemes increased as linguistic level increased and that the morphemes were acquired at somewhat different rates. To determine the order of acquisition, Johnston and Schery (in press) used two criterion measures: 1) Brown's (1973) 90% occurrence in obligatory contexts, and 2) the use of a particular morpheme one or more times by at least 50% of the subjects at a given linguistic level. The results showed that the language-deficient children, when compared with the normal children in the studies by Brown (1973) and deVilliers and deVilliers (1973), reached criterion at a later linguistic level. However, the same order of acquisition appeared as that found in the two earlier studies of normal children.

Information on the development of morphology in normal children has come from the use of three methods: longitudinal studies, cross sectional studies, and elicitation techniques. Except for the Johnston and Schery (in press) study, comparisons between deficient and normal populations generally have been limited to the five regular inflections studied by Berko (1958), whereas Brown (1973) has identified 14 grammatical morphemes in his longitudinal summary, and even these 14 do not represent all of the morphemes in English. Both the deVilliers and deVilliers (1973) and the Johnston and Schery (in press) studies demonstrate the validity of cross sectional research in morphology and, as mentioned earlier, utilize a research strategy for using normal language data to study specific aspects of language development.

Since it is frequently possible to identify obligatory contexts for grammatical morphemes, the problem of sampling variation can be more successfully controlled than in the study of syntax. That is, obligatory contexts allow criteria other than mere occurrence since the child must use a morphological form in certain contexts if he has productive control of that form. In addition, obligatory contexts allow the study of grammatical morphemes in natural discourse rather than by the elicitation methods of experimental studies. This is an important consideration because many deficient populations respond poorly to highly structured experimental tasks. Finally, the experimental studies which compare normal and deficient morphological development need to provide clear mental age or linguistic level for establishing when the morphemes are likely to appear and to consider specific linguistic criteria such as MLU as possible methods for matching deficient and normal groups.

COMPREHENSION AND IMITATION

Until recently, the analysis of spontaneous production data has focused on the structure of the child's utterances, first by distribution analysis and later by integrated grammars that attempt to characterize the linguistic knowledge necessary to produce these structures. In addition to the analysis of structure through production data, there is the analysis of structure through the study of comprehension and imitation. The use of production data for determining underlying competence in child language acquisition has often been criticized because it is contaminated with many performance variables such as motivation, memory, and disruptions natural to discourse (Chomsky, 1964; Smith, 1970). Methods for studying competence in young children that do not involve verbal production are extremely difficult to develop. With the recent interest in semantics, the use of comprehension tasks has become widespread, particulary in adult research (Carroll and Freedle, 1972).

The study of comprehension in normal language acquisition really begins with the early diary studies, which include many insightful observations (Leopold, 1939; Lewis, 1951; Piaget, 1962). More recently, Shipley, Smith, and Gleitman (1969) presented children with commands of varying linguistic complexity and which required nonverbal responses. Their results showed that for young children, understanding was similar to the utterances they produced. For older children, understanding seemed to be somewhat more advanced than their spontaneous speech indicated. Huttenlocher (1974) has recently reported the early results of the first longitudinal study of language comprehension. This research provides a rich elaboration of specific linguistic developments that parallel the general mental development described by Piaget (1962) for the first 2 years. One of the more important findings is that children during the 2nd year respond appropriately to many words which they do not produce. In addition, there is no apparent overgeneralization in comprehension, as has been often noted in production (E. Clark, 1973a).

Other studies involving comprehension have considered its relationship to imitation and production. For example, in the often cited Fraser, Bellugi, and Brown (1963) study, imitation was found to precede comprehension while comprehension was found to precede production. Several studies have replicated this basic design, with both supportive (Lovell and Dixon, 1965), and/or contradictory or ambiguous results (Fernald, 1972; Keeney and Wolfe,

1972). For example, the Fernald (1972) study found that comprehension and production were equivalent when irrelevant responses were not counted as errors, while Keeney and Wolfe (1972) found in the case of verb number inflection, that production may precede comprehension. What these studies indicate, of course, is that the relationship between imitation, comprehension, and production is not well understood, particularly as they interact with one another while the child is acquiring language.

In a series of training studies by Guess and Baer (1973) retarded subjects were used to demonstrate that learning to understand a linguistic form may be independent of learning to produce it. That is, when subjects were trained to understand or to use, in this case, the plural morpheme, little generalization was noted from comprehension to production, or vice versa. Miller and Yoder (1973) have reported a methodological study to determine if different response measures provide equivalent information regarding linguistic comprehension in mentally retarded children. The three modes tested were: 1) pointing to pictures which depicted linguistic materials, 2) acting out the content of linguistic materials through object manipulation, and 3) sentence imitation. They found that sentence imitation was not an adequate measure of comprehension in retarded children. These findings point to the importance of testing measures developed in normal research before they are considered reliable indicators of linguistic functions in deficient populations.

Elicited imitation has often been used as an independent means of assessing underlying competence for both normal (Brown and Fraser, 1963; Scholes, 1970) and deficient children (Lackner, 1968; Menyuk, 1964; Menyuk and Looney, 1972). Slobin and Welsh (1973) described the use of elicited imitation and discussed its shortcomings and advantages. Since the interpretation of any utterance is heavily dependent upon context, children often cannot imitate utterances that they have previously produced spontaneously (Slobin and Welsh, 1973). In addition, imitation is also susceptible to all the constraints affecting performance. However, the fact that children in repetition tasks filter any linguistic sequence through their own internalized systems allows the researcher through systematic construction of stimulus materials to analyze important aspects of linguistic processing. For example, the ways in which children recode sentences in which phonological, syntactic, or semantic aspects have been manipulated as the independent variable can reveal much about their productive strategies.

In a well designed study to determine the strategy children use to retain or delete certain words, Scholes (1970) had children between 3 and 4 years imitate word strings varying in length from three to five words. The word strings were either well formed, semantically anomalous but well formed, or syntactically ill formed. In addition, a second set of strings substituted nonsense items for content words or for function words. Moreover, stress was controlled by presenting the strings auditorily without suprasegmental diction.

Contrary to the suggestions of Brown and Bellugi (1964) that young children use telegraphic speech because content words are stressed and carry the most information, Scholes (1970) found that the child retains content words primarily because they have familiar word structure and semantic roles that allow them to stand out in a string of words. That is, children seem to know that articles, for example, are not terribly important items regardless of their grammatical relations. Menyuk and Looney (1972) found similar results for language-deficient children.

Historically, imitation has often been considered to be an important developmental process that precedes production and, in some cases, comprehension, in the learning of linguistic and social systems (Bandura and Walters, 1963; Guillaume, 1968; Piaget, 1962). More recently, proponents of generative grammar have argued forcefully that underlying structures rather than their surface representations provide the primary linguistic data and that these underlying structures are not available to imitation (Chomsky, 1959; McNeill, 1970). Moreover, two recent studies that compared the function of imitative and spontaneous utterances in young children found that spontaneous speech was more advanced than imitative speech, suggesting that imitation as a learning process is not progressive (Ervin-Tripp, 1964; Kemp and Dale, in press).

Bloom, Hood, and Lightbown (1974) have reported a longitudinal study of imitation with six normal children who were making the transition from single words to two-word utterances. They determined the extent and consistency of imitation and compared both imitative and spontaneous utterances in a number of lexical and grammatical contexts. They found that some children used imitation as a process for language learning while others did not. Moreover, for those children who did imitate, imitation was used differentially; that is, some used imitation to acquire new lexical items while others used imitation to learn semantic relations between lexical items. Finally, the imitating children seemed to imitate only those lexical items or relational structures that they were in the process of learning. Once an imitative item was used spontaneously, the item was seldom if ever imitated again. In this sense, imitation was found to be progressive for those children who used it.

The recent work related to understanding, imitation, and production is of obvious interest to those concerned with the study of language-deficient children. Imitation has been the primary and, in some cases, the exclusive method used in almost all language training despite the fact that its role in language learning is only partially understood. In fact, some normal children do not use it as a strategy for learning language at all. However, when normal children do imitate, they filter linguistic structures through their linguistic systems and, in addition, seem to imitate only those structures that they are in the process of learning (Bloom, Hood, and Lightbown, 1974). These findings underscore the necessity for knowing the structures that the child is in the process of learning before materials used in imitative training are developed.

Frequently, it has been assumed that language-deficient children understand far more than they can produce or that they often imitate utterances which they do not comprehend. The comprehension-production "gap" is not well understood, even in normal children (Bloom, 1974; Ingram, 1974). The hypothesis that deficient children imitate utterances that they do not understand finds no support in the literature on normal children (Bloom, Hood, and Lightbown, 1974; Slobin and Welsh, 1973).

SEMANTICS AND COGNITION

Recent developments in linguistic theory suggest that syntax and semantics are interdependent and inseparable (Chafe, 1970; Fillmore, 1968; McCawley, 1968). These developments are reflected in the works of Bloom (1970), Bowerman (1973), Brown (1973), and Schlesinger (1971), which show that any complete description of the form of an utterance is heavily dependent on its content or meaning. Moreover, with this new emphasis on meaning, three complementary aspects of child language research are developing: 1) the analysis of semantic meaning or intention, 2) the exploration of the relationship between language and other mental development, and 3) the study of the strategies by which the child acquires an integrated linguistic system.

The most extensive study of the semantic intentions which characterize particular linguistic levels has been Brown's (1973) summary analysis of the first two levels of this development (I = 1.75–2.25 mean morphemes per utterance; II = 2.25–2.75 mean morphemes per utterance). Using 12 samples from five languages, including English, he defined the relations of multiword utterances found in stage I according to semantic rather than grammatical criteria. The important finding was that a small number of basic two-term relations accounted for the majority of the utterances produced at this linguistic level. There were eight basic two-term relations and seven additional two-term relations that appeared consistently but with very low frequency. Moreover, all of the children expanded the two-term relations using the same two strategies. The first strategy was to add a term to a two-term relation utterance by combining two two-term relations and deleting the redundant term. For example, "Eve eat" (agent-action) and "eat lunch" (action-object) were combined to form "Eve eat lunch" (agent-action-object) with the redundant term "eat" deleted.

The second strategy was to expand one term, always the noun phrase, into a two-term relation. For example, "eat lunch" (action-object) could be expanded to "eat Eve lunch" (action-possessive-possession), with the object term expanding to include the possessor-possession relationship. Brown

(1973) has proposed a law of cumulative complexity which essentially states that the number of relations in a sentence is a good measure for specifying complexity at this level. The fact that multiword utterances increase as MLU increases indicates very little about how these increments are made. The cumulative complexity index is an important step toward quantifying what lies behind these increments.

The law of cumulative complexity predicts, then, that a three-term relation such as "Eve eat lunch" (agent-action-object) is more complex than either of the two-term relations of which it is composed ("Eve eat"—agent-action—and "eat lunch"—action-object) for the very reason that the three-term relation includes both of the two-term relations plus something new, namely, a third relation (agent-object). The importance of the cumulative complexity principle is that it allows one to predict that if the child can construct $x + y$, then the child also knows x and y independently. Conversely, it does not predict that if the child knows x and y, he is also able to construct $x + y$. This principle has particular relevance for the study of deficient language since there is now evidence suggesting that deficient children have a deficit in the number of different constructions which they can generate from a basic set of two- (or more) term relations (Morehead and Ingram, 1973).

Once a base set of terms or content words and their semantic roles and grammatical relations are learned, the child in level II amplifies the meanings learned in level I by adding a set of grammatical morphemes. Brown (1973) has also provided a rather extensive analysis of the meanings of the 14 grammatical morphemes which he studied. These grammatical morphemes add to the existing lexicon and their basic relations number, tense, aspect, notions of specificity and containment or support. For example, the prepositions "in" and "on" differentiate more precisely containment and support as locational aspects of space.

Although Piaget (1962) emphasized that the major meanings expressed in early language acquisition were derived from early mental development occurring during the first 2 years, this concept only recently appeared in child language research when attempts were made to characterize the semantic intentions of the child. In addition, Piaget (1962) also proposed that language was only one aspect of the general symbolic capacity to represent objects and events that were not available in immediate perception and ongoing actions. The first proposition has received much attention in the recent literature (Bloom, 1973; Bowerman, 1974; Brown, 1973; E. Clark, 1974; H. Clark, 1973b; Cromer, 1974a; Morehead and Morehead, 1974; Schlesinger, 1974; Sinclair, 1971, 1973; Slobin, 1973). Its importance for the study of linguistically deficient children is that it allows methods and procedures for developing precursor measures prior to the appearance of syntax and the availability of MLU and other complexity measures. For example, Morehead and Morehead (1974) have suggested that infant tests (e.g., Mehrabian and Williams, 1971; Uzgiris and Hunt, 1966) designed from Piaget's (1952) work on

sensorimotor intelligence, along with detailed descriptions of early presyntactic and symbolic development (Brown, 1973; Lezine, 1973; Morehead and
Morehead, 1974; Sinclair, 1971, 1973), can be used to attain presyntactic
levels of linguistic development because imitation substages are reliable predictors of both general mental development and early symbolic development.

The second proposal by Piaget (1962)—that language is part of a larger
representational or symbolic system which also includes perception, deferred
imitation, imagery, symbolic play, drawing, and dreaming—has only recently
received attention in normal language acquisition research (Bloom, 1974;
Bowerman, 1974; Cromer, 1974a; Greenfield, Smith, and Laufer, in press;
Morehead and Morehead, 1974). However, the proposal has generated research as well as training studies with language-deficient children. For example, Inhelder (1966) and de Ajuriaguerra (1966), using Piagetian tasks, found
that children with a delayed rate of linguistic development showed a specific
deficit in other aspects of representational development although these children frequently had normal base intellectual development. In addition,
Lovell, Hoyle, and Siddall (1968) reported that for linguistically deficient
children, the shorter their MLU, the less time they spent in symbolic play.
Finally, Morehead (1972) reported preliminary data from one austistic child
which suggested that training in one area of prelinguistic representational
behavior such as symbolic play may facilitate other aspects of representational development including language.

Few experimental studies have attempted to relate specific linguistic
structures to general cognitive development. The studies that have been done
are generally derived from the Genevan position that although cognitive and
linguistic systems develop according to their own laws, cognitive operations
will provide the basis for explaining language. Three studies have been carried
out to test whether linguistic abilities are determined by different levels of
cognitive operations such as reversibility (Ferreiro and Sinclair, 1971; Inhelder, 1969; Sinclair, 1969). Conservation studies have been used to determine when a child is capable of "conserving" the quantity of a substance that
remains the same as it transforms from one state to another. For example, in
the standard water beaker test, the child is asked to judge whether beakers of
equal dimension contain identical quantities of water. After the water from
one of the glasses is poured into a tall narrow beaker of equal volume, the
child is again asked for a judgment. Typically, children younger than 6 years
fail to conserve; children between 6 and 7 are ambiguous or in transition;
children 7 years and older conserve. The cognitive operation allowing success
on conservation tasks is reversibility, an operation by which the child is able
not only to follow transformations through successive states but also to
follow the reverse order of transformations to their previous state or states
and/or point of origin.

Sinclair (1969) explored the relationship between the conservation of
liquids and seriation and the comprehension and production of three linguistic aspects likely to be affected by the presence or absence of conserva-

tion. The three aspects were: 1) lexical specificity (e.g., "thin" instead of "little"), 2) comparative rather than absolute terms (e.g., "more" or "less" instead of "most" or "least"), and 3) coordinated sentences (e.g., "This one is shorter but thicker than that one"). In the comprehension task children were asked to find a pencil that was shorter but thicker, while in the production task they were asked to describe objects differing in two dimensions such as a short, thick pencil and a long, thin pencil. The children were divided into three groups on the basis of conservation testing: 1) those who failed to conserve, 2) those in transition, and 3) those who succeeded. Sinclair (1969) found few differences between the three groups on the comprehension task but a clear parallel between conservation level and the use of related linguistic structures. More specifically, conserving children tended to be lexically specific, to use comparative rather than absolute terms, and to coordinate two dimensions in their descriptions, while nonconserving children did not. Two related studies, one reported by Inhelder (1969) using seriation and another by Ferreiro and Sinclair (1971) using temporal order, found similar results.

The results of these studies show a correlation only between linguistic structures and operational level. However, Sinclair (1969) also reported an additional study which showed that training with certain linguistic structures does not bring about a corresponding change in operational structures although training may increase the child's attention to the relevant dimensions in a conservation task. These findings support the Piagetian (1970) view that cognition develops independent of language at least until the operational stage, which begins at around 7 years. This view is consistent with evidence from the only two studies of linguistically deficient children which, as mentioned earlier, found these children to have normal operational or intellectual development but to be deficient in other aspects of representation such as imagery (de Ajuriaguerra, 1966; Inhelder, 1966).

Although operational structures such as reversibility have no obvious analogue in language, other concepts, particularly those related to space, may have. For example, Piaget and Inhelder (1967) have described three major developmental periods during which the child moves from topological to projective to Euclidean notions of space. Parisi and Antinucci (1970) used this work on spatial development to determine whether the order in which locative terms developed would parallel the order of spatial concept development. They found the predicted order of acquisition for locative terms in Italian, but they did not directly compare their subjects' levels of cognitive and linguistic development. Johnston (1973) confirmed the Parisi and Antinucci (1970) findings that topological locatives are learned prior to projective-Euclidean terms with an English sample. In addition, she found some evidence that a child's use of locatives such as "in front of," "behind," and "between" could be predicted from his performance on spatial tasks.

H. Clark (1973b) has also proposed an interesting hypothesis regarding the development of spatial and temporal terms based on the assumption that these terms are a natural outgrowth of the child's construction of a perceptual space derived from the orientation of his own body in space. For example, the normal position of a child's body in space has three reference planes and several related directions which can be assigned positive or negative values: 1) ground level with upward positive and downward negative, 2) vertical left and right orientation with front and back being assigned positive and negative values, respectively, and 3) vertical front and back with right and left both assigned positive value. Using a cumulative complexity measure similar to Brown's (1973) but including positive and negative values (with positive values being learned first), Clark postulated that there is a strong relationship between spatial terms and the child's perceptual system and between spatial and temporal terms. There is some experimental evidence to support this position in recent work by Donaldson and Wales (1970) and E. Clark (1971). No related studies exist using language-deficient populations.

The determination of linguistic structures that characterize a particular level of linguistic development has consumed much of the recent research effort in child language development. There are now significant advances in discovering the heuristic methods or self-instruction techniques used by the child in acquiring linguistic structures. To understand this new direction in child language research, it is necessary to exemplify the different ways in which the term heuristic or *strategy* is used. Piaget (1971) has cited many examples indicating that all mental development, including language, is an outgrowth of the basic biological principles of organization and adaptation. Organization refers to the integration of subsystems into an equilibriated structured whole, while adaptation refers to the assimilation of information to mental structures and the accommodation of these structures to that information.

Slobin (1973) rephrased this basic principle and applied it to the acquisition of linguistic structures as "new forms first express old functions and new functions are first expressed by old forms." To exemplify the first half of this principle (i.e., that new forms first express old content), Brown's (1973) data show that inflected verb forms mark the same semantic distinctions as those marked by the earlier appearing uninflected forms. Thus, uninflected progressive forms such as "I go now" change to the inflected form by adding "-ing" to the verb and produce "I going now," with the content of the two utterances remaining the same. Chukovsky (1968), a Russian poet and writer, spent many years collecting examples of new content being expressed first in old forms—to cite a few: "Can't you see I'm barefoot all over" and, while looking in a mirror, "I pretty-mire myself." A fundamental use of the term strategy, then, defines a set of heuristics, probably biologically based, used by the child in constructing both cognitive and linguistic systems.

Since there are important developments in sensorimotor behavior or early cognition during the first 2 years that predate the onset of language, it has been assumed that at least early linguistic development—if not the entire development leading to a full coordination of language and thought at around 12 years (Piaget, 1963)–depends in part on strategies specific to mental development that precede it (Brown, 1973; Lezine, 1973; Morehead and Morehead, 1974; Sinclair, 1971, 1973).

There are some recent data that give support to this assumption. For example, using a seriation and embedding task that required young children to manipulate objects, Greenfield, Nelson, and Saltzman (1972) found three action strategies that correspond to the early relations that appear in syntactic development. Goodnow and Levine (1973) also found similar parallels between copying shapes and the rule-governed behavior found in child language. Finally, E. Clark (1973b) reported three experiments which indicate that young children's interpretations of early appearing prepositions such as "in," "on," and "under" are influenced by nonlinguistic strategies related to spatial concepts as well as by the actual semantic coding of these lexical items. Since all language-deficient populations share the feature of extreme delay in the onset as well as acquisition time of language, these studies suggest rather explicit ways to test the hypothesis that onset delay may be caused by the deficient child's inability to reapply strategies used in early cognition to the acquisition of language.

A third use of the term strategy refers to the notion that there are probably specific sets of strategies for different physical and social systems to be learned by the child. Even though cognitive development is generally felt to underlie important aspects of linguistic development, particularly those related to meaning, it is not generally assumed that these two systems evolve according to the same set of laws (Chomsky, 1965). Slobin (1973) has postulated an important set of universals specific to language and corresponding "operating principles" or strategies based on an impressive compilation of cross cultural studies. For example, children universally pay close attention to word and morpheme order whether or not the language they are learning uses word order as a primary means of expressing relations and/or meaning. Ervin-Tripp (1973) has also provided an excellent discussion of possible linguistic strategies used by the very young child. She includes in her discussion many examples which amplify the basic operating principles outlined by Slobin (1973).

The term strategy has also been used in the study of spontaneous speech samples to describe specific heuristics used by children. Several investigators have found that early two-word constructions appear in two distinct forms (Bloom, 1970; Brown, 1973; Schlesinger, 1971). The first form represents a closed semantic set pertaining to reference rather than relations, in that the meaning of the construction is derived from either of the two words rather than from the relation between them. These early constructions include the nominative or existence (e.g., "that ball"), recurrence (e.g., "more milk"), and nonexistence (e.g., "no cookie"). The second form differs from the first in that neither word in early two-word constructions carries the meaning of the utterance. Rather, it is the relation between the two that signifies the semantic intention of the construction. Examples of the second form include agent-action (e.g., "Daddy walk"), attributive (e.g., "big ball"), and agent-object (e.g., "Mommy sock").

Bloom (1973) has suggested that different children may use different strategies in making the transition from successive single words to early two- and three-word constructions and that these strategies are reflected in the two distinct forms in which early syntax appears. In her own longitudinal study, she found that some children begin with referential constructions or a system of formal markers, such as "more milk," while others begin with relational constructions or a system of grammatical categories and their relations. Bloom (1973) attributed the selection of a particular strategy to the complex interactions between cognitive development and linguistic experience. However, Morehead and Morehead (1974) have suggested that relational syntax may derive from logical-mathematical knowledge whereas referential syntax derives from physical knowledge. If this correspondence between cognitive and linguistic systems holds, then it can be assumed that relational syntax represents a more advanced strategy because logical-mathematical knowledge develops later and is more complex than physical knowledge. Brown (1973) also suggests that rate of language learning is closely related to general factors in intelligence.

Brown (1973) has found that once children develop relational syntax, they all use the same two strategies for expanding two-word or two-term relations. As mentioned earlier, one strategy was to develop a new two-term relation by combining two already existing two-term relations and deleting the redundant term, while the second strategy was to expand one of the terms in a two-term relation. An interesting point to emphasize here is that these two strategies were found consistently in different children learning *different* first languages.

Distinct strategies also have been found in experimental studies using older children and complex linguistic structures. Cromer (1970) has developed three sets of sentences in which the relationship between surface structure and the underlying grammatical relations is not always apparent. Moreover, in these sentences the only clue for recovering the meaning of the deep structure is in the adjective. The first set of sentences have adjectives like "happy" and "willing" and a surface structure subject which always corresponds to the deep structure subject. Thus, in a sentence like "The duck is happy to bite," it is the named animal that always does the biting. The second set of sentences, in which the surface structure subject does not correspond to the deep structure subject, used adjectives like "easy" and "fun." Thus, in the sentence "The wolf is easy to bite," it is the unnamed animal that does the biting. In the third set of sentences the relation between deep and surface structure subjects is ambiguous and depends on context for resolution. Thus, in a sentence like "The wolf is nice to bite," it is not clear who does the biting.

Using normal children between the ages of 5 and 11 on a comprehension task where puppets manipulated by the child signified the agent or the object effected, Cromer (1974b) found two distinct stages with a transitional period separating the two. Children with a mental age younger than 6.3 years always indicated the named animal as the puppet doing the biting. These children in this first stage seemed to use a primitive rule implying that the surface subject was always considered to be the deep subject. For the transitional period, children with a mental age greater than 6.3 years inconsistently selected interpretations common to the first and second stages for all three sets of sentences. This intermediate level suggests that the children realized that different interpretations were possible but failed to relate the appropriate surface structure adjectives to their corresponding deep structure interpretations. Finally, the second stage attained by children with a mental age between 7 and 11 years allowed correct interpretations for all sentences. Cromer (1972a) also found that mentally retarded children of comparable mental age pass through the same developmental sequence as do normal children.

Cromer (1972a, 1972b, 1974b) then developed a set of sentence frames derived from various transformations on the original sets of sentences to test the hypothesis that children may learn these adjectives by hearing them in related transformations. Some transformations allow subject adjectives but not object adjectives, and vice versa. For example, the subject adjective "glad" is allowed in "I am always glad to see you" while the objective adjective "fun" is not allowed in "I am always fun to see you." Also, "Seeing you is fun" is possible while "Seeing you is glad" is not. Nonsense words were substituted for adjectives in a number of related transformation frames, and the sentences were presented using a picture card technique to normal children, mentally retarded children, and normal adults who had been previously classified as stage I, transitional, or stage II subjects. The subjects were shown pictures of, for example, a dog with a bone and told, "The dog said, 'I'm always *risp* to get a bone,' " with the embedded sentence always stated twice. The picture was then removed, and as in the earlier experiments, the child was asked to manipulate two puppets while being asked, "Now show me, who does the biting in this: 'The wolf is *risp* to bite'?"

Using the nonsense words in different transformational frames, Cromer (1974b) found that normal children used strategies appropriate to their level or stage of linguistic processing; that is, stage I subjects always assumed that the surface structure subject performed the action, transitional subjects assumed that either surface or deep structure subject performed the action but were not sure which one, and stage II subjects assumed that the deep structure subject always performed the action.

An interesting difference was found for both mentally retarded children and normal adults in that both groups used only the stage I strategy of assuming that the surface structure subject performed the action (Cromer, 1972a, 1974b). Cromer (1974c) provides an intriguing explanation of these results, suggesting that the deep structure subject strategy used by the stage II older normal children may reflect a universal strategy of always seeking the marked form, a form which is often introduced to modify more basic linguistic information or the unmarked form (see Greenberg, 1966, for a discussion of marked versus unmarked forms). Moreover, he goes on to argue that if this is a specific linguistic rather than a general cognitive strategy, there might be a loss of the use of this strategy in subjects beyond the critical period for first language learning. Thus, older retarded and normal adult subjects may no longer have this strategy available to them. It will be recalled, however, that both older retarded and normal adult subjects comprehend real adjectives that require the deep structure strategy in sentences like "The wolf is happy to bite."

What Cromer (1974c) seems to have found is one viable explanation for why the language of older mentally retarded children develops at a much slower rate than that of normals and why adults are not as efficient as young children in learning second languages—the most economical linguistic strategies simply may not be available to them. These findings and their interpretations have important implications for language-deficient children other than the retarded since they provide a rationale and a method for studying the development or lack of development of these strategies in other populations.

Finally, two points of caution need to be made regarding the concept of strategy as it has been discussed here. First, the study of strategies is always confounded by the level of the child's development as well as the kind of performance used to reveal specific strategies. As demonstrated by Piaget's (1970) work and the research by Cromer (1974c), particular strategies are closely tied to level or stage of cognitive or linguistic development. In fact, Genevan research has depended heavily on strategies as a way of inferring cognitive structures that differentiate stages of development. That the kind of performance task used is affected by the child's level of knowing any complex system such as language has been dramatically demonstrated in a recent study by deVilliers and deVilliers (1972). They found that children younger than 3 years were incapable of making judgments about word order despite the apparent universal use of adult word order by children, including those tested, at a much earlier age.

Second, if heuristics can be defined as self-instruction, then there is by implication in higher mental functions some intentional plan or, in the language of computer programming, "executive routines" (Neisser, 1967). It is this aspect of strategy use that is missing from the experiments discussed earlier. In Piaget's (1971) theory self-regulation is an important aspect of behavior which appears by the end of the child's 1st year. Intentionality or self-instruction, then, is clearly available before the onset of language. To include this aspect of acquiring language, Antinucci and Parisi (1973) have developed in their theory of child language development a concept of linguistic intentionality called the performative.

Following the lead of Chomsky (1965), it can be assumed that in learning any complex system the normal child will follow the most efficient and economical strategies available to him. Otherwise, it would be difficult to explain the rate at which normal children acquire language. It remains to be determined, however, why normal children go about learning language in the exact ways that they do. Nevertheless, it can be determined whether or not linguistically deficient children use the same strategies as normal children use. Given the tremendous delay in onset and acquisition time for deficient populations, a best guess is that they do not. In fact, Cromer's (1972a, 1974b) work with retarded children and normal adults suggests that strategies specific to certain linguistic structures may not be available at the time the structures are to be acquired or that these strategies may even fail to develop, forcing the child to use less efficient methods for acquiring more advanced linguistic structures.

SUMMARY

In this chapter I have attempted to include studies which tell us something about the nature of language acquisition in deficient populations as well as those studies in normal language that indicate new directions for research. We now have considerable evidence in both language and cognition that deficient children do not organize these systems in ways that are fundamentally different from those used by normal children. This general finding suggests, to me at least, that new research should focus on the acquisition process rather than on the organization of linguistic systems. For this reason, a substantial portion of this chapter has dealt with comprehension and imitation, the relationship of cognition to language, and finally, the strategies that children may use in acquiring language. It is this last aspect, that of language acquisition strategies, that seems to be the most potentially productive area for future research.

ACKNOWLEDGMENT

I wish to thank Judith Johnston for her critical reading of this chapter and Ann Morehead for her stylistic and substantive suggestions.

REFERENCES

de Ajuriaguerra, J. 1966. Speech disorders in childhood. In C. Carterette (ed.), Brain Function: Speech, Language and Communication, pp. 117–140. University of California Press, Los Angeles.
Antinucci, F., and D. Parisi. 1973. Early language acquisition: A model and

some data. *In* C. Ferguson and D. Slobin (eds.), Studies in Child Language Development, pp. 607–619. Holt, Rinehart and Winston, New York.

Bandura, A., and R. Walters. 1963. Social Learning and Personality Development. Holt, Rinehart and Winston, New York.

Bellugi, U., and E. Klima. 1972. The roots of language in the sign talk of the deaf. Psychol. Today June: 61–64.

Berko, J. 1958. The child's learning of English morphology. Word 14: 150–177.

Bever, T. G. 1970. The cognitive basis for linguistic structures. *In* J. R. Hayes (ed.), Cognition and the Development of Language, pp. 279–362. John Wiley & Sons, New York.

Bloom, L. 1967. A comment on Lee's "Developmental sentence types: A method for comparing normal and deviant syntactic development." J. Speech Hear. Disord. 32: 293–296.

Bloom, L. 1970. Language Development: Form and Function in Emerging Grammars. MIT Press, Cambridge, Mass.

Bloom, L. 1973. One Word at a Time: The Use of Single-Word Utterances. Mouton, The Hague.

Bloom, L. 1974. Talking, understanding, and thinking. *In* R. Schiefelbusch and L. Lloyd (eds.), Language Perspectives–Acquisition, Retardation, and Intervention, pp. 285–311. University Park Press, Baltimore.

Bloom, L., L. Hood, and P. Lightbown. 1974. Imitation in language development: If, when and why. Cog. Psychol. 6: 380–420.

Bloom, L., P. Lightbown, and L. Hood. 1974. Structure and variation in child language. Unpublished manuscript. Department of Psychology, Columbia University, New York.

Bloomfield, L. 1933. Language. Holt, Rinehart and Winston, New York.

Bowerman, M. 1973. Early Syntactic Development: A Cross-Linguistic Study with Special Reference to Finnish. Cambridge University Press, Cambridge.

Bowerman, M. F. 1974. Development of concepts underlying language. *In* R. Schiefelbusch and L. Lloyd (eds.), Language Perspectives–Acquisition, Retardation, and Intervention, pp. 191–209. University Park Press, Baltimore.

Bradbury, B., and E. Lunzer. 1972. The learning of grammatical inflections in normal and subnormal children. J. Child Psychol. Psychiatry 13: 239–248.

Braine, M. 1963. The ontogeny of English phrase structure: The first phase. Language 39: 1–14.

Brown, R. 1973. A First Language: The Early Stages. Harvard University Press, Cambridge, Mass.

Brown, R., and U. Bellugi. 1964. Three processes in the acquisition of syntax. Harvard Educ. Rev. 34: 133–151.

Brown, R., and C. Fraser. 1963. The acquisition of syntax. *In* C. Cofer and B. Musgrave (eds.), Verbal Behavior and Learning: Problems and Processes, pp. 158–201. McGraw-Hill, New York.

Carroll, J., and R. Freedle (eds.). 1972. Language Comprehension and the Acquisition of Knowledge. Winston, Washington, D.C.

Chafe, W. 1970. Meaning and the Structure of Language. The University of Chicago Press, Chicago.

Chomsky, N. 1957. Syntactic Structures. Mouton, The Hague.

Chomsky, N. 1959. A review of B. F. Skinner's "Verbal Behavior." Language 35: 26–58.

Chomsky, N. 1964. Formal discussion. *In* U. Bellugi and R. Brown (eds.), The Acquisition of Language. Monogr. Soc. Res. Child Dev. 92: 35–39.

Chomsky, N. 1965. Aspects of the Theory of Syntax. MIT Press, Cambridge, Mass.

Chomsky, N., and M. Halle. 1968. The Sound Pattern of English. Harper, New York.

Chukovsky, K. 1968. From Two to Five. University of California Press, Berkeley.

Clark, E. 1971. On the acquisition of the meaning of before and after. J. Verb. Learning Verb. Behav. 10: 266–275.

Clark, E. 1973a. What's in a word: On the child's acquisition of semantics in his first language. In T. Moore (ed.), Cognitive Development and the Acquisition of Language, pp. 65–110. Academic Press, New York.

Clark, E. 1973b. Non-linguistic strategies and the acquisition of word meaning. Cognition 2: 161–182.

Clark, E. 1974. Some aspects of the conceptual basis for first language acquisition. In R. Schiefelbusch and L. Lloyd (eds.), Language Perspectives–Acquisition, Retardation, and Intervention, pp. 105–128. University Park Press, Baltimore.

Clark, E., and O. Garnica. 1974. Is he coming or going? On the acquisition of diectic verbs. J. Verb. Learning Verb. Behav. 13: 559–572.

Clark, H. 1973a. The language-as-fixed-effect fallacy: A critique of language statistics in psychological research. J. Verb. Learning Verb. Behav. 12: 335–359.

Clark, H. 1973b. Space, time, semantics and the child. In T. Moore (ed.), Cognitive Development and the Acquisition of Language, pp. 28–64. Academic Press, New York.

Cooper, R. 1967. The ability of deaf and hearing children to apply morphological rules. J. Speech Hear. Res. 10: 77–85.

Cromer, R. 1970. Children are nice to understand: Surface structure clues for the recovery of a deep structure. Brit. J. Psychol. 61: 397–408.

Cromer, R. 1972a. The learning of linguistic surface structure cues to deep structure by educationally subnormal children. Amer. J. Ment. Defic. 77: 346–353.

Cromer, R. 1972b. The learning of surface structure clues to deep structure by a puppet show technique. Q. J. Exp. Psychol. 24: 66–76.

Cromer, R. 1974a. The development of language and cognition: The cognition hypothesis. In B. Foss (ed.), New Perspectives in Child Development, pp. 185–252. Penguin Books, Harmondsworth, Middlesex.

Cromer, R. 1974b. Child and adult learning of surface structure cues to deep structure using a picture card technique. J. Psycholing. Res. 3: 1–14.

Cromer, R. 1974c. Are subnormals linguistic adults? In N. O'Connor (ed.), Language and Cognitive Deficit. Butterworths, London.

deVilliers, P., and J. deVilliers. 1972. Early judgments of semantic and syntactic acceptability by children. J. Psycholing. Res. 1: 299–310.

deVilliers, P., and J. deVilliers. 1973. A cross-sectional study of the acquisition of grammatical morphemes in child speech. J. Psycholing. Res. 2: 267–278.

Donaldson, M., and R. Wales. 1970. On the acquisition of some relational terms. In J. Hayes (ed.), Cognition and the Development of Language, pp. 235–268. John Wiley & Sons, New York.

Dunn, L. 1965. Peabody Picture Vocabulary Test. American Guidance Service, Minneapolis.

Ervin-Tripp, S. 1964. Imitation and structural change in children's language.

In E. Lenneberg (ed.), New Directions in the Study of Language, pp. 163–189. MIT Press, Cambridge, Mass.

Ervin-Tripp, S. 1973. Some strategies for the first two years. *In* T. Moore (ed.), Cognitive Development and the Acquisition of Language, pp. 261–286. Academic Press, New York.

Fernald, C. 1972. Control of grammar in imitation, comprehension and production: Problems of replication. J. Verb. Learning Verb. Behav. 11: 606–613.

Ferreiro, E., and H. Sinclair. 1971. Temporal relations in language. Int. J. Psychol. 6: 39–47.

Fillmore, C. 1968. The case for case. *In* E. Bach and R. Harms (eds.), Universals in Linguistic Theory, pp. 1–87. Holt, Rinehart and Winston, New York.

Fraser, C., U. Bellugi, and R. Brown. 1963. Control of grammar in imitation, comprehension and production. J. Verb. Learning Verb. Behav. 2: 121–135.

Ginsberg, H. 1972. The Myth of the Deprived Child: Poor Children's Intellect and Education. Prentice-Hall, Englewood Cliffs, N.J.

Goodnow, J., and R. Levine. 1973. The grammar of action: Sequence and syntax in children's copying. Cog. Psychol. 4: 82–98.

Graham, J., and L. Graham. 1971. Language behavior of the mentally retarded: Syntactic characteristics. Amer. J. Ment. Defic. 75: 623–629.

Greenberg, J. 1966. Language Universals. Mouton, The Hague.

Greenfield, P., K. Nelson, and E. Saltzman. 1972. The development of rulebound strategies for manipulating seriated cups: A parallel between action and grammar. Cog. Psychol. 3: 291–310.

Greenfield, P., J. Smith, and B. Laufer. Communication and the Beginnings of Language. Academic Press, New York. In press.

Guess, D., and D. Baer. 1973. Some experimental analysis of linguistic development in institutionalized retarded children. *In* B. Lakey (ed.), The Modification of Language Behavior, pp. 1–34. Charles C Thomas, Springfield, Ill.

Guillaume, P. 1968. Imitation in Children. The University of Chicago Press, Chicago.

Huttenlocher, J. 1974. The origins of language comprehension. *In* R. Solso (ed.), Theories in Cognitive Psychology. Halstead Press, New York.

Ingram, D. 1974. The relationship between comprehension and production. *In* R. Schiefelbusch and L. Lloyd (eds.), Language Perspectives–Acquisition, Retardation, and Intervention, pp. 313–334. University Park Press, Baltimore.

Inhelder, B. 1966. Cognitive development and its contribution to the diagnosis of some phenomena of mental deficiency. Merrill-Palmer Q. 12: 299–319.

Inhelder, B. 1969. Memory and intelligence in the child. *In* D. Elkind and J. Flavell (eds.), Studies in Cognitive Development, pp. 337–364. Oxford University Press, New York.

Jakobson, R., G. Fant, and M. Halle. 1952. Preliminaries to Speech Analysis. MIT Technical Report 13, Cambridge, Mass.

Johnston, J. 1973. Spatial notions and the child's use of locatives in an elicitation task. Presented at the Stanford Child Language Research Forum, April 1–3, Stanford, Cal.

Johnston, J., and T. Schery. The use of grammatical morphemes by children with communication disorders. *In* D. Morehead and A. Morehead (eds.), Language Deficiency in Children: Selected Papers. University Park Press, Baltimore. In press.

Keeney, T., and J. Wolfe. 1972. The acquisition of agreement in English. J. Verbal Learning Verbal Behav. 11: 698–705.

Kemp, J., and P. Dale. Spontaneous imitations and free speech: A developmental comparison. Child Dev. In press.

Lackner, J. 1968. A developmental study of language behavior in retarded children. Neuropsychologia 6: 301–320.

Lee, L. 1966. Developmental sentence types: A method for comparing normal and deviant syntactic development. J. Speech Hear. Disord. 31: 311–330.

Leopold, W. 1939. Speech Development of a Bilingual Child: A Linguist's Record. Vol. 1. Northwestern University Press, Evanston, Ill.

Lewis, M. 1951. Infant Speech: A Study of the Beginnings of Language. Harcourt, Brace, New York.

Lezine, I. 1973. The transition from sensorimotor to earliest symbolic function in early development. *In* Early Development, pp. 221–232. Vol. 51. Association for Research in Nervous and Mental Disease, Williams & Wilkins, Baltimore.

Lovell, K., and B. Bradbury. 1967. The learning of English morphology in educationally subnormal special school children. Amer. J. Ment. Defic. 71: 609–615.

Lovell, K., and E. Dixon. 1965. The growth of the control of grammar in imitation, comprehension and production. J. Child Psychol. Psychiatry 5: 1–9.

Lovell, K., H. Hoyle, and M. Siddall. 1968. A study of some aspects of the play and language of young children with delayed speech. J. Child Psychol. Psychiatry 9: 41–50.

MacNamara, J. 1972. Cognitive basis of language learning in infants. Psychol. Rev. 79: 1–13.

McCarthy, D. 1954. Language development in children. *In* L. Carmichael (ed.), Manual of Child Psychology, pp. 492–630. John Wiley & Sons, New York.

McCawley, J. 1968. The role of semantics in grammar. *In* E. Bach and R. Harms (eds.), Universals of Linguistic Theory, pp. 124–169. Holt, Rinehart and Winston, New York.

McNeill, D. 1966. Developmental psycholinguistics. *In* F. Smith and G. Miller (eds.), The Genesis of Language: A Psycholinguistic Approach, pp. 15–84. MIT Press, Cambridge, Mass.

McNeill, D. 1970. The Acquisition of Language: The Study of Developmental Psycholinguistics. Harper & Row, New York.

Mehrabian, A., and M. Williams. 1971. Piagetian measures of cognitive development up to age two. J. Psycholing. Res. 1: 113–126.

Menyuk, P. 1963. Syntactic structures in the language of children. Child Dev. 34: 407–422.

Menyuk, P. 1964. Comparison of grammar of children with functionally deviant and normal speech. J. Speech Hear. Res. 7: 109–121.

Menyuk, P. 1969. Sentences Children Use. MIT Press, Cambridge, Mass.

Menyuk, P., and P. Looney. 1972. A problem of language disorder: Length versus structure. J. Speech Hear. Res. 15: 264–279.

Miller, J., and D. Yoder. 1973. Assessing the comprehension of grammatical form in mentally retarded children. Presented at the Third Congress of the International Association for the Scientific Study of Mental Deficiency, September, The Hague.

Miller, W., and S. Ervin. 1964. The development of grammar in child language. *In* U. Bellugi and R. Brown (eds.), The Acquisition of Language. Monogr. Soc. Res. Child Dev. 92: 9–34.

Moores, D. F. 1974. Nonvocal systems of verbal behavior. *In* R. Schiefelbusch and L. Lloyd (eds.), Language Perspectives—Acquisition, Retardation, and Intervention, pp. 377–427. University Park Press, Baltimore.

Morehead, D. 1972. Early grammatical and semantic relations: Some implications for a general representational deficit in linguistically deficient children. *In* D. Ingram (ed.), Papers and Reports on Child Language Development, pp. 1–12. Committee on Linguistics, Stanford, Cal.

Morehead, D., and D. Ingram. 1973. The development of base syntax in normal and linguistically deviant (deficient?) children. J. Speech Hear. Res. 16: 330–352.

Morehead, D., and A. Morehead. 1974. From signal to sign: A Piagetian view of thought and language during the first two years. *In* R. Schiefelbusch and L. Lloyd (eds.), Language Perspectives—Acquisition, Retardation, and Intervention, pp. 153–190. University Park Press, Baltimore.

Neisser, U. 1967. Cognitive Psychology. Appleton-Century-Crofts, New York.

Newfield, M., and B. Schlanger. 1968. The acquisition of English morphology by normal and educable mentally retarded children. J. Speech Hear. Res. 11: 693–706.

Parisi, D., and F. Antinucci. 1970. Lexical competence. *In* G. Flores d'Arcais and W. Levelt (eds.), Advances in Psycholinguistics, pp. 197–210. North Holland, Amsterdam.

Piaget, J. 1952. The Origins of Intelligence in Children. Humanities Press, New York.

Piaget, J. 1962. Play, Dreams, and Imitation in Childhood. Norton, New York.

Piaget, J. 1963. Le language et les operations intellectuelles. *In* Problems de Psycholinguistics. Symposium de l'association de psychologie scientifique de langue francaise. Presses University France, Paris.

Piaget, J. 1970. Piaget's theory. *In* P. Mussen (ed.), Carmichael's Manual of Child Psychology, pp. 703–732. John Wiley & Sons, New York.

Piaget, J. 1971. Biology and Knowledge. The University of Chicago Press, Chicago.

Piaget, J., and B. Inhelder. 1967. The Child's Conception of Space. Norton, New York.

Powers, M. 1957. Clinical and educational procedures in functional disorders of articulation. *In* L. Travis (ed.), Handbook of Speech Pathology, pp. 769–804. Appleton-Century-Crofts, New York.

Rosenbaum, P. 1967. IBM Grammar II. IBM Research Report no. 2.

Schlesinger, I. 1971. Production of utterances and language acquisition. *In* D. Slobin (ed.), The Ontogenesis of Grammar, pp. 63–101. Academic Press, New York.

Schlesinger, I. M. 1974. Relational concepts underlying language. In R. Schiefelbusch and L. Lloyd (eds.), Language Perspectives—Acquisition, Retardation, and Intervention, pp. 129–151. University Park Press, Baltimore.

Schlesinger, I., and K. Meadow. 1972. Sound and Sign: Childhood Deafness and Mental Health. University of California Press, Berkeley.

Scholes, R. 1970. On functors and contentives in children's imitations of word strings. J. Verb. Learning Verb. Behav. 9: 167–170.

Shatz, M., and R. Gelman. 1973. The development of communication skills: Modifications in the speech of young children as a function of listener. Monogr. Soc. Res. Child Dev. 38: 1–38.

Shipley, E., C. Smith, and L. Gleitman. 1969. A study in the acquisition of language: Free responses to commands. Language 45: 322–342.

Shriner, T. 1967. A review of mean length of response as a measure of expressive language development in children. J. Speech Hear. Disord. 34: 61–67.

Sinclair, H. 1969. Developmental psycholinguistics. In D. Elkin and J. Flavell (eds.), Studies in Cognitive Development, pp. 315–336. Oxford University Press, New York.

Sinclair, H. 1971. Sensorimotor action patterns as a condition for the acquisition of syntax. In R. Huxley and E. Ingram (eds.), Language Acquisition: Model and Methods, pp. 121–130. Academic Press, New York.

Sinclair, H. 1973. Language acquisition and cognitive development. In T. Moore (ed.), Cognitive Development and the Acquisition of Language, pp. 9–25. Academic Press, New York.

Slobin, D. 1973. Cognitive prerequisites for the development of grammar. In C. Ferguson and D. Slobin (eds.), Studies in Child Language Development, pp. 175–208. Holt, Rinehart and Winston, New York.

Slobin, D., and C. Welsh. 1973. Elicited imitation as a research tool in developmental psycholinguistics. In C. Ferguson and D. Slobin (eds.), Studies in Child Language Development, pp. 485–497. Holt, Rinehart and Winston, New York.

Smith, C. 1970. An experimental approach to children's linguistic competence. In J. Hayes (ed.), Cognition and the Development of Language, pp. 109–135. John Wiley & Sons, New York.

Snow, C. 1972. Mother's speech to children learning language. Child Dev. 43: 549–565.

Stokoe, W. 1972. Semiotics and Human Sign Languages. Mouton, The Hague.

Templin, M. 1957. Certain Language Skills in Children: Their Development and Interrelationships. University of Minnesota Press, Minneapolis.

Tyack, D. 1973. The use of language samples in a clinical setting. J. Learning Disabil. 6: 213–216.

Uzgiris, I., and J. Hunt. 1966. An instrument for assessing psychological development. (Mimeo.) Psychological Development Laboratory, University of Illinois, Urbana.

Weir, R. 1962. Language in the Crib. Mouton, The Hague.

Generative Studies of Children's Phonological Disorders: A Strategy of Therapy

Arthur J. Compton, Ph.D.
Research Speech and Language Pathologist
San Francisco Hearing and Speech Center

CONTENTS

Little Joey excitedly runs up to his mother and says, "Tee goddie gwink tudie duite." Translation? "See doggie drink Susie's juice." No, Joey isn't talking Greek. He's speaking perfectly good 2-year old English, children's style. By 5 years, however, Joey's speech should sound like fairly normal English, adult style. But not all children are so fortunate, and at 5 or 6 years, one in 20 may still be talking much like Joey without apparent cause. For all practical purposes, the child attempting to communicate in the face of such an articulatory handicap might just as well be speaking another language, and the frustration suffered by child, parents, teachers, and peers alike is every bit as great.

From a linguistic standpoint, children who fail to develop normal speech are, in fact, speaking another language so far as their sound (phonological) system is concerned. The speech of such children is often clinically described

Supported by Grant HD 07185-03 from the National Institute of Child Health and Human Development.

as "infantile" or "delayed" and, popularly, as "baby talk." Such terms, while reflecting a general recognition of the continuity and similarity between deviant and early normal child speech, are grossly misleading and are in no way to be literally equated with notions of simplified or "watered down" speech anymore than the speech of the American Indians or African tribal peoples is to be considered as underdeveloped or unenriched forms of primitive noises and grunts. Thus, while children with articulatory disorders have linguistically strayed from the path of normal development, the phonological system underlying their deviant speech is generally no more impoverished or less complex than that of normal children of the same age. Rather, they are operating by a different sound system. Consequently, to modify effectively children's deviant speech, it is necessary to design therapy in accordance with their own unique patterns of speech, i.e., to move from the child's sytem to that to be learned.

The primary focus of this chapter is on the practical applications of systematic phonological analyses (generative phonology) to the diagnosis and treatment of children with phonological disorders. The theoretical foundations and clinical effectiveness of this approach have been reported previously (Compton, 1970). The clinical uses of generative phonological analyses to be discussed herein are based upon an extensive program of research at the San Francisco Hearing and Speech Center concerning normal and abnormal development of speech and the nature and treatment of children's articulatory disorders.

The general strategy of diagnosis and therapy includes the following phases: 1) recording a representative sample of the child's speech, 2) phonetically transcribing the recorded sample as closely as possible, 3) organizing the phonetic data, 4) analyzing the phonological system (determined by the patterns of articulatory deviations), 5) devising a therapy plan from the phonological analysis, 6) carrying out the therapy plan, and 7) periodically reevaluating (a repeat of the first five phases, usually about every 3 months) for the purpose of updating the therapy program.

ARTICULATORY TESTING AND PHONETIC TRANSCRIPTION

The validity and, therefore, the clinical value of the phonological analysis is crucially dependent on a representative sampling of the child's speech and an accurate and thorough phonetic transcription of the sample. To obtain a sample of the child's speech suitable for phonological analysis, it is necessary to view the child's production of sounds in a variety of different phonetic contexts or environments. In normal speech, speech sounds are produced differently in different contexts, and this is just as true of a child with defective speech. It would not be unusual, for example, for a child with an articulatory disorder to produce the "s" sound as a "t" before vowels in initial word position, as a "sh" in final position, and omit it entirely in the blends. Furthermore, because children with deviant speech typically have much more variability of pronunciation of the same sounds in identical contexts, it is important for the sampling to be sensitive to this aspect of pronunciation. Finally, for the analysis to depict accurately the child's deviant phonological system, the sample must typify his characteristic or usual pronunciation.

Ideally, the phonological analysis should be based on a sample of spontaneous, conversational speech. This format, however, presents two problems. First, the running speech of the children with whom we are concerned is largely unintelligible and, hence, inaccessible to analysis. Second, there is the very practical obstacle of obtaining a manageable sample of running speech containing all of the sounds in their multiple contexts as well as the variant pronunciations of these sounds within the same contexts. The solution I have adopted is to elicit the necessary inventory of sounds by having the children name a series of pictures. By tape-recording the child's responses and transcribing them afterwards, the several sounds making up each response can all be tested at once. This permits the test items to be held to a minimum, since the sounds to be tested can be compacted into a relatively small set of carefully constructed picture stimuli (approximately 80–90 pictures. Consequently, the evaluation time can be greatly reduced (one 45-min session is generally sufficient); this is particularly important for young children who have relatively short attention spans and fatigue easily. Transcribing the child's recorded responses (as opposed to transcribing on the spot) also provides an opportunity for more than one hearing of the items as well as corroboration with others, thereby markedly increasing the accuracy of the phonetic transcription and, hence, the phonological analysis.

Constructing the Articulatory Test

While many articulation tests are available, none have been designed for the kind of phonological analysis to be presented and are therefore largely unsuited for this purpose. However, with a little ingenuity, the investigator can readily devise his own set of picture stimuli, or perhaps, modify the available test materials to obtain an adequate phonological sample. The test described here has been developed and refined over a period of several years during the course of approximately 100 evaluations of 5- and 6-year-old children. During this time, the design and details of construction of the test have been substantially worked out. However, specific picture stimuli are still periodically revised or replaced to achieve greater familiarity and ease of recognition for children with many divergent ethnic, social, and environmental backgrounds. A list of the stimulus items comprising the present form of the test is provided in Table 1.

The picture stimuli do not constitute a test in the conventional sense of the term, i.e., a standardized set of materials used to derive a score. Rather, the stimuli are intended to elicit from children responses that will provide

Table 1. Experimental picture word list for assessing children's phonological disorders[a]

1. Dog	22. Teeth	43. Plant	64. Grasshopper
2. Ball	23. Television	44. Mop	65. Splash
3. Shoes	24. Giraffe	45. Juice	66. Fork
4. Zebra	25. Breathe	46. Mother	67. Frog
5. Zipper	26. Bed	47. Cob	68. This or that
6. Blocks	27. Pig	48. Present	69. Mouth
7. Skate	28. Three	49. Flag	70. Sprinkle
8. Shirt	29. Snake	50. Santa Claus	71. Rabbit
9. Wall	30. Spider (web)	51. Vegetables	72. Thank you
10. Brush	31. Slide	52. Rouge	73. Gum
11. Cheese	32. Yes	53. Pen	74. Yawn
12. Crib	33. Witch	54. Stove	75. Rug
13. Nurse	34. Swing	55. Thumb	76. These or those
14. Nose	35. Church	56. Tractor	77. Duck
15. Ring	36. Lamp	57. Hat	78. Bridge
16. Fish	37. Cage	58. Thread	79. Tub
17. Clown	38. Glove	59. Cup	80. Smooth
18. Gun	39. Violin	60. Leaf	81. Sun
19. Knife	40. String	61. Rake	82. Vase
20. Feather	41. Scratch	62. Drum	83. Beige
21. Smoke	42. Horse	63. Treasure	84. Pan

[a]These items are mainly illustrative of the nature of the test, since the particular pictures depicting the stimulus items are perhaps as crucial as the items themselves.

data suitable for phonological analysis.[1] Nonetheless, the stimuli are designed to make systematic observations of articulatory performance for the purpose of evaluation, and I continue to use the term test, recognizing that I am doing so more broadly than the term is sometimes used.

The articulatory test is composed of 84 items, carefully selected to elicit all of the sounds of English in a variety of different phonetic contexts, while maximally conserving the total number of picture stimuli (and responses) required. For example, initial /d/ is elicited by the picture words "dog" and "duck" (items 1 and 77 of Table 1) at the same time that final /g/ and /k/ are being elicited. Thus, in choosing a second item to represent final /g/ (single consonants occur at least twice in each context), the choice of "pig" (item 27) also provides a test of initial /p/ and would be preferable to a word such as "dig" which duplicates the initial /d/ already contained in "dog" and "duck." Some duplication is unavoidable, but the strategy is clearly the most

[1] Actually, an implicit "score" of articulatory severity is derived from a phonological analysis of a child's responses which appears in the form of the number and type of deviant phonological rules. A future goal of the study is to develop an index of communicative disruption resulting from the various kinds of deviant rules. Clearly, this is a more meaningful way of scoring than present practices of simply counting deviant sounds.

efficient way of limiting the test items without sacrificing necessary information.

All vowels are sampled several times in different environments, although the construction of the test focuses more heavily on the multiple contexts of the consonants and consonant clusters, since they are more subject to abnormality and contextual deviancy than are the vowels. In the few instances in which children have disordered vowel systems, the problem is generally massive, and a specialized test is devised to assess thoroughly their deviant patterns.

Each consonant is represented at least twice in initial and final word position. Most consonants also occur at least once in intervocalic position (between vowels), although in this environment they usually follow the pattern of their initial or final counterparts, depending on the stress pattern (marking the syllable boundary) of the words in which they occur. All of the initial position blends (/st, dr, bl, skr/ etc.) occur one or more times. Also represented are some of the more common consonant clusters in intervocalic and final positions, such as /kt/ as in "tractor," /nt/ as in "present," /ŋk/ as in "sprinkle," etc.

Each response is elicited twice, to provide an estimate of the child's consistency or stability of pronunciation of the same sounds in identical environments. In addition to the sounds elicited specifically by the test, much fortuitous sampling also results from the children's misnaming of items and interjected conversational speech. In fact, throughout the test, samples of conversational speech are deliberately encouraged whenever the child displays some interest in particular test items. These samples, generally intelligible from their context, are a valuable supplement to the overall validity of the analysis, because they provide a cross check against the child's production of sounds in the single word responses.

The stimulus pictures are mounted on 5 X 7 inch cards with any special instructions for elicitation printed on the back. Because of the impossibility of clearly representing a few English sounds with pictures familiar to most children (or by verbal prompting, for that matter), there is sometimes no alternative but to provide the child with a spoken model. This is usually the case, for example, with such items as "rouge," "vase," and "beige" (items 52, 82, and 83) and is an unavoidable fact of the language. Generally, however, by a trial-and-error process, easily recognized pictures can be found for most sounds, often contrary to our preconceived notions. Uncluttered pictures and simple drawings frequently make better stimuli than photographs and other authentic renditions of adult realism.

Administering the Articulatory Test

The articulatory evaluation generally can be completed within a 1-hr session, allowing a few minutes at the beginning of the period to gain rapport with the

child and about 30–45 min to administer the test items. The child's responses should be recorded on a good fidelity tape recorder, since poor quality reproduction not only loses important information but is also very difficult to transcribe. The testing procedures for the initial evaluation are as follows.
1. Encourage the child to speak at his normal talking level. Provided the microphones are fairly sensitive, they will pick up most children's speech, even if they are not naturally loud talkers, so long as they are speaking within 15–20 inches of the microphone. Beware of whispered speech, which is very difficult to transcribe, and yelled speech, which is usually distorted.
2. Present each stimulus picture without providing a spoken model. In most instances, it is possible to lead the child to the desired response by structuring the way in which you present the stimulus, for example: "Humpty Dumpty sat on a (wall)," "When we take in air, we (breathe)," etc. The object of the evaluation is to get the child's natural or usual form of spontaneous pronunciation. If, after a little ingenuity, you are still unable to elicit the desired, unstimulated response and must provide a model, then say the word in a natural and undramatized way.
3. Have the child repeat the name of each stimulus picture twice. Usually it is necessary to remind a child to say the word a second time for the first few items until he gets the idea, and then he will do so spontaneously without prodding during the rest of the evaluation.
4. During the evaluation, most children will show some particular interest in some of the pictures. When this happens, encourage the child to speak freely for a short period to provide a sampling of his connected speech.
5. As the child names the pictures, watch for any unusual articulatory gestures or mannerisms. Such visual cues are often a valuable supplement during later transcription, since there are occasional discrepancies between the visual appearance of a sound and the auditory consequences, i.e., a sound may be visually distorted but acoustically normal or seen in one way but heard differently.
6. While administering the evaluation, set aside one sample (picture) for each defective sound in the child's speech. At the end of the evaluation, present these items again, but this time provide a spoken model to allow an estimate of the child's ability to produce the sounds with stimulation.

For all subsequent reevaluations, exactly the same procedures are followed, except that the last step is omitted and five additional picture stimuli are added for each sound the child has been working on during therapy. The additional stimuli provide more in-depth information for evaluating the child's progress.

Transcribing the Recorded Evaluation

A good command of phonetic transcription is both a skill and a tool, fundamental to making a systematic analysis of the child's deviant phonological system. It is a key to open the door into the child's world of sound, and without it, we remain locked out.

Before doing the analysis, it is not clear which phonetic characteristics of the child's speech should be included as a part of his phonological system and which details should be discarded as atypical variants.[2] Consequently, it is important to transcribe as much phonetic detail as possible, so that significant patterns are not lost. Such practices, for example, as designating certain variant sounds as 'distortions' can only hide or obscure systematic patterns and have little clinical value for assessing the child's speech and planning a therapy program.

With a little practice, a good command of phonetic transcription can be easily achieved. In fact, by doing nothing more than simply listening closely to a recorded sample of a child's speech, you are likely to be amazed at the amount of phonetic detail you are able to hear. For the most part, the chief obstacle is not in hearing or discriminating phonetic differences but in having a symbol available to record what you already hear. For practical purposes of clinical evaluation, the symbols or notations used are insignificant so long as we consistently transcribe the differences we hear in the same way. It is better to invent a notation to record some phonetic detail than to ignore or pass it by because we do not have a conventional symbol available. However, as a convenient reference, a list of useful transcription notations is provided in Table 2. These notations, used in conjunction with the symbols of the International Phonetic Alphabet, should prove quite adequate for transcribing most of the phonetic characteristics present in children's speech.

The transcription should include the entire utterance and not just those sounds which are deviant, since the analysis is to take into account both normal and abnormal speech production. When a child misarticulates a sound, it is important to take into account whether he does so all of the time or whether he has the option of producing it correctly. An estimate of the relative frequency of correct-incorrect productions of each sound is also invaluable clinical information.

In writing down the phonetic transcription, each transcribed response may be numbered for easy reference and must include the corresponding picture name or translation. Because the child's speech is likely to be largely unintelligible, it is particularly important to note the order in which the stimuli are given, so that the responses can be later identified during transcription. It is also important to designate specifically: 1) utterances which occur as conversational speech, 2) responses which require a spoken model, and 3) any other qualifying information which may have some bearing upon the analysis.

[2] Child speech, like adult speech, is subject to false starts, slips of the tongue, and other such unsystematic variations which do not constitute a part of the linguistic system and, consequently, should not be included in the analysis. These variants are usually quite conspicuous because they are both sporadic and irregular and stand out as exceptions.

Table 2. Some useful phonetic notations for transcribing children's speech

---

Strong aspiration is denoted by ' following a symbol, i.e., [k'æt]

Nonaspiration is denoted by = following a symbol, i.e., [k=æt]

Nasalization is denoted by ~ above a symbol, i.e., [kæ̃t]

Rounding is denoted by ○ around a symbol, i.e., [ⓙ ɪp]

Unrounding is denoted by □ around a symbol, i.e., [w̅ ɛt]

Lateralization is denoted by ↔ above a symbol, i.e., [ʃ̑ɪp]

Lengthening is denoted by : after a symbol, i.e., [fɪʃ:]

Hissing or *whistling* is denoted by ᵂ above a symbol, i.e., [s̆ ɪp]

Fronting of a sound from its usual place of articulation is denoted by an arrow ← pointing forward and *backing* of a sound, by an arrow → pointing backward, i.e., [k̠ æt]

Abrupt termination is denoted by > following a symbol, i.e., [fɪʃ>]

Unreleased stops are denoted by ⌐ following a symbol, i.e., [kæt ⌐]

Syllabic consonants are denoted by . under a symbol, i.e., [mɪtn̩]

Juncture (slight pause) between two sounds is denoted by + between the symbols

Primary stress is denoted by ' above a syllable, and *secondary stress* is denoted by ˆ above a syllable

Pitch (inflection) is denoted by the numerals 1, 2, or 3 written above the utterance; for example, 1 3 above an utterance indicates rising pitch, whereas 3 1 designates falling pitch

Partially articulated sounds are denoted by an offset symbol, i.e., [kæ^t]

When discrimination of a sound is ambiguous, the alternate possibilities are written one above the other, i.e., $\begin{bmatrix} & d \\ mæt & \end{bmatrix}$

In transcribing the recorded evaluation, two or three hearings of each utterance are usually required. Beyond the third or fourth hearing, we have generally exceeded our limits of objective perceptual discrimination, and little else is gained from repeated listenings, save frustration. It is also important to recognize the frailty of human perception and be aware that our ears may sometimes play tricks on us. What we hear is very often markedly influenced by our perceptual set and expectations. In transcribing unintelligible children's speech, for example, I have often had the shocking experience of seeing my careful and 'accurate' transcription completely devastated, upon realizing that the response I had just transcribed meant something entirely different than I had thought. Oller and Eilers (in press) too have demonstrated that phonetic transcriptions of children's speech are subject to much more variability when the transcribers must guess the meaning of an utterance as opposed to being supplied with it. Consequently, because of the potential element of subjectivity always present in human perception, generally, and in speech perception, specifically (regardless of expertise), it is advisable that two transcribers work independently and then meet jointly to resolve any discrepancies, discarding any instances in which no consensus can be reached.

Organizing the Phonetic Data

To facilitate the analysis, all of the child's productions of each sound for each phonetic context are tabulated by frequency of occurrence. Vowels are omitted, unless there is evidence of abnormality. For example, suppose initial /f/ had been produced normally three times and, five times, was substituted by [p].[3] This information would be extracted from the 'raw' transcription by tallying each phonetic realization of initial /f/ on a summary form listing all of the consonants and blends by their positional contexts. All of the child's productions for each sound would be so tabulated, also designating any instances in which the sounds were contained in a stimulated response or occurred in conversational speech. The analysis is then derived from this summarized, phonetic data, since the patterns of errors in the child's speech are much more easily pinpointed and stand out more vividly than attempting to wade through the unorganized jungle of phonetic symbols in the original transcriptions.

General Remarks on the Nature of Phonological Analysis

Broadly speaking, there are roughly 45–50 speech sounds in English, but as far as actual talking is concerned, this is a gross understatement. The actual task of a child learning to produce the sounds of language obviously far exceeds a mastery of perhaps 50 specific sounds. Otherwise, his job would be relatively simple and straightforward, as would ours in describing it, and there would be little point in pursuing a study of the sound system of language; we would not be studying a system but merely a handful of sounds and when they were acquired.

Suppose, for example, the word "kick" were recorded and then played backwards. Would we still hear "kick"? The answer is no, for the "k" sound beginning the word is not the same as the one which ends it, and such is the case for any other "sound" we might try. Even at the beginnings of words, the "same" sound is not the same, as illustrated by the words "keep," "cup," and "coupe" in which the initial /k/ is drawn progressively farther back in the mouth (point of tongue contact with the velum) under influence of the vowels. Furthermore, the [k] in "coupe" has more lip rounding because of the influence of the rounded vowel [u], and should an /s/ be added immediately before a /k/, as in "scoop," it becomes an unaspirated [k=] .

---

[3] Throughout this chapter, the distinction between symbols enclosed by / / and [ ] is as follows: / / denotes the implicit version of a sound which may be thought of as roughly equivalent to the "stored" or "internalized" representation of a sound in its unspoken form, and [ ] designates the overt, phonetic shape that an internalized "sound" takes on when it is actually spoken.

These are but a few of the varying forms of /k/, and if we were to continue examining other contexts and expanding our search to other sounds, we would soon discover that English (or any other language) is composed of, not 50, but literally hundreds of different sound variations. Does this mean that a child somehow must commit to memory all of these many sounds in their specific phonetic contexts during the course of learning to talk? Fortunately not, for the sounds of speech do not vary independently of each other but, instead, are organized into various intersecting classes which follow systematic patterns of phonetic realization. For example, /g/ as well as /k/ (the class of velar stops) is subject to the same vowel influences of articulatory placement and lip rounding, and /s/ has no special claim on /k/, for all of the voiceless stops (/p,t,k/) become unaspirated following /s/. The child, then, does not fall victim to hundreds of separate phonetic entities but, rather, quickly discovers and gains control of the unifying principles underlying them.

The sounds of speech are multiply related to one another and fall into various intersecting classes (natural groupings) on the basis of certain shared attributes. For example /m/ is simultaneously a member of the class of nasal sounds (/m,n,ŋ/) with respect to the attribute of nasality and the class of bilabial sounds (/p,b,m/) by virtue of its place of articulation. Accordingly, speech sounds are not indivisible entities but are composed of various subcomponents or attributes, commonly called features. Some of these features are the carriers of linguistic contrast in that they provide the basis for distinguishing among the utterances of a language. The difference, for example, between "bat" and "mat" is generally attributed to the presence or absence of nasality in the initial segment and the difference between "bat" and "pat," to the presence of absence of voicing. Features carrying discriminating information of this sort are often said to be phonemic (as opposed to phonetic), i.e., distinctive features.

Many other features characterizing speech sounds do not play a contrastive role, as far as distinguishing meaning among utterances, but serve to render them as "natural" or "native" sounding. They are the details or "particulars" of pronounciation of sounds in specific phonetic contexts, as in the previous example of the voiceless stops which incorporate the feature of unaspiration following /s/. Such features, although not serving a contrastive linguistic function are, nonetheless, noticeably conspicuous when violated, as witnessed in the speech of children with articulatory disorders and nonnative speakers. Hence, the notion of linguistically nondistinctive is not to be equated with perceptually indistinct.

Furthermore, some of the noncontrastive features of English may be linguistically distinctive in other languages (the contrast between aspiration and nonaspiration in Hindi, for example) as well as in the speech of children still learning to talk and children with phonological disorders. As an example, many children who omit the /s/ in the blends still apply the rule for

Table 3. Representation of the contrastive features underlying the consonants of English

	p	b	t	d	k	g	m	n	ŋ	f	v	θ	ð	s	z	ʃ	ʒ	tʃ	dʒ	r	l	w	j
Place[a]	1	1	4	4	6	6	1	4	6	2	2	3	3	4	4	5	5	5	5	5	4	6	5
Voice	–	+	–	+	–	+	+	+	+	–	+	–	+	–	+	–	+	–	+	+	+	+	+
Nasal	–	–	–	–	–	–	+	+	+	–	–	–	–	–	–	–	–	–	–	–	–	–	–
Round																						+	
Consonantal	+	+	+	+	+	+	+	+	+	+	+	+	+	+	+	+	+	+	+	+	+	–	–
Friction	–	–	–	–	–	–	–	–	–	+	+	+	+	+	+	+	+	+	+	–	–	–	–
Stop	+	+	+	+	+	+	+	+	+	–	–	–	–	–	–	–	–	+	+	–	–	–	–

[a]The places of articulation features are defined as follows: place$_1$, bilabial; place$_2$, labial dental; place$_3$, lingual dental; place$_4$, lingual alveolar; place$_5$, palatal; and place$_6$, velar.

unaspirating the voiceless stops, so that a word such as "spin" pronounced [p=ɪn], is contrastive in their phonological system with the word "pin" pronounced [pɪn], the distinction being marked by the presence or absence of aspiration in the initial segment.

Returning now to the 45-odd speech sounds of English from a somewhat different perspective, it is perhaps clearer that they are not the actual sounds we speak but the skeletons of speech upon which the details of reality must be added. They are unspoken abstractions which embody the essential features of linguistic contrast. The various phonological principles we learn during childhood serve to relate these underlying features to the particular surface (noncontrastive) features appropriate to the actual pronunciation of sounds in specific phonetic contexts.

A characterization of the contrastive features underlying the consonants of English in their abstract or unspoken form is given in Table 3. While theoretically founded, the feature system presented here is motivated mainly by very practical considerations concerned with explicitly describing normal and abnormal speech of children in the most simple and straightforward way possible. Aside from a few minor differences, the feature system closely corresponds to the traditional classifications of speech sounds which, for the most part, are fully adequate for characterizing the phonological systems of children and have the additional advantage of being readily understood. I have not adhered to a strictly binary feature classification (where features can only assume a value of + or −, indicating their presence or absence), and the features relating to place of articulation are represented by one of six values, each designating one of the major points of articulatory contact of the consonants of English. The manner features, however, are specified in binary form, since they are more readily accommodated by a binary classification.

Each column of the table designates the particular set of feature values or specifications appropriate for a specific consonant. Notice that each consonant differs by at least one feature from every other consonant, which corresponds to the fact that each consonant has a separate or unique identity, i.e., they are linguistically contrastive. At the same time, however, all of the consonants have one or more features in common with various other consonants, which in turn gives rise to a variety of multiple groupings (natural classes) by virtue of the shared features they possess. If, in fact, the resultant groupings appropriately delineate those classes of sounds, which conform to actual phonological regularities (patterns), they may be said to constitute natural classes.

PHONOLOGICAL ANALYSIS OF CHILDREN'S MISARTICULATIONS

The major assumption on which the phonological analysis is founded is that the sounds of speech do not function independently but, instead, have an intricate complex of relationships with one another. These relationships manifest themselves as systematic patterns that in turn reflect the organization of the phonological system. In other words, the existence of observable patterns presupposes the existence of an underlying organization that is internally consistent, for recurring patterns do not just happen. Rather, they happen because they are a result of a system which generates them, and consequently, patterning is a kind of surface reflection of the abstract (underlying) structural relationships that characterize the system. Thus, to characterize the structural properties or relationships of the system is the only way to explicitly describe the patterns that the system produces (the output). The patterns are a product. They cannot exist except as they are a consequence of the structure of the system which generates them.

The purpose of the analysis is to characterize explicitly the relational principles which underlie or give rise to the observable, deviant productions in the speech of children with phonological disorders. The method of analysis and specific form in which the phonological principles (rules) are expressed can be best demonstrated by examining an actual analysis of a child's speech. The subject, Frank B., was 5 years old at the time of the initial evaluation and had a severe phonological disorder. Frank's speech was approximately 80% unintelligible, but his IQ was slightly above average, and he had no evidence of hearing loss or other physical anomalies which would cause his speech to be abnormal. Tables 4 and 5 present a description of Frank's pronunciations of the consonants and blends at the time of his first evaluation.

The second and third columns of Table 4 give his pronunciations of initial and final consonants for the corresponding ones shown in column one. For example, the first row of column two indicates that initial /p/ is produced normally (designated by [p]). Similarly, the same row of column three indicates that final /p/ may be either released (designated by [p]) or unreleased (designated by [p']) with about equal frequency (frequency of occurrence is indicated by the number following the symbols). Table 5 gives Frank's pronunciations of the consonant blends in initial position, the second and fourth columns designating his pronunciations of the corresponding blends shown in the first and third columns. Thus, the first row of column two shows that the /pr/ blend is produced as a [p] with the /r/ portion of the blend omitted and, as in Table 4, the number after the symbol indicates frequency of occurrence.

Notice, first of all, that a simple counting of the various deviant productions shown in Tables 4 and 5 yields more than 60 different types of misarticulations. Presented in this form, however, these misarticulations constitute nothing more than a collection of observations, for they are only the surface manifestations of the child's underlying phonological system. Our task, then, is to discover the regularities (patterns) inherent in these surface observations, which then will enable us to direct therapy toward the principles giving rise to the misarticulations.

Table 4. Phonological description of Frank's pronunciations of initial and final consonants for the first evaluation[a]

Underlying sound	Child's productions (initial position)	Child's productions (final position)
/p/	[p] 9	[p] 3, [pˀ] 3
/t/	[t] 8, [k] 2	[t] 7, [tˀ] 6
/k/	[k] 8	[k] 5, [kˀ] 7
/b/	[b] 5	[b] 1, [bˀ] 1, [pˀ] 3, [p] 4
/d/	[d] 9, [g] 2	[dˀ] 1, [tˀ] 5, [t] 3
/g/	[g] 4	[g] 2, [kˀ] 5, [k] 4
/m/	[m] 5	[m] 7, ϕ 1
/n/	[n] 6	[n] 8
/ŋ/	—	[ŋ] 5, [^{n}n] 1
/f/	[f] 5	[f] 7
/s/	[s] 9, [ʃ] 2	[s] 11, [s:] 1
/ʃ/	[ʃ] 4, [s] 4	[ʃ] 1, [s] 8
/θ/	[t] 5	[s] 4
/tʃ/	[tʃ] 6	[s] 4, [ʃ] 1
/v/	[v] 2, [w] 2	[f] 2, [pˀ] 2, [p] 1
/z/	[s] 4	[s] 5 [zˢ] 1
/ʒ/	—	[s] 4
/ð/	[d] 4	[s] 3
/dʒ/	[dʒ] 5	[s] 5
/h/	[h] 6	—
/w/	[w] 5	—
/l/	[l] 3, [j] 2, ϕ 7	[l] 4
/r/	[w] 8	—
/j/	[j] 4	—

[a]Numbers specify frequency of occurrence.

Table 5. Phonological description of Frank's initial position consonant blends for the first evaluation[a]

Underlying form	Child's productions	Underlying form	Child's productions
/pr/	[p] 2	/pl/	[p] 2
/br/	[b] 6	/bl/	[b] 2
/tr/	[tʃ] 4	/kl/	[k] 4
/dr/	[dʒ] 4	/gl/	[g] 2
/kr/	[k] 3	/fl/	[f] 5
/gr/	[g] 2	/sl/	[s] 4, [ʃ] 1
/fr/	[f] 3	/sp/	[p=] 2
/θr/	[t] 3	/st/	[t=] 2
/spr/	[p=] 4	/sk/	[k=] 3
/str/	[dʒ] 3	/sm/	[m] 2
/skr/	[k=] 4	/sn/	[n] 4
/spl/	[p=] 2	/sw/	[s] 1, [f] 4

[a]Numbers specify frequency of occurrence.

The first step of the analysis is to begin examining the child's deviant productions for patterns encompassing related sounds which consistently reoccur in specific phonetic environments. For example, observe that /t,d/ (the class of alveolar stops) are occasionally replaced by the corresponding pair of sounds [k,g] (the velar stops) when they occur in initial position before vowels, but when they occur before /r/ in the /tr,dr/ blends, they are realized as the cognate pair of sounds [tʃ,dʒ] (the affricates). Furthermore, in each case in which the sounds of one class are produced as those of another class, the voicing feature of the sounds being substituted is preserved, i.e., t→k and t→tʃ are voiceless while d→g and d→dʒ are voiced.

Observe further that in final position, the misarticulations of /t,d/ are not specific only to the alveolar stops. Instead /b,d,g/, the class of voiced stops, are all generally produced as their corresponding voiceless cognates [p,t,k], and the entire class of stops /p,b,t,d,k,g/ may also be realized as unreleased. Although nonreleased stops may occur as a normal variant of English in final position, their use in Frank's speech was much more prevalent and usually resulted in the illusion that they were omitted entirely. The differences in the phonological principles giving rise to the deviant productions of /t/ and /d/ in initial and final positions illustrate the relative independence between these environments; that is, there is likely to be little correspondence or "cross over" between the phonological principles underlying the misarticulations in initial and final positions.

The preceding examples illustrate the general strategy by which phonological regularities are discovered in a child's speech, and as we continue our search, other such regularities will emerge. The next step of the analysis is to translate these patterns into an organized collection of phonological principles, i.e., a generative phonology. Tables 6 and 7 present an analysis of the underlying principles characterizing all of Frank's misarticulations shown in Tables 4 and 5. The analysis of initial consonants and blends is shown in Table 6, and the analysis of final consonants is given in Table 7. An explication of each of the rules shown in Tables 6 and 7 follows.

Rule 1 The alveolar stops /t,d/ are replaced by the corresponding velar stops [k,g], the arrow indicating the direction of replacement or change. Thus, /t/ is produced as [k] and /d/ is produced as [g]. The slash, "/", is to be interpreted as "in the phonetic environment of." The "#" symbol following the slash is a linguistic boundary marker which, in this case, designates the beginning of a word, and the "_" following the boundary marker specifies the position in which the sound occurs, i.e., initial position in this rule.[4] The "opt" (optional) restriction indicates that the rule may be applied optionally, that is, other pronunciations are possible; as the rules are presently formu-

---

[4] I cannot overemphasize that all of the stated phonological rules that appear throughout this chapter are to be interpreted only as abstract characterizations of "psychologically real" phonological relations or principles. This claim is in no way to be equated with a claim of the psychological, physiological, or neurological reality of the operations used to generate the phonological descriptions.

Table 6. Phonological analysis of Frank's initial consonants and blends for the first evaluation[a]

Phonological rules

1. $\begin{bmatrix} t \\ d \end{bmatrix} \rightarrow \begin{bmatrix} k \\ g \end{bmatrix}$ /#_ opt. 10%

2. $\begin{bmatrix} p \\ t \\ k \end{bmatrix} \rightarrow \begin{bmatrix} p= \\ t= \\ k= \end{bmatrix}$ /s_ oblig. (not a deviant rule)

3a. $\begin{bmatrix} t \\ d \end{bmatrix} \rightarrow \begin{bmatrix} t\int \\ d_3 \end{bmatrix}$ /_r oblig.

3b. [t=] → [d₃] /_r oblig.

4. [v] → [w] /#_ opt. 50%

5. $\begin{bmatrix} \theta \\ \delta \end{bmatrix} \rightarrow \begin{bmatrix} t \\ d \end{bmatrix} \Big/ \begin{array}{l} \text{\#\_ oblig.} \\ \text{\_r oblig.} \end{array}$

6. [z] → [s] /#_oblig.

7. [s] → [∫] /#_ opt. 20%

8. [∫] → [s] /#_ opt. 50%

9. [l] → $\begin{bmatrix} \phi \\ j \\ \phi \end{bmatrix}$ $\begin{array}{l} \text{/\#\_ opt. 60\%} \\ \text{/\#\_ opt. 10\%} \\ \text{/cons.\_ oblig.} \end{array}$

10. [r] → $\begin{bmatrix} w \\ \\ \phi \end{bmatrix}$ $\begin{array}{l} \text{/\#\_oblig.} \\ \\ \text{/cons.\_oblig.} \end{array}$ } (ordered after rules 3a, 3b, and 5)

11. [s] → $\begin{bmatrix} f \\ \\ \phi \end{bmatrix}$ $\begin{array}{l} \text{/\_w opt. 75\%} \\ \\ \text{/\_cons. oblig.} \end{array}$ } (ordered after rules 2 and 9)

12. [w] → φ /f_ oblig.

[a]Unless otherwise specified, all initial consonants occur in the context preceding a vowel. Percentages are estimates of how often the rules apply. Opt., optional rules; oblig., obligatory rules.

lated, optional may be interpreted to mean that the sounds also can occur normally. The percentage values following the rules are estimates of how often the rules apply and are derived from the frequency tabulations given in Tables 4 and 5. Consequently, the percentage value following rule 1 indicates that the rule applies only about 10% of the time, whereas about 90% of the time /t,d/ occur normally. These percentage estimates, while only approximations, are often quite helpful for determining the relative status of various deviant rules and for evaluating a child's progress during therapy. For example, if a rule applied 80% of the time were subsequently reduced to 20% through therapy, the resulting 60% difference would provide an approximate index of clinical progress.

Notice that the phonological principle characterized by rule 1 does not apply to the /t/ and /d/ sounds individually but to the class of sounds of which they are members. The actual principle underlying the substitution of /t/ and /d/, then, is that stop consonants produced in place$_4$ (alveolar) are shifted back in place of articulation to place$_6$ (velar), with all other features remaining unchanged, i.e.,

$$\begin{bmatrix} \text{stop+} \\ \text{place}_4 \\ \text{voice} \pm \end{bmatrix} \rightarrow \begin{bmatrix} \text{stop+} \\ \text{place}_6 \\ \text{voice} \alpha \end{bmatrix}$$

The α variable assigned to the voicing feature on the righthand side of the rule is a notational convention indicating that this feature assumes the same

Table 7. Phonological analysis of Frank's final consonants for the first evaluation[a]

Phonological rules

13. $\begin{bmatrix} b \\ d \\ g \end{bmatrix} \rightarrow \begin{bmatrix} p \\ t \\ k \end{bmatrix}$ /_# opt. 90%

14. $[\text{stop+}] \rightarrow \begin{bmatrix} \text{stop+} \\ \text{release-} \end{bmatrix}$ /_# opt. 50%

15. $[v] \rightarrow \begin{bmatrix} f \\ b \end{bmatrix} \begin{matrix} =50\% \\ =50\% \end{matrix}$ /_# oblig.

16. $\begin{bmatrix} t\int \\ dʒ \end{bmatrix} \rightarrow \begin{bmatrix} \int \\ ʒ \end{bmatrix}$ /_# oblig.

17. $\begin{bmatrix} \int \\ ʒ \end{bmatrix} \rightarrow \begin{bmatrix} s \\ z \end{bmatrix}$ /_# $\frac{[\overline{\text{voice-}}]}{[\text{voice+}]}$ opt. 90% oblig.

18. $\begin{bmatrix} \theta \\ ð \end{bmatrix} \rightarrow \begin{bmatrix} s \\ z \end{bmatrix}$ /_# oblig.

19. $[z] \rightarrow \begin{bmatrix} z_s \\ s \end{bmatrix} \begin{matrix} =20\% \\ =80\% \end{matrix}$ /_# oblig.

[a]Percentages are estimates of how often the rules apply. Opt., optional rules; oblig., obligatory rules.

voicing specification (+ or −) as that specified on the lefthand side. The above feature specification of rule 1 more explicitly captures this principle (shift in place), and strictly speaking, all phonological rules should be specified by means of features. However, I have taken the liberty of abbreviating the rules (by using the more familiar phonological symbols) for the sake of simplifying the presentation to achieve easier readability, but it is nonetheless important to read into these abbreviations the actual feature changes being depicted.

Rule 2 The voiceless stops /p,t,k/ are realized as unaspirated stops whenever they occur in the phonetic context immediately following /s/, i.e., the /s/ blends. The "oblig" (obligatory) restriction indicates that the rule always applies. This is actually a normal rule of English, except that Frank omits the /s/ in the blends (by rule 11), and thus, his unaspirated stops appear in initial position (unlike English), rendering them noticeably conspicuous.

Rule 3a The alveolar stops /t,d/ are produced as the affricates [tʃ,dʒ] but only in the context before /r/. Consequently, a word such as dry would be pronounced as [dʒai] (the /r/ portion of the blend is omitted by rule 10).

Rule 3b This rule is actually a varying form of rule 3a and accounts for Frank's pronunciation of the /str/ blend. This rule arises from rule 2 which changes the /t/ portion of the blend to [t=] (unaspirated), and the [t=] is realized as [dʒ] by rule 3b. Therefore, Frank's pronunciation of a word like "straw" would come out as [dʒɔ] (the /s/ portion of the blend is lost by rule 11, and the /r/ is again omitted by rule 10).

Rule 4 Initial /v/ is optionally produced as [w] about half the time.

Rule 5 The lingual-dental (place$_3$) fricatives /θ,ð/ are always substituted by the alveolar stops [t,d], and likewise, the voiceless member /θ/ always occurs as [t] before /r/ in the /θr/ blend.

Rule 6 Initial /z/ is always produced as [s].

Rule 7 Initial /s/ is realized as [ʃ] about 20% of the time. This rule also may apply to the output of rule 6, thereby allowing both [s] and [ʃ] as alternate pronunciations of /z/.

Rule 8 Initial /ʃ/ is produced as [s] about half the time. Observe that this rule is the inverse of rule 7, thereby suggesting at first glance that Frank is simply unable to discriminate between /s/ and /ʃ/. In other words, bidirectional substitution patterns as s⟷ʃ generally signal a lack of discrimination and, consequently, would be accounted for by identical feature specifications of the sounds in question rather than by phonological rules. However, the discrepancy between the frequency of occurrence of the substitutions, s → ʃ = (20%) versus ʃ → s = (50%), suggests they are not truly bidirectional, and this conclusion is further borne out by the later clinical results (to be covered in the next section).

Rule 9 /l/ is either omitted (about 60%) or occurs as [j] (about 10%) in initial position and is always omitted in the blends.

Rule 10 /r/ is always realized as [w] in initial position and always omitted in the blends. Because rules 3a, 3b, and 5 are all contingent upon the /r/ context that is deleted by rule 10, the application of this rule must be reserved until they have been applied and the rules are, therefore, said to be ordered.[5] Thus, even though /r/ never emerges to the surface in the blends, it still exerts its influence upon the consonants /t,d,θ/ which precede it, that is, /r/ exists as an underlying reality in Frank's phonological system even though the /r/ is never overtly represented in his speech.

Rule 11 /s/ may be produced as [f] in the context before /w/ and is always omitted before the consonants in the /s/ blends. This rule is also ordered and must apply after rules 2 and 9. Rule 2 requires the /s/ context (to derive the unaspirated stops) before the removal of /s/ by rule 11. This consequent ordering serves to preserve the underlying or abstract reality of /s/ (in the blends) which has no concrete realization except for the /sl/ blend. The pronunciation of the /sl/ blend arises from rule 9, which deletes the /l/ portion, and the /s/ is then subject to rule 7, which may optionally change the /s/ to [ʃ].

Rule 12 This rule is ordered to apply following rule 11 and deletes the /w/ from the /sw/ blend after the /s/ is changed to [f] by rule 11. "Sway," thereby, would be pronounced as [fe], "swing" as [fɪŋ], etc.

Rule 13 (Table 7) This is a devoicing rule which substitutes the final voiceless stops for their corresponding voiced cognates about 90% of the time.

Rule 14 All stop consonants in final position may be optionally realized as unreleased stops approximately half the time. This rule is specified in features to avoid a cumbersome listing of all of the sounds included in the class of stops. It also serves to reemphasize that all the rules presented here are to be "mentally" translated into their feature equivalents and interpreted as such.

Rule 15 Final /v/ is always produced as either [f] or [b]; the percentage values following these two alternate realizations specify their approximate distribution. Notice that when [f] is substituted, this rule, like rule 13, works as a devoicing rule. However, when [b] is substituted, the voicing feature is held constant and the fricative and stop features are switched. However, the voicing of [b] is then generally lost by the subsequent application of rule 13. The following alternate pronunciations of the word "move" illustrate the various combined effects of rules 13, 14, and 15.

[muf] (by rule 15)
[mub] (by rule 15)
[mubˀ] (by rules 15 and 14)
[mup] (by rules 15 and 13)
[mupˀ] (by rules 15, 14, and 13)

[5] When all possible sequences of application of the same rules result in the same output, the rules are said to be unordered. However, if the output varies with order, then the particular order that yields the correct output must be specified, and the rules constitute an ordered set.

Rule 16 The final affricates /tʃ,dʒ/ are always replaced by the palatal fricatives [ʃ,ʒ].

Rule 17 The final, palatal fricatives /ʃ,ʒ/ are substituted by the alveolar fricatives [s,z]. The further specification, [voice-], following the rule is a convention for singling out the voiceless member of the pair of sounds, and thus, the rule is to be interpreted as optionally applying to /ʃ/ about 90% of the time. Similarly, the obligatory restriction associated with [voice+] designates the rule always applies to /ʒ/. Observe, too, that the palatal fricative substitutions arising from rule 16 are likewise subject to this rule.

Rule 18 The final, lingual dental fricatives /θ,ð/ are always replaced by the alveolar fricatives [s,z].

Rule 19 The final, voiced, alveolar fricative /z/ is almost always realized as its voiceless cognate [s] with an occasional occurrence of a voiced onset designated by [ᶻs]. This rule also applies to the output of rules 17 and 18, and the combined effect of these three rules results in converting all of Frank's nonlabial, friction sounds into [s], with the exception of the nominal occurrence of [ʃ] permitted by rule 17. Note, also, that rule 19, along with rules 13 and 15, almost entirely blocks the occurrence of all voiced consonants in final position, therefore suggesting these three rules may encompass a more general principle of consonantal devoicing in Frank's speech. The clinical results to follow lend some support to this hypothesis.

CLINICAL APPLICATIONS OF THE PHONOLOGICAL ANALYSES

The basic assumption underlying the clinical use of phonological analyses is that the elimination of any specific articulatory error effects a change in the principle giving rise to that error. Hence, all of the other articulatory errors arising from that principle also will be eliminated without having to work directly with them. Therefore, by selecting specific key sounds which will have the greatest impact upon the organizational structure of the child's deviant phonological system, the effects of therapy will be maximized. To illustrate the strategy and results of this approach, we again return to Frank B. and follow the successive stages of his phonological development during the course of his therapy program.

Frank is one of 18 children who have participated in the clinical research program and serves only as a typical case in point. He was enrolled for two 45-min sessions of individual therapy twice a week and attended for approximately 1.5 years. At that time he was dismissed from therapy with essentially normal speech. As noted earlier, his speech was about 80% unintelligible at the time of the initial evaluation, and the resulting phonological analysis presented in Tables 6 and 7 serves as the starting point for planning his therapy program. Every 2–3 months thereafter, his speech was reevaluated to reappraise and update his therapy. The analyses accompanying these reevaluations are given in Tables 8 through 13 and constitute a record or history of Frank's changing phonological system as it evolved throughout the period of therapy. A discussion of the therapy plan and the consequent changes in his phonological system for each reevaluation period follows.

Reevaluation Period 1

This period covers the intervening time between the initial evaluation and the first reevaluation during which Frank had attended 20 therapy sessions. Throughout this period, the clinician worked with Frank on the production of initial /z/, the initial /sp/ blend, and final /b/, and all direct therapy was always limited to just these sounds. Thus, aside from possible extraneous influences outside of therapy, any resulting changes in his phonological system would reflect the effects of the specific key sounds included in his therapy program.

The choice of initial /z/ was directed toward rule 6 (refer to Table 6) to eliminate the substitution of [s], which in turn would also block the substitution of [ʃ] stemming from rule 7. Notice that Frank also substitutes [s] for /z/ in final position (rule 19, Table 7), and at the time, I had hypothesized that the selection of initial /z/ therefore might have some influence on final /z/ as well. This sort of cross over between initial and final environments, however, has since turned out to be unfounded, but the example itself serves to illustrate the clinical value inherent in systematic phonological analyses, namely, that the approach makes it possible to test our hypotheses and thereby prevents us from perpetuating our misconceptions.

The /sp/ blend was selected to eliminate the omission of /s/ in the blends (rule 11, Table 6), the rationale being that the production of [s] in the single context of the /sp/ blend would result in eliminating the pattern of omission of /s/ in all the other blends. The appearance of /s/ before the consonants (in the blends), then, also would provide the appropriate environment for the unaspirated, voiceless stops, thus removing them from their displaced, initial position context (arising from the combined effects of rules 2 and 11).

The selection of final /b/ provided a means of working with the (excessive) nonreleasing of the stop consonants (rule 14, Table 7) as well as with the devoicing of the voiced stops (rule 13, Table 7), i.e., the substitution of the voiceless stops for their voiced cognates. Notice that the selection of a voiceless consonant would have precluded the possibility of working simultaneously with rules 13 and 14.

The analysis of Frank's phonological system at the end of the first therapy period is shown in the first column of Tables 8 and 9. Notice, first of all, that of the 19 rules shown in these tables, 12 have remained unchanged (NC beneath a rule number designates a rule that has not changed from the previous evaluation). Based on Frank's therapy program, however, we would not have predicted that any of these rules should be affected (save possibly

Table 8. Phonological analysis of Frank's initial consonants and blends for the first and second reevaluations[a]

Phonological rules (reevaluation 1)	Phonological rules (reevaluation 2)
1. No longer present	1. ——
2. NC $\begin{bmatrix} p \\ t \\ k \end{bmatrix} \rightarrow \begin{bmatrix} p= \\ t= \\ k= \end{bmatrix}$ /s_ oblig.	2. Unnecessary to specify due to change of rule 11
3a. NC $\begin{bmatrix} t \\ d \end{bmatrix} \rightarrow \begin{matrix} t\int \\ d_3 \end{matrix}$ /_r oblig.	3a. No longer present
3b. NC $[t=] \rightarrow [d_3]$ /_r oblig.	3b. No longer present
4. NC $[v] \rightarrow [w]$ /#_ opt. 50%	4. NC $[v] \rightarrow [w]$ /#_ opt. 50%
5. NC $\begin{bmatrix} \theta \\ \eth \end{bmatrix} \rightarrow \begin{bmatrix} t \\ d \end{bmatrix} / \begin{matrix} \#\_ \text{ oblig.} \\ \_r \text{ oblig.} \end{matrix}$	5. NC $\begin{bmatrix} \theta \\ \eth \end{bmatrix} \rightarrow \begin{bmatrix} t \\ d \end{bmatrix} / \begin{matrix} \#\_ \text{ oblig.} \\ \_r \text{ oblig.} \end{matrix}$
6. $[z] \rightarrow [z{:}s]$ /#_ oblig.	6. No longer present
7. No longer present	7. ——
8. NC $[\int] \rightarrow [s]$ /#_ opt. 50%	8. No longer present
9. NC $[l] \rightarrow \begin{bmatrix} \phi \\ j \\ \phi \end{bmatrix} \begin{matrix} /\#\_ \text{ opt. 60\%} \\ /\#\_ \text{ opt. 10\%} \\ /\text{cons.}\_ \text{ oblig.} \end{matrix}$	9. $[l] \rightarrow \phi$ /cons._ opt. 15%
10. NC $[r] \rightarrow \begin{bmatrix} w \\ \phi \end{bmatrix} \begin{matrix} /\#\_ \text{ oblig.} \\ /\text{cons.}\_ \text{ oblig.} \end{matrix}$	10a. $[r] \rightarrow \begin{bmatrix} \fbox{r} \end{bmatrix}$ /#_ opt. 50%
	10b. $[r] \rightarrow [l]$ $\begin{matrix} /\text{cons.} \\ /\text{labial+}\_ \text{ opt. 60\%} \end{matrix}$
11. $[s] \rightarrow \begin{bmatrix} f \\ \phi \end{bmatrix} \begin{matrix} /\_w \text{ opt. 75\%} \\ /\text{cons.}\_ \text{ opt. 20\%} \end{matrix}$	11. $[s] \rightarrow [f]$ /_w opt. 75%
12. NC $[w] \rightarrow \phi$ /f_ oblig.	12. NC $[w] \rightarrow \phi$ /f_ oblig.

[a]Unless otherwise specified, all initial consonants occur in the context preceding a vowel. Percentages are estimates of how often the rules apply. NC designates a rule that has not changed from the previous evaluation. Opt., optional rules; oblig., obligatory rules.

Table 9. Phonological analysis of Frank's final consonants for the first and second reevaluations[a]

Phonological rules (reevaluation 1)	Phonological rules (reevaluation 2)
13. $\begin{bmatrix} b \\ d \\ g \end{bmatrix} \rightarrow \begin{bmatrix} b^1 & p \\ d^1 & t \\ g^1 & k \end{bmatrix}$ / # opt. 90%	13. $\begin{bmatrix} b \\ d \\ g \end{bmatrix} \rightarrow \begin{bmatrix} b^1 & p \\ d^1 & t \\ g^1 & k \end{bmatrix}$ / # opt. 50%
14. [stop+] → stop+ release− / # opt. 20%	14. No longer present
15. [v] → $\begin{bmatrix} f \\ b \end{bmatrix} \begin{matrix} =50\% \\ =50\% \end{matrix}$ / _ # oblig. NC	15. [v] → $\begin{bmatrix} f \\ b \end{bmatrix} \begin{matrix} =25\% \\ =50\% \end{matrix}$ / # opt. 75%
16. $\begin{bmatrix} t\int \\ d_3 \end{bmatrix} \rightarrow \begin{bmatrix} \int \\ 3 \end{bmatrix}$ / _ # oblig. NC	16. $\begin{bmatrix} t\int \\ d_3 \end{bmatrix} \rightarrow \begin{bmatrix} \int \\ 3 \end{bmatrix}$ / # oblig. NC
17. $\begin{bmatrix} \int \\ 3 \end{bmatrix} \rightarrow \begin{bmatrix} s \\ z \end{bmatrix}$ / _ # $\begin{matrix} \overline{[voice-]} \text{ opt. } 90\% \\ [voice+] \text{ oblig.} \end{matrix}$ NC	17. $\begin{bmatrix} \int \\ 3 \end{bmatrix} \rightarrow \begin{bmatrix} s \\ z \end{bmatrix}$ / # $\begin{matrix} \overline{[voice-]} \text{ opt. } 90\% \\ [voice+] \text{ oblig.} \end{matrix}$ NC
18a. [θ] → [s] / _ # opt. 60%	18a. [θ] → [s] / _ # opt. 60% NC
18b. [ð] → [v] / # oblig.	18b. [ð] → [v] / # oblig. NC
19. [z] → $\begin{bmatrix} z_s \\ s \end{bmatrix} \begin{matrix} =20\% \\ =80\% \end{matrix}$ / _ # oblig. NC	19. [z] → $\begin{bmatrix} z_s \\ s \end{bmatrix} \begin{matrix} =20\% \\ =80\% \end{matrix}$ / # oblig. NC

[a]Percentages are estimates of how often the rules apply. NC designates a rule that has not changed from the previous evaluation. Opt., optional rules; oblig., obligatory rules.

rule 19), so that this result is not surprising. Considering the remaining seven rules which have changed, rules 1 and 7 are gone entirely, indicating that the deviant productions previously specified by these rules are no longer present in Frank's speech. It is unlikely that the therapy program had any direct bearing upon the disappearance of these rules. Rather, both were already quite infrequent options (compare rule 1 = 10% and rule 7 = 20%, Table 6), and it is more likely they were already in their terminal stages when therapy was begun.

It is also significant that rule 8 ($\int$ → s) remains unchanged and survives rule 7 (s → $\int$), thus confirming the independence of these two rules, as opposed to the possibility of a discrimination failure between /s/ and /$\int$/ which was discussed in the earlier analysis.

Rule 6 shows that initial /z/ is now always initiated with voicing which is maintained slightly longer than normal (the notation ":" designates lengthening) and then subsequently devoiced, i.e., [z:s]. This is a definite positive change that can be directly attributed to the work with initial /z/ during therapy. As previously noted, the therapy with initial /z/ did not have any effect on final /z/ (rule 19), thus arguing for their separate identity. Had this not been the case, then the two rules 6 and 19 could have been collapsed into a single rule to represent a common phonological principle underlying the substitutions.

Rule 11 indicates that /s/ is now omitted only about 20% of the time before consonants whereas, prior to therapy, it was always omitted in this context. Thus, by working with only the single /sp/ blend, the production of /s/ before all the other consonants has also been effectively established.

The effects of therapy with final /b/ upon rules 13 and 14 are shown in Table 9. As indicated by rule 13, all of the final voiced stops are now initiated with voicing during their beginning phase, although the voicing is not generally sustained during the release phase. Rule 14 shows a decrease in the occurrence of unreleased stops by approximately 25% from the initial evaluation.

The change in form of rule 18 from the initial evaluation does not seem to be related to Frank's therapy program, other than possibly as some indirect consequence of working with final /b/. Notice that there are two essential changes, one quantitative and the other qualitative. First, there is a decrease in the substitution of [s] for /θ/ by about 40% with a corresponding increase in the occurrence of /θ/. Second, the substitution of [z] for /ð/ is replaced by [v], which in turn is pronounced as either [f] or [b] by the subsequent application of rule 15. The replacement of [v] for [z] represents a disruption in the previously congruent pattern of substitution ([s,z] for /θ, ð/), thus necessitating the split of rule 18 (Table 7) into two separate rules.

Reevaluation Period 2

This period includes the time between the first and second reevaluations in which Frank attended 16 therapy sessions. The therapy program was based on his grammar for the first reevaluation, as shown in the first column of Tables 8 and 9. His therapy program included initial /z/, the initial /sp/ blend, the initial /tr/ blend, initial /l/, and final /g/. The initial /z/ and the /sp/ blend are carryovers from his first therapy program, and final /g/ is likewise a continuation of the therapy with final voicing and unreleasing of stops that was previously covered by final /b/. The switch from final /b/ to /g/ was made for experimental purposes only to determine whether a back stop (place$_6$) might be more effective in combatting rules 13 and 14, but otherwise the clinical rationale was exactly the same as that already discussed for final /b/. The addition of the /tr/ blend was directed toward rules 3a and 3b to eliminate the substitution of the affricates [tʃ,dʒ] for the alveolar stops /t,d/ in the context before /r/. This selection also made it possible to simultaneously work with the pattern of omitting /r/ in the blends, which is specified by rule 10. The other new addition to Frank's program of initial /l/ was chosen to eliminate the omission and occasional substitution of [j] for initial /l/ (refer to rule 9).

The resulting changes in Frank's phonological system are shown in the second column of Tables 8 and 9. Rules 4, 5, 12, 16, 17, 18a, 18b, and 19 remain unchanged again, not unexpectedly, since the therapy program did not encompass these rules.

Rule 2 is no longer specified since the unaspirated stops now always appear in their appropriate context as a result of the complete elimination of the omission of /s/ before consonants (note rule 11).

Rules 3a and 3b are no longer present, and this result is attributed to the therapy with the single /tr/ blend, coupled with the elimination of the /s/ deletion before /t/ in the /str/ blend (rule 11) which had provided the context for rule 3b. Furthermore, the speed with which these rules were eliminated from Frank's grammar dramatically highlights the effectiveness of focusing therapy upon the principles underlying a child's deviant phonological system, rather than "guesswork" therapy aimed at surface misarticulations.

Rule 6, the devoicing of initial /z/, has now been totally expelled as a result of therapy with this sound.

The disappearance of rule 9, the substitution of [s] for /ʃ/, was an unexpected loss which cannot be directly attributed to the therapy program, since no specific work was included for this substitution.

The change in rule 9 resulting from therapy with initial /l/ indicates that the omission (and occasional substitution of [j]) of initial /l/ no longer occurs. Additionally, the obligatory deletion of /l/ in the consonantal blends has now decreased to a marginal 15%. This latter result, too, is attributed to the therapy with initial /l/ and also, perhaps, to the reinforcement provided by working with /r/ (also a liquid) in the context of the /tr/ blend.

Rule 10 has been divided into two parts to characterize more clearly the two different phonological processes which are now operating. First, the therapy with /r/ in the context of a blend has "spilled over" to the initial /r/, which now occurs normally about half the time or, alternately, as an un-rounded variant of /r/ (designated by ɹ̣) as shown in rule 10a. Second, the deletion of /r/ in the blends has been completely eliminated by working only with the /tr/ blend. However, a curious side effect has arisen in which [l] may be substituted for /r/, but only in the context following the labial consonants /p,b,f/. This substitution is depicted by rule 10b, and the only obvious interpretation is that it is an artifact of the therapy program resulting from working with /l/. This sort of interaction between the liquids /r/ and /l/ has also shown up in two other children in the clinical program, and thus is not totally unique to Frank. The example itself emphasizes the importance of keeping close track of the effects of our therapy so that we do not overlook such new artifactual patterns which may arise in the process of "correcting" a child's deviant speech.

Rule 11 specifies that the substitution of [f] for /s/ before /w/ continues, but the omission of /s/ before consonants no longer occurs. Consequently, the pattern of omitting /s/ in all of the blends has been completely eradicated by the therapy with the single /sp/ blend.

Rule 13 (Table 9) has undergone a positive change, stemming from the therapy with final /g/. As before, the voiced stops still may be produced with a voiced onset which is lost when the sounds are released, but the application of the rule has decreased by approximately 40% from the first reevaluation. Thus, the voiced stops are now occurring normally about half the time. Furthermore, rule 14 is no longer present, again attributed to therapy with final /g/ which has resulted in eliminating the pattern of nonreleasing of the stop consonants.

The change in rule 15 from obligatory to optional indicates that /v/ occurs normally (with voicing) about 25% of the time with an accompanying decrease in the substitution of [f] for /v/ (devoicing) by approximately 25%. Although no specific therapy was included for final /v/, the change might be interpreted as an indirect consequence of the advent of voicing of the final stops. Recall that [b], the alternate substitution of /v/, had generally been replaced by [p] (devoiced) by rule 13. However, in its present form, this rule now only applies about 50% of the time and even then, the devoicing is only partial, i.e., v → b (by rule 15) and then b → b⁷p (by rule 13). Notice too that the changes in rules 13 and 15 similarly affect the surface pronunciations of final /ð/, which is also replaced by [v] (by rule 18b), even though rule 18b remains unaltered.

Reevaluation Period 3

During this period Frank attended 19 therapy sessions. His therapy program was derived from the grammar for the second reevaluation, which is given in the second column of Tables 8 and 9. His therapy included the initial /bl/ and /br/ blends, final /g/, and final /dʒ/. The /bl/ blend was selected to eliminate the nominal omission of /l/ in the blends (rule 9) and, at the same time, to provide a contrast with the /br/ blend, which was chosen to combat the substitution of [l] for /r/ following the labial consonants (rule 10b). As previously noted, rule 10b was newly introduced into Frank's phonological system during the second reevaluation period. The combined effects of therapy with the /bl/ and /br/ blends were intended to dispel this rule before it became firmly established. Final /g/ remains as a continuation of previous therapy directed at the devoicing of final stops (rule 13).

The new addition of final /dʒ/ was selected to eliminate the substitution of the palatal fricatives [ʃ,ʒ] for the affricates /tʃ,dʒ/ (rule 16). The choice of the voiced (as opposed to the voiceless) affricate was also intended as a clinical experiment to determine whether its introduction would have any impact upon the general pattern of fricative devoicing in Frank's speech. Since the affricates are a kind of amalgamation of the stop and fricative features, the /dʒ/ should also reinforce the voiced stops, but the inclusion of

Table 10. Phonological analysis of Frank's initial consonants and blends for the third and fourth reevaluations[a]

Phonological rules (reevaluation 3)	Phonological rules (reevaluation 4)
1. —	1. —
2. —	2. —
3a. —	3a. —
3b. —	3b. —
4. [v] → [w] /#_ opt. 50% NC	4. [v] → [w] /#_ opt. 50% NC
5. NC $\begin{bmatrix} \theta \\ \eth \end{bmatrix}$ → $\begin{bmatrix} t \\ d \end{bmatrix}$ /#_ oblig. _ɹ oblig	5. $\begin{bmatrix} \theta \\ \eth \end{bmatrix}$ → $\begin{bmatrix} t \\ d \end{bmatrix}$ /#_ [voice−] opt. 75% _ɹ [voice+] opt. 40%
6. —	6. —
7. —	7. —
8. —	8. —
9. No longer present	9. —
10a. [ɾ] → [ɾ] /#_ opt. 50% NC	10a. No longer present
10b. No longer present	10b. —
11. [s] → [f] /_w opt. 75% NC	11. [s] → [f] /_w opt. 75% NC
12. No longer present	12. —

[a]Unless otherwise specified, all initial consonants occur in the context proceding a vowel. Percentages are estimates of how often the rules apply. NC designates a rule that has not changed from the previous evaluation. Opt., optional rules; oblig., obligatory rules.

final /g/ in Frank's therapy program precluded any direct test of this part of the hypothesis.

The effects of the therapy program on Frank's phonological system are depicted by the analysis given in the first column of Tables 10 and 11. Rules 4, 5, 10a, 11, 18a, and 18b remain unaltered during this period.

Rule 9 is no longer present, indicating that the therapy with the /bl/ blend has successfully eliminated the residual omission (approximately 15%) of /l/ following the consonants in the blends.

Table 11. Phonological analysis of Frank's final consonants for the third and fourth reevaluations[a]

Phonological rules (reevaluation 3)	Phonological rules (reevaluation 4)
13. No longer present	13. ——
14. ——	14. ——
15. [v] → [b] / _# opt. 50%	15. No longer present
16. $\begin{bmatrix} tʃ \\ dʒ \end{bmatrix}$ → $\begin{bmatrix} ʃ \\ ʒ \end{bmatrix}$ / _# $\begin{bmatrix} \text{voice−} \end{bmatrix}$ opt. 70% $\begin{bmatrix} \text{voice+} \end{bmatrix}$ opt. 10%	16. [tʃ] → [ʃ] / _# opt. 20%
17. [ʒ] → [z] / _# opt. 60%	17. NC [ʒ] → [z] / _# opt. 60%
18a. NC [θ] → [s] / _# opt. 60%	18.[b] $\begin{bmatrix} θ \\ ð \end{bmatrix}$ → $\begin{bmatrix} f \\ v \end{bmatrix}$ / _# $\begin{bmatrix} \text{voice−} \end{bmatrix}$ opt. 60% $\begin{bmatrix} \text{voice+} \end{bmatrix}$ opt. 75%
18b. NC [ð] → [v] / _# oblig.	
19. [z] → [s] / _# opt. 40%	19. NC [z] → [s] / _# opt. 40%

[a]Percentages are estimates of how often the rules apply. NC designates a rule that has not changed from the previous evaluation. Opt., optional rules; oblig., obligatory rules.
[b]Rules 18a and 18b of the third reevaluation have been collapsed into a single rule (18) for the fourth reevaluation.

Rule 10b (the substitution of [l] for /r/ after labial consonants) has dropped from Frank's phonological system, and this result is attributed to the combined effects of therapy with the /bl/ and /br/ blends.

Rule 12 (the omission of /w/ in the /sw/ blend) has completely disappeared, and this loss seems to be unrelated to Frank's therapy program.

The devoicing of final stops as specified by rule 13 has been eliminated as a result of therapy with final /g/ and possibly supplemented by the final voiced affricate /dʒ/.

Rule 16 has undergone a marked change, particularly for the voiced affricate /dʒ/, which occurs normally approximately 90% of the time. The therapy with final /dʒ/ has similarly affected its voiceless cognate, /tʃ/, which now appears normally 30% of the time.

Perhaps the most significant development in Frank's speech is the breakthrough in the voicing of final fricatives which is reflected by the changes in rules 15, 17, and 19. This result is interpreted as a consequence of working with final /dʒ/, and it is perhaps no accident that the advent of voicing of the final fricatives coincides with the elimination of devoicing of the final stops. Also to be noted is the total disappearance of the substitution of [s] for /ʃ/ (rule 17) even though no specific therapy was included for this substitution.

Reevaluation Period 4

Frank attended 25 therapy sessions during this period. His therapy program, derived from the analysis shown in the first column of Tables 10 and 11, included initial /ð/, final /v/, final /θ/, and final affricates /tʃ,dʒ/. The initial /ð/ was directed at rule 5 to work with the substitution of the alveolar stops [t,d] for lingual dental fricatives /θ,ð/. The final /v/ was chosen to eliminate the substitution of [b] for /v/ (rule 15), and the selection of final /θ/ was intended to work with the substitution of [s] for /θ/ Rule 18a. The final affricate /dʒ/ is a continuation of the previous therapy program directed at the substitution of the palatal fricatives [ʃ,ʒ] for the affricates /tʃ,dʒ/. Recall that the substitution of [ʒ] for /dʒ/ had been nearly eliminated by working with /dʒ/, but the effect of this therapy upon the voiceless cognate /tʃ/ was less extensive. Thus, to speed up the suppression of the [ʃ] substitution for /tʃ/, final /tʃ/ was also added to this phase of the therapy program as an adjunct to final /dʒ/.

The phonological analysis of Frank's speech at the conclusion of this period is presented in the second column of Tables 10 and 11. Rules 4, 11, 17, and 19 remain the same. Although no specific therapy was directed toward rule 19 (the devoicing of final /z/), I had anticipated that the effects of working final /dʒ/ might again extend to /z/, but this result was not forthcoming.

Rule 5 shows a substantial decrease in the substitution of [t,d] for /θ, ð/ resulting from therapy with final /ð/. This decrease was more pronounced for the voiced member /ð/, which now occurs normally over 50% of the time.

Rule 10a (the unrounding of initial /r/) is no longer present, and the absence of this rule has no obvious connection to the therapy program during this period.

Rule 15 (the substitution of [b] for /v/) has been completely eradicated as a consequence of the therapy with final /v/.

The change in rule 16 shows that the combined effects of working with /tʃ/ and /dʒ/ has eliminated the substitution of [ʒ] for /dʒ/ and decreased the substitution of [ʃ] for /tʃ/ by approximately 50%.

Rule 18 represents a revision of rules 18a and 18b, which have been collapsed into a single rule. The substitutions for /θ, ð/ covered by this rule have had a rather curious evolution during Frank's therapy. At the outset, the substitutions followed a symmetrical pattern in which the pair of alveolar fricatives [s,z] were substituted for /θ, ð/ (refer to rule 18, Table 7). Then, at the end of the first reevaluation period, this pattern congruency was disrupted when [z] was replaced by [v] as a substitution for /ð/. This change was depicted by splitting rule 18 into two parts, i.e., rules 18a and 18b shown in column one, Table 9. These two rules then remained unchanged until the fourth reevaluation period, when the substitution of [s] for /θ/ was replaced by [f]. The replacement of [f] for [s] thus gives rise to a new symmetrical pattern in which the pair of labial dental fricatives [f,v] may occur as substitutions for /θ, ð/. Rule 18 incorporates this change. Notice that except for the switch in the substitution of [s] to [f], there was no apparent clinical gain, since the actual percentage of substitutions for /θ/ remained the same. There was, however, a 25% decrease in the substitution of [v] for the /ð/. This is attributed to the therapy with final /θ/.

Reevaluation Period 5

During this period, Frank attended 16 therapy sessions, and his program was based on the analysis given in the second column of Tables 10 and 11. His therapy included initial /ð/, final /θ/, and final /tʃ/, all of which were continuations from the preceding period. The initial /sw/ blend was also added to work with rule 11 (the substitution of [f] for /s/ before /w/).

The changes in Frank's phonological system for this period are shown in the first column of Tables 12 and 13. Rules 4, 16, 17, and 19 were unaltered, and of these rules, no changes had been expected, with the exception of rule 16. Thus, the therapy with final /tʃ/ had no effect upon the residual substitution of [ʃ] for /tʃ/ (rule 16) persisting from the previous period.

Rule 5 shows a 30% decrease in the substitution of [d] for /ð/ resulting from the work with initial /ð/, but the corresponding substitution of [t] for /θ/ remains unaffected.

Rule 11 (the substitution of [f] for /s/ before /w/) has been eliminated as a consequence of therapy with the /sw/ blend.

The change in rule 18 indicates a decrease of approximately 40% in the substitution of [f] for /θ/ resulting from the therapy with final /θ/. There

Table 12. Phonological analysis of Frank's initial consonants and blends for the fifth and sixth reevaluations[a]

Phonological rules (reevaluation 5)	Phonological rules (reevaluation 6)
1. —	1. —
2. —	2. —
3a. —	3a. —
3b. —	3b. —
4. [v] → [w] /#_ opt. 50% NC	4. No longer present
5. $\begin{bmatrix} \theta \\ \eth \end{bmatrix} \rightarrow \begin{bmatrix} t \\ d \end{bmatrix} \Big/ \begin{array}{l} \#\_ \overline{[\text{voice}-]} \text{ opt. } 75\% \\ \_\text{r} [\text{voice}+] \text{ opt. } 10\% \end{array}$	5. No longer present
6. —	6. —
7. —	7. —
8. —	8. —
9. —	9. —
10a. —	10a. —
10b. —	10b. —
11. No longer present	11. —
12. —	12. —

[a]Unless otherwise specified, all initial consonants occur in the context preceding a vowel. Percentages are estimates of how often the rules apply. NC designates a rule that has not changed from the previous evaluation. Opt., optional rules.

was, however, no consequent change in the substitution of [v] for /ð/. This latter result parallels that obtained for the initial lingual dental fricatives /θ, ð/, in which the voiceless member of the pair showed a similar resistance to change. This sort of resistance to carryover from one member of the pair to the other has also occurred with many of the other children in the clinical program. Perhaps, then, a single phonological principle does not underly the substitutions of this class of sounds; in which case, rules 5 and 18 are incorrectly formulated. This interpretation, however, is linguistically inconsistent with the phonological patterns exhibited in children's speech. An alternate possibility is that the relatively infrequent occurrence of these sounds in English limits their exposure (outside of therapy), thus minimizing the effects of therapy. This interpretation also would explain the persistence of the

Table 13. Phonological analysis of Frank's final consonants for the fifth and sixth reevaluations[a]

Phonological rules (reevaluation 5)	Phonological rules (reevaluation 6)
13. —	13. —
14. —	14. —
15. —	15. —
16. [tʃ] → [ʃ] /_# opt. 20%	16. No longer present
17. [ʒ] → [z] /_# opt. 60%	17. [ʒ] → [z] /_# opt. 60%
18. $\begin{bmatrix} \theta \\ ð \end{bmatrix} \rightarrow \begin{bmatrix} f \\ v \end{bmatrix} /\_\#\ \frac{[\overline{\text{voice}^-}]\ \text{opt. }20\%}{[\text{voice}+]\ \text{opt. }75\%}$	18. [ð] → [v] /_# opt. 75%
19. [z] → [s] /_# opt. 40% NC	19. No longer present

[a]Percentages are estimates of how often the rules apply. NC designates a rule that has not changed from the previous evaluation. Opt., optional rules.

misarticulation of final /ʒ/ long after the misarticulation of /ʃ/ had disappeared from Frank's speech i.e., reevaluation period 3.

Reevaluation Period 6

This was the final period of Frank's therapy program, and he attended 24 sessions. His therapy was based on the analysis presented in the first column of Tables 12 and 13. From this analysis, it is apparent that most of the remaining phonological rules apply only to single sounds which constitute a residue of misarticulations left over from previous therapy. Consequently, this phase of Frank's program was geared mainly to "cleaning up" these lingering, isolated misarticulations. His therapy included initial /v/ (rule 4), initial /θ/ (rule 5), final /tʃ/ (rule 16), final /θ/ (rule 18), and final /z/ (rule 19).

The effects of therapy on the remaining phonological rules are shown in the analysis given in the second column of Tables 12 and 13. Rules 4, 5, 16, and 17 have been successfully eliminated. The substitution of [f] for final /θ/ (rule 18) was also eliminated, but as in the previous period, the therapy with final /θ/ had no effect upon final /ð/. Rule 17 (the substitution of [z] for /ʒ/) continues unchanged, but no therapy was directed toward this rule. Since final /ð/ and final /ʒ/ occur so infrequently in English, the continued presence of these misarticulations (rules 17 and 18) in Frank's speech could hardly justify any further therapy and he was dismissed.

General Remarks

Frank began therapy with a severe phonological disorder that rendered his speech almost totally unintelligible, and he was dismissed from therapy 17 months later with essentially normal speech. He was selected for inclusion here as representative of the 18 children who have participated in the clinical research project. His progress was no more dramatic or exceptional than any of the other children. The results of these clinical studies indicate that by directing therapy toward the underlying principles of a child's deviant phonological system, even severe articulatory disorders can be eradicated within a period of 1.5 years or less. This is to be contrasted with traditional approaches in most clinics and schools, where therapy typically extends for periods of 3 years or more for children with disorders of comparable severity.

The case study of Frank illustrates the general strategy for translating a phonological analysis into a motivated plan of therapy. I would like to emphasize, however, that the analysis itself is not a recipe for therapy. Rather, it is more like a map to aid us in choosing the best route to reach a destination. In the process of selecting the specific, key sounds to include in therapy, we are formulating our working hypotheses of the most effective routes to follow in correcting a child's speech. The effects of therapy on the child's speech constitute a test of these hypotheses. With each child, we are conducting a research project, the results of which allow us to further refine our hypotheses and thereby improve the effectiveness of therapy. In this sense, then, the dichotomy between therapy and research is totally without foundation.

THE STRUCTURE OF THE NORMALLY DEVELOPING PHONOLOGICAL SYSTEM

The study of abnormal phonological development encompasses the study of normal development, since what constitutes abnormal must be defined in relation to normal. Thus, an integral part of the research program includes the study of the normal acquisition of speech, beginning with the first meaningful utterances at about 1 year and extending through the 3rd year, the age at which most children have fairly well mastered the sound system of their language.

Preliminary linguistic analyses have been completed with six children. These analyses are based on longitudinal samples of the children's speech which have been phonetically transcribed by the parents, all of whom were trained in doing close phonetic transcription. The transcriptions are recorded in a small, easily carried notebook resembling a sort of running diary. The samples are transcribed on the spot and are generally recorded daily, scattered throughout the children's waking hours as they go about their routine of daily living.

The results of this phase of the study indicate two distinct but simultaneous phases of phonological development, although neither phase is independent of the other.

First, the children do not seem to learn to perceive and produce individual sounds as units, one by one. Rather they learn specific attributes or features of sounds sequentially, which in turn provide the basis of discrimination or contrast for the particular set of sounds they are able to use at any given point in time. Thus, in some stages, new sounds can be accommodated within a child's feature system without the addition of new features. A child who has a contrast between /p,b,t/ (a contrast between bilabial and alveolar place of articulation and between voicing and nonvoicing) already has the necessary features for adding /d/. However, at this stage, his system will not yet accommodate /m/ until the feature of nasality has been acquired. However, once he does so, /n/ can also be admitted with no further features being required.

"True" problems of discrimination among sounds, therefore, are tied to incomplete feature acquisition, as opposed to the absence or inappropriate use of phonological rules which operate upon the features. Unlike many theories of feature acquisition, however, the results of our studies clearly demonstrate that features are not "blanketly" admitted into a child's system, but instead are closely tied to phonetic context. For example, the contrast between voicing and nonvoicing of stop consonants usually appears much earlier in initial position than final position, whereas the "same" contrast among friction sounds generally occurs first in final position.

In the second phase of phonological development, the children seem to learn implicit rules which operate on the set of features they have acquired at any given point in time, thus resulting in highly regularized patterns of sound usage. One child, for example, during a period of 2 months, consistently lengthened all vowels before nasal consonants, even though the nasal consonants themselves were often omitted in her overt speech.

RELATIONSHIP BETWEEN NORMAL AND ABNORMAL PHONOLOGICAL DEVELOPMENT

Because of the lack of systematic studies of normal speech development (or abnormal development, for that matter), the question of whether or not articulatory disorders are manifestations of arrested "early normal" development or are deviant patterns unparalleled in normal development, has been subject to little more than unfounded speculation. However, as the present study continues, there is increasing evidence that the deviant phonological patterns found in children who develop abnormal speech almost exactly parallel those which are present at one or another stage of normal development. Some of the more prevalent developmental generalizations follow.

1. The first utterances are consonant-vowel syllables with final consonants and unstressed syllables omitted. This result is specific to beginning development, although several of the children with defective speech exhibited the same pattern as their predominant form of speech.
2. The first consonants are voiceless stops /p,t,k/ (often unaspirated) occurring in initial word position. This is also specific to beginning development, but the persistent substitution of unaspirated stops for aspirated ones was still present in approximately 70% of the children with defective speech.
3. The first friction consonants are voiceless (/f,θ,s,ʃ/) and develop in final word position prior to initial word position. Again, this is specific to beginning development, but it also corresponds to the ease of successful acquisition by the children in therapy.
4. Substitutions of consonants are more likely to occur along the continuum of place of articulation, as opposed to manner of articulation, with the substitutions generally being a shift to a more forward (in the mouth) place of articulation.
5. When substitutions in manner of articulation occur, place of articulation is usually held constant, the most common place being at the upper gum ridge (alveolar) above the teeth, i.e., [t] for /s/, [n] for /l/, [d] for /z/, etc.
6. Changes in order or reversing of sounds (metathesis) is a common phonological process of sound change, i.e., "doggie" pronounced as "goddie," "mop the floor" as "mof the ploor," etc. (a consistently reoccurring but not so obvious phonological process).
7. Consonants in initial word position often take on similar characteristics or even become identical to other consonants that follow under the influence of the latter (assimilation), i.e., "top" pronounced as "pop," "cat" as "tat," "jacket" as "gacket," etc. (The reverse process of later consonants being influenced by earlier ones also occurs, but with less frequency.)
8. Many seeming pronunciation oddities (exceptions) can be traced back to earlier stages of development and constitute a sort of subclass of misarticulations or a "residue" of the past which persist, even though the normal phonological patterns have since become firmly established.

While the preceding generalizations are by no means exhaustive of the results found to date, they do provide the illustrative force to support the hypothesis that the same or quite similar phonological processes are operating when children develop speech normally as well as when they fail to do so.

A THEORY OF THE ACQUISITION OF PHONOLOGICAL DISORDERS

The child with a phonological disorder does not deviate from normal phonological development but in fact perpetuates it. A child acquiring speech normally goes through various stages of omission and sound substitution patterns that are subsequently dropped or replaced by others as he moves from one phase of development to the next. The child with defective speech, however, seems to be operating according to some sort of "rigidity" principle by which he "hangs on to" and thus accumulates these patterns of omissions and substitutions which otherwise would be discarded in moving from one stage to another.

In so doing, children with defective speech also may develop various idiosyncratic phonological patterns (often bizarre, but nonetheless quite innovative), perhaps as an attempt to compensate for a phonological system that fails to meet their communicative needs by rendering them unintelligible. Consequently, the speech of a 5- or 6-year-old child with an articulatory disorder is not simply a case of "arrested" early normal development resembling that of a 2-year-old child. Rather, it is a highly integrated system of omission and sound substitution patterns every bit as complex as the phonological system of a child with normal speech of the same age. In this sense, then, such a child is not operating by a simplified or "primitive" phonological system but has more nearly developed a different phonological system comparable to speaking another language.

ACKNOWLEDGMENT

I wish to thank Maribeth Lynn for her clinical services and valuable criticism during the preparation of this chapter.

REFERENCES

Compton, A. J. 1970. Generative studies of children's phonological disorders. J. Speech Hear. Disord. 35: 315–339.
Oller, D. K., and R. E. Eilers. Phonetic expectation and transcription validity. Phonetica. In press.

PERCEPTION –
AUDITION

Distinctive Features: A Measure of Consonant Perception

Sadanand Singh, Ph.D.
Professor of Hearing and Speech Sciences
Ohio University

CONTENTS

INTRODUCTION

In recent years there has been considerable advancement in our knowledge of the acoustic, articulatory, and linguistic properties of speech sounds. The details of these properties, considered crucial for phonemic determination by acoustic analysis, articulatory mappings, and linguistic derivations of rules, have been precise to the extent that they can be successfully utilized to synthesize speech of high intelligibility and reasonable naturalness. In the history of such scientific investigation, there is very little insight regarding man, the processor of speech. Questions relating to the behavior of man as a processor of speech have not yet been answered in explicit terms. For example: How are speech sounds perceived? What are the perceptual attributes of these speech sounds? What weights do these properties carry in a normally functioning person's perception of speech in varying listening conditions? How does the perception differ between adults and children, normal and hearing-impaired, native speakers and foreign speakers, etc.? These questions are of utmost importance to those who deal with deviations and impairments in hearing and speech. An attempt at answering these questions entails gaining insight into the interaction of the human speech processing system with the speech stimuli. This paper deals with the above questions in the framework of a theory of speech perception with two major procedural advancements: 1) designation of a priori features to predict perceptual responses, and 2) extraction of a posteriori features from these responses.

A PRIORI DESIGNATION OF A FEATURE SYSTEM TO PREDICT PHONEME PERCEPTION

Prediction of One Set of Perceptual Responses by One Feature System

The use of a given feature system was not adequately explained in a number of studies investigating the perceptual reality of distinctive features. These investigators used one or more competing sets of a priori feature systems to predict listeners' responses to speech sounds. These feature systems are being referred to as a priori because the experimenters determined how the data would be classified prior to analysis. The merit of these studies is that they have tested the perceptual importance of a given feature system as a whole and also the relative importance of a feature in a given feature system. These tests have been conducted to determine the rank order of the perceptual strength of the distinctive features in: 1) condition of acoustic distortion (e.g., noise and filtering) of the stimuli (Miller and Nicely, 1955); 2) cross linguistic settings (Singh and Black, 1966); 3) the recall of speech sound in short-term memory (Klatt, 1968; Wickelgren, 1966); 4) the utilization of choice reaction time as a measure of distinctive feature differences between phonemes (Cole and Scott, 1972; Weiner and Singh, 1974); and 5) judgment of pairs and triads of speech stimuli utilizing various psychological methods for eliciting perceptual responses (Singh, 1970b, 1971; Singh and Becker, 1972; Wang and Bilger, 1973). While all of the above studies prove unambiguously that all features of a given system are not of equal importance, they do not agree regarding the explanatory powers of a given feature system.

Miller and Nicely (1955) Before presenting their experimental results, Miller and Nicely expressed dissatisfaction with the prevalent method of reporting perceptual responses as a function of noise and frequency distortions. They reported: "One limitation of the existing studies, however, is that results are given almost exclusively in terms of the articulation scores, the percentages of the spoken words that the listener hears correctly. By implication, therefore, all of the listeners' errors are treated as equivalent and no knowledge of the perceptual confusions is available." (p. 388) Thus, instead of eliciting right/wrong or all-or-none types of responses, Miller and Nicely elicited total confusions occurring among the 16 English consonants studied in the context of the vowel /a/ spoken and listened to by five female North American speakers in 17 signal-to-noise (S/N) ratios and filter conditions. Five features with acoustic and articulatory bases (Jakobson, Fant, and Halle, 1951; Singh, in press (a)) were chosen by Miller and Nicely for predicting the perceptual confusions of consonants. The main questions asked in this experiment were:

1. How well does this feature system explain the confusions of consonants?
2. Does each of these five features transmit equal amounts of information?
3. Are these five features independent of each other?

Miller and Nicely used a statistical procedure, a measure of covariance, described by Shannon and Weaver (1963), which allowed them to provide a parametric answer to each of the above questions.

Information transmission is a measure of the mathematical relationship between the stimulus, the amount of noise in the system, and the response. This statistic has been described as mean logarithmic probability. That is, if the input variable x can assume the discrete values $i = 1, 2, \ldots, k$ with probability P_i, and the output variable y can assume the values $j = 1, 2, \ldots, m$, then the number of decisions needed to specify the particular stimulus-response pair is mean logarithmic probability xy where P_{ij} is the probability of the joint occurance of input i and output j. This probability is high if the noise in the system is low. A measure of covariance of input with output is given by the following equation:

$$T(x,y) = -\sum_{i,j} P_{ij} \log_2 \frac{P_i P_j}{P_{ij}}$$

where T is the transmission of information from stimulus x to response y; P_i is n_i/n; P_j is n_j/n; and P_{ij} is n_{ij}/n. The n_i is the frequency of stimulus i; n_j is the frequency of response j; and n_{ij} is the frequency of the joint occurrence of stimulus i and response j in a sample of n observations.

In any one of the 17 Miller and Nicely confusion matrices, the 16 consonants at the left of the matrix represent stimuli and the 16 at the head represent responses. Each cell represents the number of times a given stimulus had been perceived as a given response. The diagonal, obviously, is the number of correctly perceived items, and the errors are scattered off the diagonal. Miller and Nicely computed the transmitted information for each of the 17 experimental conditions for both the phonemes (composite channel) and the features (component channels). They subdivided each of the 17 confusion matrices into the voice communication network of five component channels where four channels were assigned binary codes, for example,

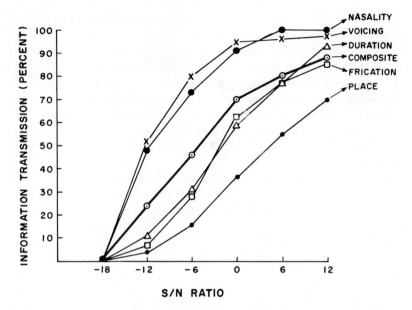

Figure 1. Information transmission for nasality, voicing, duration, composite, frication, and place as a function of six S/N ratios. (Data plotted from Miller and Nicely, 1955.)

voicing (0,1), nasality (0,1); and one channel place was assigned a tertiary code (0,1,2).

In Figure 1 the effects of six S/N ratios (abscissa) is shown on the rate of information (ordinate) for the five features and the phoneme. The features nasality and voicing show greater strengths (represented by greater amount of information transmission) than the features duration, frication, and place of articulation. Information rate of the composite channel (phoneme) is placed between these two sets of groups for features.

The results of low-pass and high-pass filter conditions are shown in Figures 2 and 3, respectively. These figures reveal that the features nasality, voicing, and frication had a higher rate of information under the low-pass conditions while the features duration and place of articulation had the higher rate of information in the high-pass filter conditons. These comparisons are more meaningful when they are plotted to determine the cross over points for each of the five features as well as the composite channel. The implication derived from such cross over is that the two systems are contributing approximately equal amounts of information for the intelligibility of the criterion measure.

Figure 4 shows the comparison of the cross over points of the five different features and the composite channel. It is clear in this figure that these points are different for the different criterion measures. In this figure the cross over point for frication is at 750 Hz (4A); for place of articulation at 1,900 Hz (4B); for duration at 2,200 Hz (4C); for composite transmission

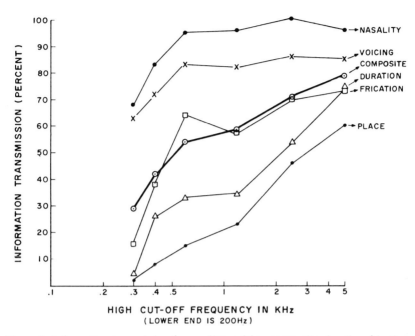

Figure 2. Information transmission for nasality, voicing, composite, duration, frication, and place as a function of six low-pass bandwidths. (Data plotted from Miller and Nicely, 1955.)

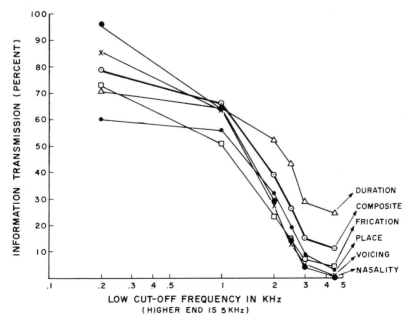

Figure 3. Information transmission for duration, composite, frication, place, voicing, nasality, as a function of six high-pass bandwidths. (Data plotted from Miller and Nicely, 1955.)

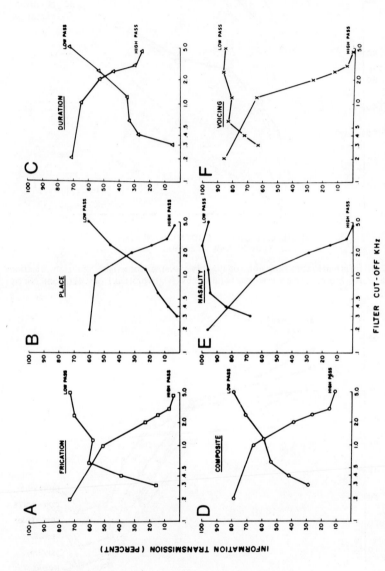

Figure 4. Low- and high-pass cross over points for information transmission values frication (A), place of articulation (B), duration (C), composite (D), nasality (E), and voicing (F).

at 1,250 Hz (4D); for nasality at 450 Hz (4E); and for voicing at 500 Hz (4F). Thus, the cross over points for nasality, voicing, and frication are below and for place and duration are above the cross over point for composite channel.

Cross talk and feature importance   Miller and Nicely showed clearly that a multichannel (feature) system describes auditory functions for phoneme processing more precisely and in greater detail than a composite channel (phonemic) system does. Since the multichannel system was considered important, they devised a statistical procedure to evaluate a given distribution of features. A comparison of the maximum possible composite channel information (an outcome of an errorless system) with the sum of the maximum possible feature channel information reflects the efficiency of the system. If the difference between the two information channels is zero, then the system is said to be perfect. However, because of the welcome presence of redundancy in human language, this perfection is not possible.

The maximum possible information for a composite channel was 4.0 bits, and the sum of the maximum information for the five features was 4.89 bits. Thus, there was a difference of 0.89 bits, indicating approximately 22% redundancy or cross talk for the whole system and an average of approximately 4% (22%/5) for each of the five features. Depending on the number of stimuli used in an experiment and the number of channels or features used to code these stimuli, the factor of redundancy may increase or decrease. Unfortunately, at this juncture, there is no known measure of "ideal" or "expected" redundancy against which a computed measure can be compared.

The results of the Miller and Nicely experiment showed that the different features did not hold similar ranks in speech perception. The rank order of the features was: 1) nasality (62%), 2) voicing (59%), 3) duration (41%), 4) frication (40%), and 5) place of articulation (27%). More importantly, the low- and high-pass filters and the different levels of noise affected these features differently.

Singh and Black (1966)   In this experiment the one-language hypothesis of Miller and Nicely was extended to a cross language experiment. The speakers and listeners of Hindi, English, Arabic, and Japanese spoke and identified an identical set of 26 consonants in the contexts of two vowels. The purpose was to establish a common set of parameters or features across the four languages. The focal point of interest was to investigate the universal application of a selected group of consonant features in speech perception. The quantitative method utilized in this study was the same as described in Miller and Nicely (1955). The Miller and Nicely feature system was extended from five to seven distinctive features for accommodating the distinctions of a larger set of consonants. The object was to find the rank order of the strengths of the features in the error responses of the listeners and their similarity in the different language groups.

The percentage of information transmission in the 16 speaking-listening conditions is shown in Table 1. A single rank order in this study was obtained

Table 1. Percentage of information transmitted in bits per stimulus for all features and for each feature separately

Condition	All	Voicing	Nasality	Aspiration	Friction	Place	Duration	Liquid
Hindi-Hindi	75.27	60.83	89.89	44.14	54.42	78.35	52.88	54.07
Hindi-English	69.80	50.62	94.94	41.80	52.59	76.29	42.25	61.23
Hindi-Arabic	70.04	67.18	93.43	29.59	57.47	76.29	41.94	85.08
Hindi-Japanese	68.10	75.20	94.94	14.55	12.00	72.68	40.27	66.80
Rank order		4	1	7	6	2	5	3
English-Hindi	64.72	34.06	100.00	26.38	25.22	68.04	36.77	39.16
English-English	75.44	62.70	95.20	28.36	58.90	77.31	54.25	85.28
English-Arabic	72.65	63.43	93.68	34.89	55.64	73.20	54.56	73.95
English-Japanese	71.78	33.53	100.00	17.50	45.67	79.38	40.73	68.98
Rank order		4	1	7	6	2	5	3
Arabic-Hindi	64.74	43.85	86.61	26.26	27.26	71.13	38.30	51.09
Arabic-English	70.53	57.80	64.14	41.30	54.83	71.65	46.50	68.19
Arabic-Arabic	73.42	48.95	97.47	34.03	43.94	76.80	50.76	86.28
Arabic-Japanese	66.68	63.74	95.20	25.03	39.06	71.65	40.27	65.20
Rank order		4	1	7	6	2	5	3
Japanese-Hindi	61.34	44.06	97.47	23.18	21.36	67.53	33.89	47.31
Japanese-English	68.65	52.91	100.00	16.89	44.35	69.59	44.68	54.27
Japanese-Arabic	62.87	50.62	94.44	57.58	31.94	65.98	40.42	62.42
Japanese-Japanese	68.04	73.53	97.47	13.07	47.81	78.35	43.00	66.80
Rank order		4	1	7	6	2	5	3
Overall average (rank order)		4	1	7	6	2	5	3

for the four listening groups: 1) nasality, 2) place, 3) liquid, 4) voicing, 5) duration, 6) frication, and 7) aspiration. Such perceptual consistencies on the level of distinctive articulatory features among 16 speaker-listener conditions of four distant languages seem to support the hypothesis of language universals or more specifically, a universal phonetic theory.

In general, the rank ordering of features in the Singh and Black experiment agreed with the rank ordering in the Miller and Nicely study for all features except voicing and place of articulation. The "universally" better performance of the place of articulation feature compared to voicing in the Singh and Black experiment raises some questions regarding the acceptance of these rank orders for all conditions. A comparison of the Singh and Black and the Miller and Nicely studies indicated that there were some variables uniquely detrimental to the recovery of place features in the Miller and Nicely experiment and not in the Singh and Black experiment.

Cross talk or redundancy The seven channels in which the voice communications network was subdivided may not be independent. The maximum possible information for the composite channel in this study was 4.70 bits, and the sum of the information transmission of the seven composite channel was 6.25 bits. The cross talk was therefore 6.25–4.70 = 1.55. Thus, the percentage of redundancy was 25% (1.55/6.25), or the average redundancy per channel was 3.6%. This was identical to the redundancy in the Miller and Nicely experiment.

Singh (1966) The Miller and Nicely study demonstrated the efficacy of distinctive features in predicting the error responses in conditions of acoustic distortion, and the Singh and Black study showed their efficacy in predicting the errors in conditions of linguistic distortions. In the Singh (1966) experiment, the effects of acoustic and linguistic distortions were investigated by using speakers and listeners of Hindi and English and by systematically distorting the phonemes on the frequency and time continua. Instead of utilizing consonants of broad phonetic categories, only stops were included in this experiment. The purpose was: 1) to test the effect of filtering and temporally segmenting speech on the intelligibility of plosive consonants as spoken and heard by native speakers of Hindi and English, 2) to determine the predictability of information transmission when three features were used to describe 12 stops, as compared with the use of five features to describe the same 12 stops, 3) to ascertain the extent of the preservation of distinctive features in the error responses, and 4) to note subjects' agreements in the responses to the plosives of the two languages.

Six plosive consonants were temporally truncated at 20, 40, 60, 80, 100, and 120 msec and subsequently passed through the following band-pass filters: 106 Hz to 425, to 850, to 1,700, to 3,400, and to 6,800 Hz; 212 Hz to 425, to 850, to 1,700, to 3,400, and to 6,800 Hz; 425 Hz to 850, to 1,700, to 3,400, and to 6,800 Hz; 850 Hz to 1,700, to 3,400, and to 6,800

102   Sadanand Singh

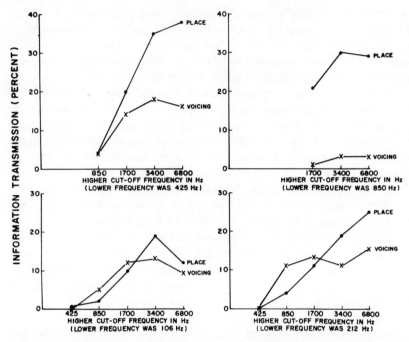

Figure 5. Information transmission for place and voicing as a function of fixed lower cutoff frequencies at 106 Hz, 212 Hz, 425 Hz, and 850 Hz. The higher cutoff frequencies were arranged in one-octave steps. The speakers and listeners were Hindi. (Based on Singh, 1966.)

Hz; 1,700 Hz to 3,400 and to 6,800 Hz; and 3,400 to 6,800 Hz. Thus, a total of 216 × 20 = 4,320 stimuli were prepared for the 10 listening subjects of each of the two languages.

In this study the analysis of the results of the confusion matrices derived from 10 listeners of each language draws heavily on a quantitative procedure originally used by Miller and Nicely and subsequently adopted in the cross linguistic study of Singh and Black. Figures 5 and 6 show the rate of information transmission for the features voicing and place as a function of higher cutoff frequencies. The lower end of the bandwidths in these conditions was fixed at 106, 212, 425, and 850 Hz. Figure 5 depicts the performance of the speakers and listeners of Hindi and Figure 6 of the speakers and listeners of English. A comparison of these figures shows opposite tendencies regarding the importance of the features place and voicing. While for the speakers and listeners of Hindi, place seemed to do better than voicing, for the speakers and listeners of English, voicing was better than place. Thus, it seems that the voicing and place dichotomy is, to a certain extent, language dependent. For English, it is voicing that dominates the feature place while for Hindi, generally, it is place that dominates the feature voicing. It may be

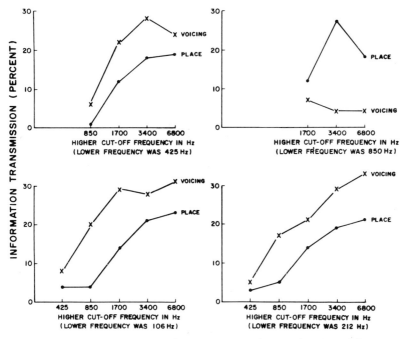

Figure 6. Information transmission for place and voicing as a function of fixed lower cutoff frequencies at 106 Hz, 212 Hz, 425 Hz, and 850 Hz. The higher cutoff frequencies were arranged in one-octave steps. The speakers and listeners were English. (Based on Singh, 1966.)

speculated here that since aspiration is phonemic in Hindi, the Hindi listeners must utilize both voicing and aspiration with divided strengths, thus weakening the feature voicing. To the contrary, since to the English listeners voicing entails both voicing and aspiration cues, they must pay more attention to it. However, there exists some independence inherent in these comparisons. When the lower ends of the frequency bands were over 850 Hz and the higher ends were over 1,700 Hz, the place of articulation was a stronger feature than voicing in both speaking and listening conditions.

Figure 7 shows the information transmitted by the features voicing and place of articulation as a function of the six levels of temporal truncations. Again, the language-dependent biases for voicing and place can be clearly seen in this figure.

Figure 8 shows the comparison of different specifications of the place of articulation feature in terms of the order in which Hindi bilabial, alveolar, and velar places were perceived as a function of frequency bandwidths. The bilabial place was the strongest feature.

Figure 9 shows the comparison of the performance of the bilabial, alveolar, and velar places as a function of temporal distortions ranging from

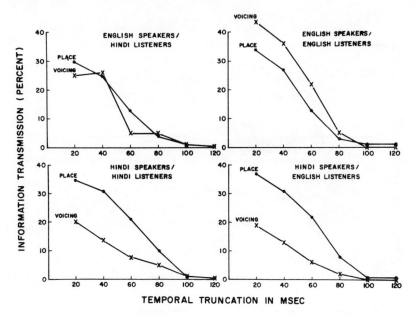

Figure 7. Information transmission for voicing and place for the four speaking-listening language groups as a function of six different durations of truncation. (Based on Singh, 1966.)

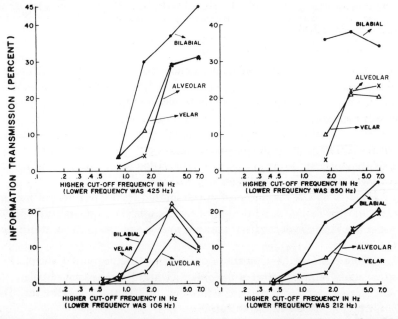

Figure 8. Information transmission for bilabial, alveolar, and velar places as a function of fixed lower cutoff frequencies at 106 Hz, 212 Hz, 425 Hz, and 850 Hz. The higher cutoff frequencies were arranged in one-octave steps. The speakers and listeners were Hindi. (Based on Singh, 1966.)

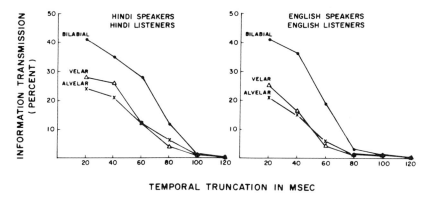

Figure 9. Information transmission for bilabial, velar, and alveolar places for Hindi speakers and listeners and English speakers and listeners as a function of six different durations of truncation. (Based on Singh, 1966.)

20 to 120 msec of truncations. For both languages the bilabial place had greater amounts of information than either the alveolar or velar places.

Cross talk or redundancy   The feature place of articulation in this study was represented in two ways. It was coded by three separate binary categories of bilabial, alveolar, and velar places in one instance and by a multicategory channel having .zero, one, and two places on a continuum in the other instance. These distinctions were drawn to test the validity of the redundancy attributed to the greater number of channels as compared with a smaller number. The sum of the maximum possible information for each of the four binary channels, voicing, bilabial, alveolar, and velar, was 3.754 bits (maximum for bilabial, alveolar, and velar places was 0.918 each, and for voicing it was 1.000), and maximum possible information for a composite channel was 2.584 bits. Thus, there was a difference of 1.170 bits. When place was treated in a multicategory system, the maximum possible information for place was 1.584 and for voicing it was 1.000, resulting in a maximum of 2.584 bits, which was equal to the information of a composite channel. Thus, if there is a precise classification of consonants into the component features, the component channels yield information equal to the information of a composite channel.

Singh (1968)   The purpose of this study was to predict the listeners' responses to multiple choice intelligibility wordlists (Black, 1957) utilizing the distinctive feature system of Singh and Black (1966). The disparity between the correct response, i.e., the stimulus word, and each of the three decoy words of the multiple choice test, was measured in terms of the number of distinctive feature differences.

The distinctive feature analysis of the error response of the multiple choice intelligibility tests is presented graphically in Figure 10. In this figure the abscissa represents the number of distinctive feature differences between the stimulus word and the three error responses, and the ordinate represents

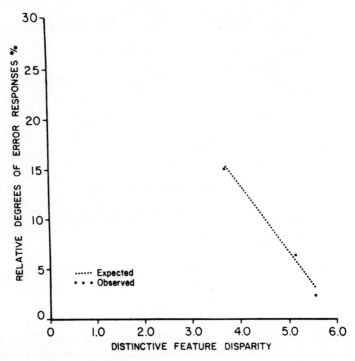

Figure 10. Plotting of relative degrees of error responses to multiple choice intelligibility test as a function of distinctive feature disparity between the stimulus and the three decoy words. (From Singh, 1968.)

the percentage of error responses—the most frequent, the second most frequent, and the least frequent. A linear relationship was reported between the number of errors among words and their distinctive feature differences. The trend shown in this figure relates to one of the several multiple choice test forms. The comparable analysis of the other two forms indicated identical trends and almost perfect correlations between multiple choice word errors and distinctive feature differences.

The linearity of the functions reported for the multiple choice tests was further investigated by incorporating data reported earlier by Miller and Nicely (1955), Singh and Black (1966), and Kile (1966). These data were procured in test situations where choices were more open. Hence there were more than three error responses and thus more than three points on the ordinates and abscissas to be compared.

The 17 confusion matrices of Miller and Nicely and the 16 confusion matrices of Singh and Black were pooled individually. Data from a similar study conducted by Kile involving consonant confusions of hearing-impaired subjects in 15 different experimental conditions were also pooled. These three pooled matrices were predicted by the Singh and Black feature system.

Figures 11–13 show the relationship between the different degrees of confusions in the listeners' responses and the distinctive feature differences between the stimulus and these error responses. A linear function was fitted between the phonemic confusions and the associated distinctive feature differences. The relative degree of error responses (ordinate) and the mean numbers of distinctive feature disparities (abscissa) correlated negatively, with the correlations of −0.878, −0.961, and −0.939 for the Miller and Nicely, Singh and Black, and Kile data, respectively.

The conclusion drawn from these high correlations and the inspection of the trend was that the degree of similarity of distinctive features is a direct predictor of the relative order of listeners' responses.

Singh (1970a) The effect of temporal truncation of 22 English consonants on the perception of six arbitrarily chosen phonetic features was

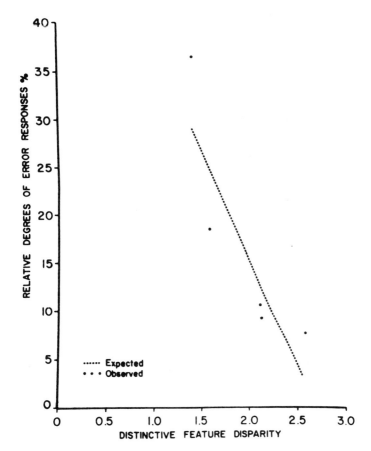

Figure 11. Plotting of relative degrees of error responses as a function of distinctive feature disparity between the stimulus and response phonemes in the Miller and Nicely (1955) data. (From Singh, 1968.)

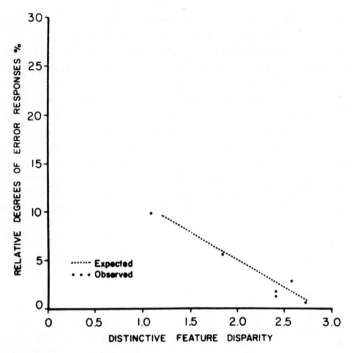

Figure 12. Plotting of relative degrees of error responses as a function of distinctive feature disparity between the stimulus and response phonemes in the Singh and Black (1966) data. (From Singh, 1968.)

determined. The features selected were affrication, plosive, voiced, voiceless, nasality, and frication. One speaker of Hindi and one of English, both male, recorded 22 consonants of English prevocalically. The initial and relatively longer portions of the syllables (including the transition of the consonant to the vowel) were truncated at the threshold of perception. The gated stimuli were photographed from an oscilloscope for measurements. Listeners of the two language groups, Hindi and English (32 in each group), were used as experimental subjects.

The results of this experiment concerning phonetic features directly are shown in Figure 14. This figure shows that when English consonants are perceived by English and Hindi listeners there is a difference in the rank ordering of features. The abscissa in this figure represents selected phonetic features, and the ordinate represents the time-to-intelligibility ratio. The time-to-intelligibility ratio was computed by dividing the critical time factor for a feature by the number of correct responses (an average for listeners of a language group). For example, for the Hindi-speaking subjects, the feature affrication yielded the smallest time-to-intelligibility ratio and the feature frication yielded the largest time-to-intelligibility ratio: the smaller the time-to-intelligibility ratio, the stronger the feature. Figure 14 also shows that for

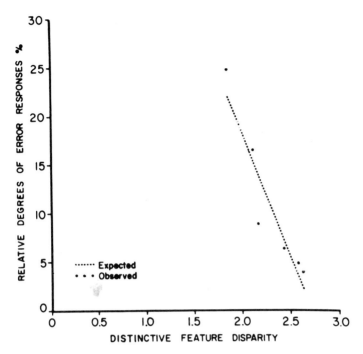

Figure 13. Plotting of relative degrees of error responses as a function of distinctive feature disparity between the stimulus and response phonemes in the Kile (1966) data. (From Singh, 1968.)

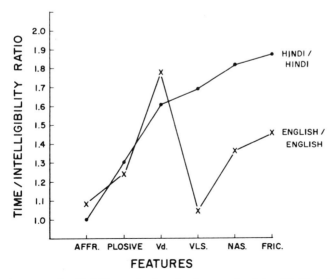

Figure 14. Time-to-intelligibility ratio for six features involving Hindi and English speakers and listeners. This ratio was obtained by dividing the smallest amount of time needed for the identification of a consonant by the percentage of identification score associated with it. (Based on Singh, 1970a.)

both language groups the feature affrication was one of the strongest features, and frication and nasality were weaker features when the temporal factor was the source of distortion. The maximal discrepancies between the two languages existed for the voiceless consonants.

Prediction of One Set of Perceptual Responses by a Number of Feature Systems

Feature systems have been proposed through various sources. These sources are primarily influenced by the affiliation and training orientation of a particular researcher. For example, a feature system proposed by a linguist may have been devised to facilitate the formulations of phonologic rules of adult speech, or a feature system proposed by a psychoacoustician may stress those acoustic "cues" of relative stability which produce predictable results, and so on. One way to verify the perceptual reality of these alternative feature systems, which all claim to describe the phoneme, is to use them as predictors for a constant set of perceptual output.

Wickelgren (1966)   Wickelgren investigated the applications of alternative distinctive feature systems in predicting errors in short-term memory for consonants. He compared three distinctive feature systems to show which system best predicts these errors. The basic assumption underlying the prediction of short-term memory errors by distinctive features was that both perception and short-term memory utilize a similar set of parameters for encoding phonemes. Wickelgren tested the hypothesis that short-term memory errors or intrusion errors in recall are committed not on an all-or-none basis but on a componential basis.

The study included two groups of consonants, one group consisting of the same 16 consonants used by Miller and Nicely and the other group consisting of all 23 consonants of English occurring at the initial position of a syllable. All syllables were of the consonant-vowel (CV) type, the vowel in each case was /a/.

The main results pertaining to the short-term memory intrusions (recall of a different consonant from the one the subject heard and wrote down) can be summarized by presenting the total percentage of correct feature recall. The feature recall was computed for three feature systems: 1) Miller and Nicely; 2) Halle (1964); and 3) Wickelgren (1966). Since the features voicing and nasality had identical specifications in all three feature systems, they resulted identical feature recall value for each system: voicing 64% and nasality 56%. The remaining three features of the Miller and Nicely system, five features of the Halle system, and two features of the Wickelgren system were the basis for the comparison of the feature systems. Recall of features in the incorrect phonemic intrusions for the Miller and Nicely feature system was 64%, for the Halle system 60%, and for the Wickelgren system 74%. Wickelgren concluded that:

the accuracy of each of the three feature systems is consistently and significantly above chance, indicating that intrusion errors in short-term memory
tend to have distinctive features in common with the presented consonant
[and that] consonants are *not* remembered in an all-or-none manner. Some of
the features of a consonant can be recalled when others cannot, producing a
systematic tendency for the errors in short-term recall to have distinctive
features in common with the correct consonant. This suggests that recall of a
consonant means recall of a set of features that defines that consonant in
memory, and each feature is recalled at least semi-independently of the other
features. (p. 397)

It is obvious in this instance, then, that the Wickelgren feature system was
a better predictor of the short-term memory intrusions than the Halle and the
Miller and Nicely feature systems. The significance of this difference was
tested by the chi-square method, and it was found that the Wickelgren system
was significantly more accurate than the Miller and Nicely feature system (at
the 0.02 level; $\chi^2 = 21.3$).

Singh (1970b) Comparisons of the three different sets of features—Singh
and Black (1966), Halle (1964), and Wickelgren (1966)—was made to investigate which of these three systems more closely approximated the judged
similarities of English consonants spoken and heard by Hindi and English
speakers. The consonants were judged in five S/N ratio conditons and four
signal level conditions in initial and final positions of a syllable. The main
difference between this experiment and that of Wickelgren is that Wickelgren's observations were intrusions in recall whereas the observations in this
experiment were a measure of similarity judgment, namely, the triadic comparison (ABX).

All responses of the distortion conditions were pooled for distinctive
feature analysis. Rank correlations were obtained between the listener's
judgment of similarity and the three distinctive feature systems independently. There were eight response matrices and three distinctive feature
matrices, involving a total of 528 rank correlations. Half of these correlations
were found significant at the 0.05 level. A comparison of the consonants in
prevocalic and postvocalic contexts showed that 59% of the correlations were
significant when judged in the prevocalic position and 43% of the correlations
were significant when judged in the postvocalic position. A greater number of
rank correlations were significant in the listening mode (60%) than in the
speaking mode (42%), implying that the auditory responses were predicted
more reliably than the productive responses. Finally, a comparison of the
three feature systems showed that the extension of the Miller and Nicely
system by Singh and Black resulted in the largest number (61%) of significant
correlations, the Halle system resulted in the second largest number (51%) of
significant correlations, and the Wickelgren system resulted in the smallest
number (41%) of significant correlations.

It may be recalled that the above findings are different from those of
Wickelgren, who reported that his system showed maximal accuracy (73%)

when compared with the Halle and the Miller and Nicely systems. It may be speculated that the basis for the differing results may be attributable to the different data collection methods involved in the Wickelgren study and the Singh (1970b) study. The responses elicited in the short-term memory and the similarity judgment paradigms have different preferences for the features.

Ahmed and Agrawal (1969)   In this study, 29 consonants of Hindi at the initial place of a CVC syllable and 31 at the final place were combined with 10 nondipthongized vowels of Hindi and were used to form the test material for listening. A total of 870 different nonsense CVC syllables were recorded for presentation by one female and two males. No syllable had the same consonant in the initial and final positions. The syllables were randomized and presented to six male listeners in nine sessions. The statistical analysis procedure used in this study was information transmission.

There were two confusion matrices, one involving the 29 consonants in the initial position of a syllable and the other involving the 31 consonants at the final position of the syllable. A feature system somewhat similar to the one used by Singh and Black was used to describe the Hindi consonants.

The results show that although some consistencies exist across positions between the rank orders of the importance of features (from most important to least important), some crucial differences are obvious. The two features nasality and aspiration showed the most pronounced differences between their ranks at the initial and final positions. Although both of these features fared well at the initial positions, with second and third rankings, respectively, they were extremely weak at the final positions, with rankings of seven and nine. Place of articulation was also an unstable feature. It ranked eighth at the initial position and fifth at the final position, indicating that contrary to the tendencies of nasality and aspiration, place is a stronger feature at the final position of a syllable.

A comparison of one Miller and Nicely condition (+12 dB S/N ratio in the 200–6,500 Hz bandwidth) and one Singh and Black condition (Hindi speakers/Hindi listeners)with the results of the present experiment, reveals a great deal of discrepancies. It must be noted, however, that these three experiments were conducted in entirely different experimental conditions. Some of the outcomes of the comparisons are as follows.

1. Initial position data in the Ahmed and Agrawal experiment agreed well with the data of Miller and Nicely.

2. There was no correlation between the Singh and Black and the Ahmed and Agrawal data.

3. No correlation was found between ranks at the initial and the final positions of a syllable in the Ahmed and Agrawal data.

4. The rank order of features of consonants depended very much on the consonants' positions in the syllable. As a particular example, place, which was found to be the hardest to hear correctly in Miller and Nicely's experiments, was found highly intelligible for various language groups in Singh and

Black's experiments and was harder to hear in the initial position than in the final position in the Ahmed and Agrawal study.

Gupta, Agrawal, and Ahmed (1969)   The procedure for this study was the same as that for the earlier experiment by Ahmed and Agrawal except that in this study the syllables were distorted by clipping the peaks of the signal. Gupta, Agrawal, and Ahmed explain the purposes of this experiment as follows.

(1) to determine the effect of clipping on the intelligibility of individual consonants and their features separately; (2) to compare the rank order of the feature system of clipped speech with that of normal speech; (3) to correlate different informations of initial consonants and final consonants, and hence to see the difference in the perception of consonants in these two positions. (p. 770)

The "effect of clipping" was computed by subtracting the information content of a feature in the clipped speech from that in normal speech. In the initial position of the syllable, maximal distortion was inflicted on place of articulation (30.85%), and minimal distortion occurred for the feature affrication (4.32%). The rank order of features, from the most susceptible to clipping distortion to the least susceptible was: place (30.85%), nasality (20.49%), liquid (17.99%), continuancy (17.33%), aspiration (9.74%), voicing (9.52%), frication (5.00%), and affrication (4.32%). In the final position of the syllable, the greatest amount of clipping effect was seen for the feature nasality and the smallest amount of clipping effect for affrication. The rank order of features, from most susceptible to least susceptible to the clipping distortions, was: nasality (30.36%), frication (26.79%), place (25.01%), liquid (23.83%), voicing (22.46%), flapped liquid (21.09%), aspiration (19.55%), continuancy (19.12%), and affrication (10.47%). Affrication was the strongest feature in the clipping condition and nasality and place were the weaker features.

By utilizing the criterion of the differential effect of clipping, a comparison was made of the initial and final positions. Figure 15 represents plottings of the effect of clipping on the eight different features that appeared at both the initial and final positions of a syllable. Two clear conclusions can be drawn from this figure. First, in general, there is a greater clipping effect on the final consonants than there is on the initial consonants. Second, place of articulation is the only feature which shows a reverse tendency to the above general conclusion. In this figure the maximal difference of the clipping effect was found for the feature frication. The effect of clipping for the initial and final consonants, as depicted in Figure 15, was correlated with a rank order correlation of 0.52. This correlation was not statistically significant. However, the rank correlation between the initial consonants of normal speech and the initial consonants of clipped speech was significant (0.78). Also, the rank correlation between the final consonants of normal speech and the final consonants of clipped speech (0.88) was significant. These last two significant

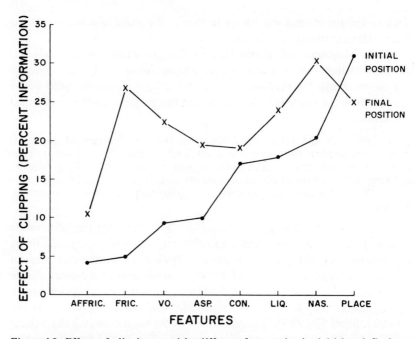

Figure 15. Effect of clipping on eight different features in the initial and final consonantal positions. The effect of clipping is the difference of transmitted information in the undistorted and clipped conditions. (Based on Gupta, Agrawal, and Ahmed, 1969, and Ahmed and Agrawal, 1969.)

correlations indicate that in spite of the clipping distortions, the position of the consonants in a syllable played a significant role in the utilization of a feature. This finding was further substantiated by the lack of any correlation between the initial and final consonants in normal speech (0.21) and between the initial and final consonants in clipped speech (0.05).

Singh (1971) The purpose of this investigation was to find whether the minimally distinct consonant pairs have different perceptual strengths and whether these strengths change under different signal-to-noise ratios and filter conditions. The minimally distinct pairs of consonants defined by the Miller and Nicely and the Halle feature systems were included in this experiment. Each stimulus-response unit of this experiment included a triad (ABX) of consonant-vowel syllables. The listeners were asked to judge whether the stimulus was more similar to the first or the second stimulus-response choice.

There were 846 similarity judgments obtained from three groups of 33 subjects in the six experimental conditons. The chi-square tests were computed for each of the minimally distinct pairs of consonants to determine whether or not the responses associated with these pairs were significantly different from one another. Fifty-nine percent (501/846) of the chi-square values showed significant differences at the 0.01 level. It was concluded, therefore, that a one-feature difference between consonants led most judges to perceive one of the members as more similar to the stimulus in 59% of the pairs. However, in 41% of comparisons, the one-feature difference did not lead to any consistent perception for the subjects.

When the similarity values between a stimulus consonant and its minimally different decoys were pooled for all subjects, the following statistical measure was used to find the distance between the stimulus and response consonants.

$$d_{ij} = \sqrt{1 - \frac{f(i/j) + f(j/i)}{n_i + n_j}}$$

In this formula d_{ij} is the distance between the stimulus and response consonants or between the stimulus i and j; $f(i/j)$ is the frequency with which stimulus j is identified as i; $f(j/i)$ is the frequency with which the stimulus i is identified as j. The n_i is the total occurrence of i; and n_j is the total occurrence of j. This measure of distance may be interpreted as follows: the greater the d_{ij} value the greater the distance. The value never exceeds one.

Figures 16 and 17 show the relative mean strength (d_{ij}) on the ordinate and distortion conditions on the abscissa. In these figures, the higher the

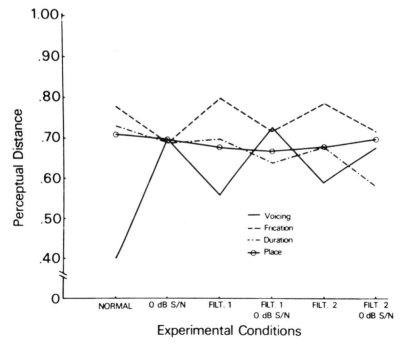

Figure 16. Perceptual strength of the features voicing, frication, duration, and place as a function of six listening conditions. The greater the distance the greater the strength. (From Singh, 1971.)

116   Sadanand Singh

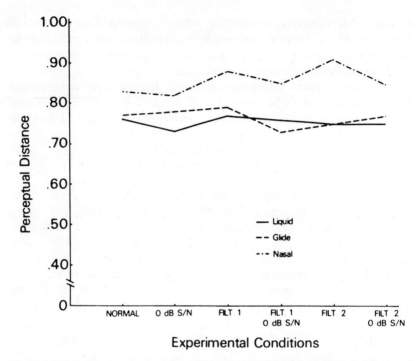

Experimental Conditions

Figure 17. Perceptual strength of the features liquid, glide, and nasality as a function of six listening conditions. The greater the distance the greater the strength. (From Singh, 1971.)

mean perceptual distance (d_{ij}) value, the greater the strength of a feature. These figures also show the following.

1. The distinguishing characteristics of the voicing feature improved in noise and deteriorated in quiet conditions.

2. The frication feature improved in quiet and deteriorated in noise.

3. The voicing feature in competition with other features in conditions of quiet was less stable.

4. The noise characteristics of frication were easily lost in the experimental noise.

5. Duration as an added cue (e.g., /s, z, ʃ, ʒ /) did improve upon the distinguishing characteristic of some of the fricatives.

6. Nasality contained the maximal distinction in all the six conditions of listening.

7. Nasality, liquid, and glide were affected very little by the filtering and noise conditions in preserving their distinctions.

Wang and Bilger (1973) The focal points of the Wang and Bilger study were: 1) which features best accounted for performance in a consonant discrimination task, and 2) whether the same features were best in a variety of contexts and listening conditions. The logic is that *if* it is possible to determine the exact nature of the perceptual features and *if* these features are invariant, *then* these features are considered natural perceptual categories.

Twenty-four initial and 19 final consonants of English (from a total list of 25 consonants) were combined with the three vowels [i a u]. Four syllable sets were constructed from these initial and final consonants, each consisting of 16 syllables. The syllable sets were called CV1, VC1, CV2, and VC2. Each of the four sets of stimuli were heard in six signal-to-noise ratio conditions (−10, −5, 0, +5, +10, and +15 dB) and four signal level conditions (50, 65, 80, and 95 dB SPL). There were three replications of each of the 24 (six S/N ratios X four signal levels) experimental conditions yielding a total of 72 experimental conditions. In the control experiment there was no noise introduced. In order to deter intelligibility, the different reductions of the signal level were utilized. Thirteen specific signal reductions were made ranging from 20 to 45 dB SPL in 5-dB steps, and from 55 to 115 dB SPL in 10-dB steps. Six subjects were used as listeners.

In the distinctive feature analysis of results of this experiment an inventory of 19 grossly overlapping features were used: 1) vocalic, 2) consonantal, 3) high, 4) low, 5) back, 6) coronal, 7) anterior, 8) voicing, 9) nasality, 10) continuancy, 11) stridency, 12) round, 13) frication, 14) duration, 15) place (Miller and Nicely), 16) place (Singh and Black), 17) place (Wickelgren), 18) sibilancy, and 19) openness. These features include a complete set of five feature systems, namely, the systems of Miller and Nicely (1955), Singh and Black (1966), Wickelgren (1966), Chomsky and Halle (1968), and Singh, Woods, and Becker (1972).

The primary statistical tool utilized in this experiment was the determination of the amount of information transmitted by these features. After computing the information content of each feature within a given feature system, Wang and Bilger separated features from most important to least important by a sequential method of analyzing transmitted information. The method is designed in such a way that as many as 11 iterations are performed to account for the maximal amount of information present in a feature system. In the first round the iterative procedure extracts the feature with maximal information content. In the second round the extracted feature is eliminated and another feature emerges (the second most important feature), and so on, until the information contribution of each feature of a system has been accounted for and until the sum of all of the partial (or individual feature) contributions adds up to 99% of the total transmitted information. This procedure is analogous to a stepwise multiple regression analysis.

The results showed that for the CV1 syllable set, of the 12 features tested, only four were consistently found to have contributed to discrimination performance. The features were voicing, sibilancy, high-anterior, and frication. For the VC1 set, except for the feature voicing, a lack of consistency was found regarding the importance of features. There was considerable agreement in terms of the relative importance of features across the six listening conditions in the CV2 syllable set. Five features were identified consistently in the iteration program: vocalic, nasality, round, high, and voicing. Because of the nature of consonants in CV1 and CV2, the first three of these features, vocalic, nasality, and round, were not represented. Thus, the only two features that could be tested across the CV1 and CV2 were high-anterior and voicing. These two features were consistently important across the syllable set. For the VC2 syllable set, the consistently important features were voicing, nasality, continuancy-open, and frication.

Utilizing the procedure of iteration, Wang and Bilger also examined comparable data from two earlier studies, one by Miller and Nicely (1955) and another by Singh and Black (1966). Eleven of the 19 features listed in the study by Wang and Bilger were used as criteria to compare the Miller and Nicely data with the Wang and Bilger data. It was found that the results of the Wang and Bilger CV1 set and the Miller and Nicely 200–6,500 Hz in 12 dB S/N ratio condition were in very close agreement. Features identified as important in both analyses were voicing, sibilancy, frication, and place. Nasality was not included in the Wang and Bilger CV1 set and therefore could not be directly compared. However, nasality was the best perceived feature in other sets of Wang and Bilger where nasal consonants were included. Sixteen of the 19 features in the Wang and Bilger study were used as criteria for comparing the Singh and Black and the Wang and Bilger data. Nasality, vocalic, voicing, and place of articulation features were distinguished in both experiments. The features frication and sibilancy were both identified in only one analysis.

On the basis of statistical analysis of these data, Wang and Bilger concluded that the distinctive articulatory and/or phonological features of consonants account for most of the transmitted information (more than 90%) in a stimulus-response condition. For example, the Singh and Black feature system accounts for 94% of the information. However, beyond certain points there were alternative features which could explain the same amount of variance. The seventh iteration revealed equal probabilities of continuancy and open features. A feature system including either continuancy or open, therefore, would yield the same result. It was concluded by Wang and Bilger that there is little support for the hypothesis that natural features or feature systems exist. This conclusion was based on their findings that several feature systems accounted equally for the transmitted information and there were no particular features or feature systems shown to be better than others across conditions and syllable sets.

The broad categories of features investigated in this experiment fell in three groups. First, nasality, voicing, and round were perceptually important in every syllable set where they were distinctive. Second, stridency and low showed opposite tendencies, since they were never found significant in any of the conditions. Third, the remaining of the distinctive features were only sometimes important for a given set.

Wang and Bilger's two conclusions—that it is possible to account for a large proportion of transmitted information in terms of articulatory and phonological features, and that natural perceptual features do not exist—entail internal inconsistencies. Most feature systems showed a high rate of transmission of information because inherent similarities exist between different feature systems. If one attempted to provide a detailed comparison of feature systems, one would find that the features of different systems share a majority of parameters (see chapter 2 in Singh, in press (b). For example, the place of articulation in the study by Miller and Nicely can be explained by the gravity and compactness features set forth by Jakobson, Fant and Halle (1951); Wickelgren's openness can be explained in terms of the description by Chomsky and Halle (1968) of stop, continuancy, and sonorancy features; and the front/back place of several multidimensional analyses (Danhauer and Singh, submitted for publication; Mitchell and Singh, 1974; Singh, Woods, and Becker, 1972; Weiner and Singh, 1974) can be explained directly by the anterior feature of the Chomsky and Halle system. Thus, the finding that all feature systems transmit a high rate of information should aid an investigator in accepting the hypothesis that these feature systems do possess natural perceptual properties.

In order to find what features were important in most conditions, the Wang and Bilger results were reinterpreted by Singh (1973). Figure 18 attempts to find the continuity of the features across the eight conditions in the Wang and Bilger results. In this figure the sets are listed in the extreme left column followed by the eight conditions in which the features were examined. At the top of the figure the 16 distinctive features (all places have been pooled) are presented. The X's in this figure represent the five top ranking features for a given condition (there are more than five X's when there were ties). NA represents the inapplicability of a feature for the experimental set. Inspection of this figure shows that the features that occurred more than 50% of the times across all sets included nasality (100%), voicing (81%), round (75%), place (69%), sibilancy (63%), and frication (56%). The emphasis here is not on visualizing the features round or vocalic, which were restricted to one consonantal set, but on visualizing features like voicing, place, and sibilancy, which appeared across all four sets.

Figure 19 shows a plotting of all of the above features except round (nasality, voicing, anterior (place), sibilancy, and continuancy (frication)) as a function of the signal-to-noise ratio. Consistent with earlier results (Singh, 1971), it can be seen here that the feature nasality was strong across most conditions. Voicing was strong only in conditions of severe noise, whereas sibilancy and place were weak in severe noise and strong in less severe noise conditions. The feature continuancy was weak across all conditions.

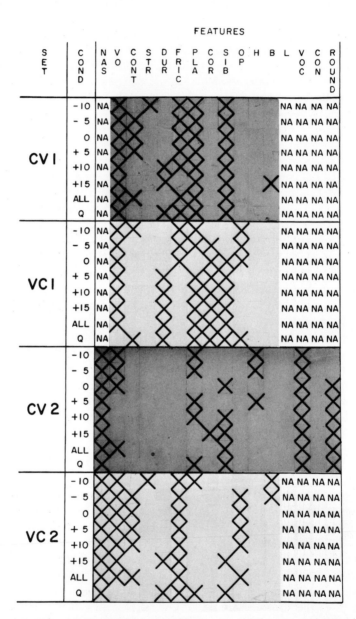

Figure 18. Tallies of five highest ranking features recovered in four syllable sets and eight test conditions. (Based on Wang and Bilger, 1973.)

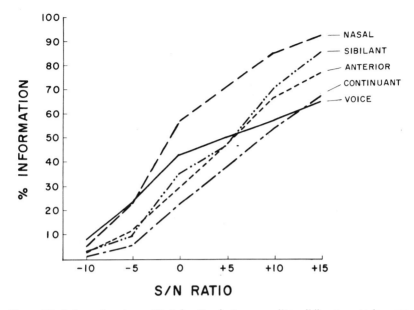

Figure 19. Information transmitted for the features nasality, sibilancy, anterior, continuancy, and voicing as a function of six S/N ratios. (Based on Wang and Bilger, 1973.)

Prediction of Different Sets of Perceptual Responses by a Number of Feature Systems

A phoneme is considered an abstract entity that man acquires at an early age. The phonetic and auditory processes are man's effort to manifest the abstraction in speaking and listening behaviors. The purpose of the experiments under the present heading is to approximate most closely the "true" or the "abstract" location of the phoneme in the repertoire of a native speaker by trying alternative strategies to approximate interphonemic similarities. The different data collection methods may involve slightly altered perceptual strategies, and a common denominator to these strategies may be considered the closest approximation to the "true" location of a phoneme in one's perceptual repertoire. The data collected in Singh, Woods, and Becker (1972) and Singh and Becker (1972) were primarily for the purpose of obtaining common perceptual properties of phonemes across three data collection methods.

Singh and Becker (1972) In this experiment four feature systems were used to predict perceptual judgments obtained using three psychological methods: 1) seven-point scaling (SF), 2) magnitude estimation (ME), and 3) triadic comparison (ABX). The feature systems chosen to be examined were 1) Miller and Nicely (1955), 2) Singh and Black (1966), 3) Wickelgren (1966), and 4) Chomsky and Halle (1968).

In order to compare the four feature systems, multiple regression weights were derived from each of the three data collection methods by fitting the features of a system on the perceptual judgments in the three data sets. For each feature system there are nine such correlations: SF/SF, SF/ME, SF/ABX, ME/SF, ME/ME, ME/ABX, ABX/SF, ABX/ME, and ABX/ABX, where the first member of the nine pairs represents the data collection used to determine weights, and the second member is the predicted set with the weighted feature systems. Multiple correlation of the three data collection methods and the four feature systems are all statistically significant at the 0.001 level of confidence (*df* for Miller and Nicely is 5,225; for Singh and Black, 8,222; for Wickelgren, 4,226; and for Chomsky and Halle, 11,221), but none of the correlations is higher than 0.663.

Further tests were performed to find whether the weights of a feature system obtained by fitting it to one data collection method would predict other data collection methods. The tau correlations of weighted feature systems and the data collection methods were all very low (≈ 0.415), and no prediction was possible by the weighted feature systems.

The tau correlations and another correlation measure utilized in this study reveals that none of the feature systems were consistently the best. These inconsistencies suggest that people either do not use features of these systems in the same way from one task to another or that multiple correlation may not be a suitable statistic for evaluating these systems.

Singh, Woods, and Becker (1972)   The raw data and the feature systems in this study were the same as in Singh and Becker (1972). However, the fitting strategy was grossly different. Instead of fitting the raw data to the distinctive feature difference of consonants by a regression analysis, the computed distances in the City-Block and Euclidean spaces derived from a multidimensional analysis (multidimensional scaling) (Kruskal, 1964a, 1964b; Shepard, 1962) were fitted to the weighted feature system.

Phoneme in perceptual space   The location of the phoneme in perceptual space can be estimated by use of a multidimensional scaling (MDS) procedure (Kruskal, 1964a, 1964b; Shepard, 1962). The problem lies in making estimates that are not tied too closely to the biases in the data collection method. The MDS technique used widely to solve such problems yields a configuration which is very loosely tied to the data at low dimensionality, and thus may be a poor representation of the subject's perceptual space. However, as the dimensionality increases, the fit becomes closer and closer to the data and, consequently, to the errors in the method used to obtain the data. At the "true" dimensionality, the MDS distances may be free from most of the errors in the data. Kruskal (1964a, 1964b) has suggested a criterion for selecting optimal dimensionality by plotting a best fit measure called "stress" as a function of dimensions. Figure 20 shows, in the lower set of graphs, a plotting of stress as a function of dimensions for each of the three data collection methods. In an ideal solution of stress, Kruskal professes an "elbow" at the optimal dimension. Since no such elbow was noticeable in our

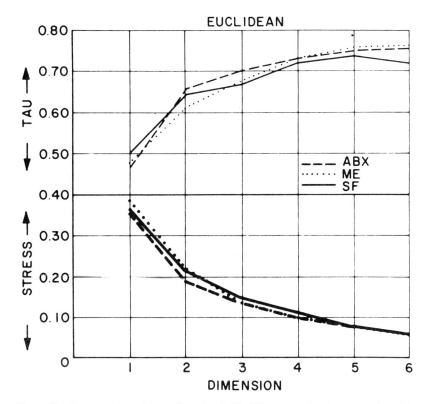

Figure 20. Stress as a function of dimension in Euclidean space (bottom curves), and tau correlation between a given dimensional space and the data (upper curves). (From Singh, Woods, and Becker, 1972.)

analysis, we devised an additional criterion for aiding the determination of optimal dimension. The criterion of tau correlation between a given dimensional space and the raw data is presented as our criterion for selecting dimensionality.

Multidimensional scaling (MDS) This analysis was performed in one to six dimensional spaces in both Euclidean and City-Block metrics. Thus, 12 MDS configurations each within the minimal stress for dimensions one through six were obtained for each of the data matrices. By combining both stress and tau correlation measures, it was determined in this study that in the City-Block space for the diadic methods (ME and SF) the consonants were perceived in three dimensional spaces, and for the triadic method (ABX) they were perceived in a four dimensional space. In the Euclidean space, however, the consonants for the diadic methods were perceived in five dimensional spaces and for the triadic method in four dimensional spaces.

The multiple correlations between a dimensional space and feature system, beta weights, normalized predictor contributions, and Freedman's *m*-ranking statistics (see Singh, Woods, and Becker, 1972, pp. 1705–1707) for the best City-Block and Euclidean spaces, indicated that of the four feature systems investigated (MN, SB, W, CH) only the Chomsky and Halle system showed consistent ranking of features over the three data collection methods. The relative importance of the features from highest to lowest, in the City-Block space, for this system, was high (1), voiced and anterior (2.5) strident (4), vocalic (5), nasal (6), coronal (7), consonantal (8), low and continuant (9.5), and back (11). In the Euclidean space the rank order was high (1), voiced (2), anterior (3), vocalic (4), nasal and strident (5.5), continuant (7), coronal (8), low (9), consonantal (10), and back (11). The rank order correlation between the relative importance of features in the City-Block and Euclidean spaces was 0.822.

INDSCAL (individual differences scaling) A further analysis of the results was based on another multidimensional analysis technique, which is designed to assign weights to the attributes (phonemes in this case) and to the individual subjects (methods in this case). This analysis was performed in two to eight dimensional spaces with several starting configurations. The solution reported was in a five dimensional space. The interpoint distances at this dimensionality correlated with the data at 0.78. These dimensions were interpreted with the features sibilancy, front/back place, plosive, voicing, and nasality.

A feature system constructed from features retrieved using INDSCAL analysis and consisting of sibilancy, front/back place, plosive, voicing, and nasality was correlated with the MDS distances. This feature system showed significant consistency (Freedman's rank) over the three data collection methods. The relative importance of the features from highest to lowest was: (1) front/back place; (2) nasality; (3) sibilancy; (4) voicing; and (5) plosive.

The conclusion drawn in this experiment was that the multidimensional analysis of similarity judgments leads to the recovery of perceptual dimensions of consonants that can be related to their articulatory or acoustic descriptions. In a few cases, however, the results may support one phonetic analysis over another. For example, the sibilants /s, z, tʃ, dʒ/ cluster together, but the stridents /f, v/ do not join the group, thus favoring the choice for the feature sibilancy over stridency. The perceptual feature place favors the phonological feature anterior more than it favors the feature high. Both anterior and high are described as "cavity features," with the difference that anterior is a vocal tract feature whereas high is a tongue-body feature. The other two tongue-body features low and back were completely unsupported as relevant perceptual features.

Role of Distinctive Features in Dichotic Processing of the Phoneme

It has been shown that speech sounds are perceived by a language-dominant left hemisphere. Since the distinctive features are considered the component of a phoneme, it is important to know: 1) whether all features have significant leaning toward the dominant hemisphere, and 2) whether some features show greater amount of dominance than other features.

Studdert-Kennedy and Shankweiler (1970)   Four dichotic tests, two for consonants and two for vowels, were constructed involving the six stop consonants and six vowels (/i, ɛ, ae, a, ɔ, u/) of English. For analysis, the stop consonants were elaborated in terms of the features voicing and place of articulation. Each consonant was considered either voiced or voiceless and also as having one of the three places: labiality, alveolarity, and velarity. The rate of percentage of information transmitted by each of these features for both the right and left ear transmission systems was determined. The comparison for the feature voicing showed that while the information value for the right ear was 49%, for the left ear it was 31%. The comparison for the feature place of articulation also showed that while the information transmission value for the right ear was 32%, for the left ear it was only 22%. It is evident in the above findings that while both features showed the feature lateralization, voicing was a stronger feature than place. It was concluded in this experiment that underlying lateralization of consonants are the independent lateralizations of their component feature. A comparison of the laterality effect on feature perception in the initial and final contexts showed that there was more prominent right ear advantage for both features for the initial consonants of a syllable than for the final consonants.

Cole and Scott (1972)   The purpose of this experiment was to investigate whether same/different reaction time judgments for pairs of syllables may be used as criteria to determine the involvement of distinctive features in processing speech stimuli. Eight consonants, specifying the features grave, diffuse, strident, nasal, continuant, and voiced, were chosen for testing. All consonants were paired with the vowel /a/. In addition to a number of same trials in both left and right ears, each of the other seven sounds were paired twice (once in each ear) with a given sound. The main finding of this experiment is a plotting of reaction time on the ordinate and the number of distinctive feature differences on the abscissa, as shown in Figure 21. In this figure, zero difference implies that the stimuli in both ears were the same. The results show that distinctive features of vowels and consonants were valid criteria to predict their discrimination when the criterion of reaction time was used. The reaction time was largest when the pairs of syllables were most similar, and the reaction time was smallest when the pairs of syllables were most dissimilar. The similarity was determined by counting the distinctive feature difference between the two pairs. The orderly effect of feature difference on the reaction time was significantly different ($F = 7.07; df = 5; P < 0.001$) when the pairs of phonemes appeared simultaneously in both ears and when the subjects were performing a discrimination task.

Blumstein and Cooper (1972)   Six English plosives were dichotically discriminated in one test and identified in other. The distinctive feature

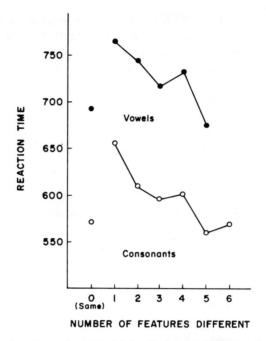

Figure 21. Reaction time values associated with feature differences between pairs of consonants and pairs of vowels. The reaction times of the same pairs of consonants and vowels are also shown. (From Cole and Scott, 1972.)

analysis of the confusions of consonants was reported for both discrimination (same/different) and identification tasks. The distinctive feature principle was operative in the discrimination task because the discrimination score was better when the pairs of consonants were two features apart than when they were one feature apart. However, the identification task showed poorer identification scores when the consonants of the dichotic task were two features different as compared to when they were one feature different. This unexpected result was explained by a proposal that the discrimination task does not involve encoding of the message in the short-term memory. The identification task involved encoding in such a manner that the feature differences must be analyzed by storing in memory prior to the completion of task. Such a procedure loads the system yielding poorer score with greater number of feature differences.

Day and Vigorito (1972) In a dichotic task temporal order judgments of synthetic syllables were investigated for plosive, liquid, and vowel categories. Day and Vigorito reported that the stops showed the right ear advantage (liquid was neutral regarding the laterality effect), and the vowel showed the left ear advantage. They drew the conclusion that stops are encoded more than liquids and vowels are.

Crystal and House (in Press) Earlier experiments by Blumstein and Cooper (1972) and by Day and Vigorito (1972) were replicated with signal modifications aimed at elucidating the role of signal level. When the syllables were masked by speech-shaped maskers, the impact of the different degrees of encoding reported by Day and Vigorito (1972) was minimized. Crystal and House equated the signal levels of the different phonetic categories and minimized the right ear advantage. Their conclusion was that "the major differences between vowels and consonants is their inherent intensities. By equalizing listening conditions certain perceptual differences among sound classes can be reduced."

A POSTERIORI STUDIES

The a priori feature systems described earlier in this chapter lack the flexibility and the provision of adding a "new" feature or eliminating a "known" feature, depending on what the perceiver's actual response strategies were. These systems also lack the essential assumption of any scientific investigation, that of testing the relevance of the known attributes without eliminating the possibility of discovering the unknown. The a priori feature systems were used because there was no suitable direct method for determining the speech perception parameters in an a posteriori fashion.

The following report discusses perceptual features of phonemes proposed a posteriorily. The data analyzed by this method were obtained from different stimulus sets, data collection methods, speaking-listening conditions, response modalities, ages, language backgrounds, and hearing disorders. The central theme of this discussion is that in spite of the above described diversities, speech perception research shows a strong tendency of invariance for certain perceptual features.

The work of experimenters whose goal was to retrieve a posteriori features of phonemes can be divided into three parts: 1) those who worked with factor analysis and some other less defined spatial model; 2) those who worked with a better defined metric and nonmetric multidimensional scaling analysis of the proximity data; and 3) those who worked with a multidimensional scaling analysis technique, found to be more suitable for speech perception research, e.g. INDSCAL. Although factor analysis and certain multidimensional analysis techniques (Torgerson, 1958) have been available for retrieving the common properties of subjects' psychological responses, not until recently have some specific techniques been developed which provide a "general solution to the problem of achieving well-defined spatial representations on the basis of measures of the degree of similarity, confusability, association, or in general psychological proximity" among stimuli of "initially obscure underlying structure" (Shepard, 1972, p. 71). The specific techniques include the Shepard-Kruskal (Kruskal, 1964a, 1964b; Shepard, 1962) method of nonmetric multidimensional scaling and the Carroll and Chang (1970) method of individual scaling.

Although the nonmetric MDS (Kruskal, 1964a, 1964b) has application to a wide variety of data, one problem with this method has been that the initial configurations of the spatial output are in an arbitrary orientation. Thus, the experimenter has to provide a known target and rotate the initial configurations. Carroll and Chang's INDSCAL ordinarily alleviates the need for rotation as the spatial points of stimuli and subjects in a given dimensional space are fixed by a least square fit.

Thus, Carroll and Chang's INDSCAL (1970) is uniquely suitable for providing a spatial representation of the speech stimuli in a number of dimensionalities where the experimenter's interpretations of the axes are strictly limited by the assumption of the orthogonality of the axes. Thus, all interpretive angles are in a 90-degree relationship. The dimensions in perceptual space are weighted according to their contributions in the subject's estimation of the proximity between stimuli. Additionally, the individual subject's private space or the individual subject's contribution to the perceptual dimensions obtained for the group is also available for scrutiny in this method.

Since the speech perception research reported here draws heavily from the INDSCAL analysis, the following four figures have been presented to

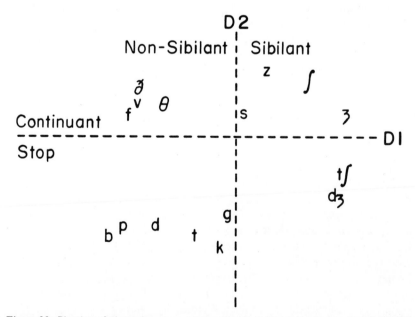

Figure 22. Plotting of dimensions one and two in a four dimensional space in a 6-dB S/N ratio condition. (From Mitchell and Singh, 1974.)

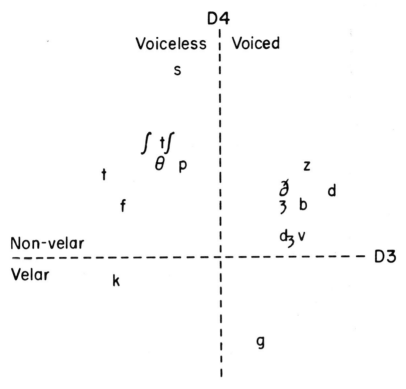

Figure 23. Plotting of dimensions three and four in a four dimensional space in a 6-dB S/N ratio conditions. (From Mitchell and Singh, 1974.)

demonstrate the three important aspects of the outcome of INDSCAL. These results are obtained from McGregor (1972) and Mitchell and Singh (1974). Figures 22 and 23 show the spatial representation of the 16 English consonants in a five dimensional space. The interpretive labels are aided by intersecting lines having 90-degree angles provided by the experimenters. Figure 24 shows the relative weights of these five dimensions (features) as a function of experimental conditions. Figure 25 shows the individual subject's weighting of the five dimensions. In the manner shown in Figure 22 the five perceptual features, one on each of the five dimensions, were obtained for the 16 consonants in the Mitchell and Singh (1974) study. The features were: voicing, sibilancy, place$_1$ (front/back), place$_2$ (velar), and continuancy. Figure 24 shows that these features assumed different weightings as a function of the S/N ratio. Actually, the feature front/back place assumed zero weight in the conditions of noise while the feature voicing gained slightly and sibilancy gained substantially in the noisy listening conditions. These five dimensions accounted for over 75% of the variance in each of the three conditions.

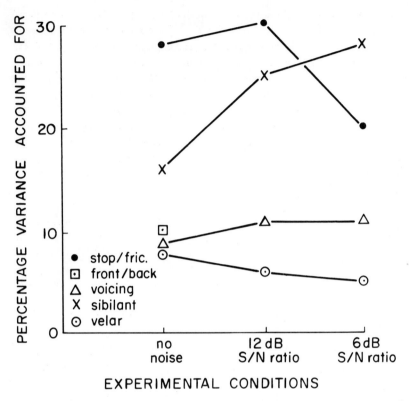

Figure 24. The relative contribution of different features in explaining the variance in the data under three experimental conditions in five dimensional space. (From Mitchell and Singh, 1974.)

Retrieval of Distinctive Features by Factor Analysis and Other Spatially Less Defined Methods

Klatt (1968) Klatt, in a reanalysis of Wickelgren's (1966) short-term memory data, used a similarity metric to determine: 1) the statistical level of significance of a feature in predicting the errors, 2) the inadequacy of a feature system utilized to explain the errors, and 3) the degree of independence of the features. Most of his results were based on the computation of a measure of deviation from the total number of cross set confusions (Dev (Ncs)). This measure is computed from binary contingency tables involving a given number of predetermined features. The initial procedure is similar to the one used by Miller and Nicely (1955). The contingency matrix consists of binary specifications of a given feature with N++ implying feature presented and feature recalled, N−− implying feature not presented and feature not recalled, N−+ implying feature not presented but recalled, and N+− implying feature presented but not recalled. An example of Ncs, the total number of cross set confusions, is the sum of the off diagonal scores (Ncs = N+− + N−+). The deviation of Ncs from its expected value for random data is considered a measure of the extent to which a feature explains phonemic errors. The rationale for such an assertion is well supported in the studies reported earlier in this chapter. It has been shown that greater confusions occur within a given feature specification category rather than across the feature category.

Dev (Ncs) was computed by subtracting the observed Ncs from the expected Ncs and by dividing the outcome by the standard deviation of the Ncs (Dev (Ncs) = ($\hat{N}cs$ − Ncs)/r). The expected $\hat{N}cs$ was computed by multiplying the appropriate row and the column sum of the contingency matrix and by dividing the outcome by a constant. The constant was a scale factor which was chosen such that the sum for all the constants for all the cells in a matrix would equal the total number of confusions.

A value of Dev (Ncs) computed to be greater than 3.0 was interpreted as highly significant. The distinctive features selected for evaluation with the associated Dev (Ncs) were: voiced (3.55), long fricative (8.27), sonorant (6.61), continuant (4.63), strident (6.70), anterior (1.89), coronal (2.24), nasal (2.01), and consonantal (1.58). When these Dev (Ncs) were condi-

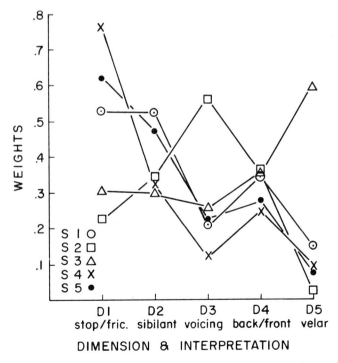

Figure 25. Weightings of five different subjects on five dimensions in the condition of no experimental noise. (From Mitchell and Singh, 1974.)

tionally computed, only the following Dev (Ncs) were found to be significant: voiced (3.55), long fricative (8.26), sonorant (4.97), and continuant (3.44). The conditional Dev (Ncs) of a feature is determined by considering the existence of the feature that precedes it. Thus, the binary features in the data with a confidence level greater than 0.99 were long fricative, continuant, sonorant, and voiced.

A further analysis by Klatt included the determination of the sufficiency of the arbitrarily selected features found to be significant or not significant in accounting for the errors in the Wickelgren data. Beyond the features listed, the feature sibilancy was added to compute the Dev (Ncs) value yielding the result 3.57, which is significant at > 0.99. This indicates that the sibilancy grouping, although not included in the initial test of the features, constitutes an important classification strategy for describing short-term memory errors.

The remainder of the analysis is based on the manipulation of the Dev (Ncs) in a convergent algorithm to modify the original feature to fit an optimal assignment of the consonants. Three optima were reported with the first optimum having Dev (Ncs) 8.34, the second optimum with a Dev-independent (Ncs) 5.76, and the third optimum with a Dev-independent (Ncs) 5.60. Only the first optimum showed resemblance with the known attributes of the phonemes. Frication was marked positively at the first optimum with the inclusion of /k g/ and with the exclusion of /v/.

Black (1970) Black used factor analysis to group consonants of English with the stated purpose that the groupings might or might not correspond with the adjectival categories plosive, fricative, lateral, glide, etc., or with systems of distinctive features. Twenty-four consonants were paired with five vowels and judged for similarity rating in the manner of magnitude estimation. Factor analysis (rotated by VARIMAX routine) was used to isolate 12 factors. Only the first four factors were such that more than one consonant had contrastively high factor loadings. The first factor was nasality with the loading of 0.91 for /m/ and /n/ each. The second factor was the slit fricative with positive factor loadings for /θ/, /ð/, /f/, and /v/ of 0.89, 0.69, 0.94, and 0.64, respectively. The third factor was a long duration fricative or grooved fricative with high factor loadings of 0.86, 0.87, and 0.93 for /s/, /z/, and /ʒ/, respectively, and a moderate factor loading of 0.45 for /ʃ/. The remainder of the factors in this study isolated one consonant per factor which may not be considered an elegant assignment of the factor to the phoneme.

Retrieval of Distinctive Features by a Distance Measure Incorporating the Notion of Optimal Dimensionality (e.g., MDS)

This section and Table 2 present results of 18 multidimensional analyses involving the perception of the consonants (Singh, in press (a)). The studies are discussed in the order in which they appear in the table. The majority of the studies were published in the last 5 years and have used the INDSCAL procedure for obtaining the perceptual features of consonants. The features

Table 2. A posteriori features of consonant perception

Study	Condition	Subject	Response	Context	Stimulus	Analysis	Na.	Vo.	Sib.	Cont.	Pla.	Son.
							Features[a]					
Wilson (1963)	1)Noise 2)Low-pass 3)High-pass	5 adults	Open choice	CV	2^4	MDS (S,W)	X	X	X[b]	X[b]		NA
Johnson (1967)	1)Noise 2)Low-pass 3)High-pass	5 adults	Open choice	CV	2^4	HCS (J)	X	X	X[b]			NA
Shepard (1972)	1)Noise 2)Low-pass 3)High-pass	5 adults	Open choice	CV	2^4	MDS (S)	X	X	X[b]	X		NA
Peters (1963)	Quiet	12 adults	Scaling	CV	2^4	MDS (T)	X[b]	X	X[a]	X[b]		NA
Shepard (1972)	Quiet	12 adults	Scaling	CV	2^4	MDS (S)	X	X	X			NA
Graham and House (1971)	Quiet	4.5-year-olds	Same/different	Word	2^4	MDS (SK)	X			X		X
Singh, Woods, and Tishman (1972)	Quiet	4.5-year-olds	Same/different	Word	2^4	MDS (SK)	X	X	X	X		X
Jeter and Singh (1972)	1)Visual 2)Auditory	1)30 adults 2)30 adults	ABX	CV	2^3	MDS (SK)	NA	X	X	X	X	NA

continued

Table 2. A posteriori features of consonant perception

Study	Condition	Subject	Response	Context	Stimulus	Analysis	Features[a] Na.	Vo.	Sib.	Cont.	Plu.	Son.
Wish (1970)	1)Noise 2)Low-pass 3)High-pass	5 adults	Open choice	CV	2^4	INDSCAL	X	X	X	X	2nd-former transition	NA
Pruzansky (1970)	Quiet		Similarity judgment	CV	2^4	INDSCAL	X	X	X	X	X	NA
Singh, Woods, and Becker (1972)	Quiet	1)1,001 adults 2)44 adults 3)18 adults	1)ABX 2)Scaling 3)ME	CV	$2^{4.3125}$	INDSCAL	X	X	X	X	X	X
Singh and Singh (1972)	1)Noise 2)Quiet 3)Peakclipping	10 adults (Hindi)	Open choice	CV VC	$2^{4.75}$	INDSCAL	X	X	X	Aspiration		X
Walden and Montgomery (1973)	Quiet	1)6 normal hearing 2)6 mild loss 3)6 severe loss	Scaling	CV	$2^{4.25}$	INDSCAL		X	X	X		X
Mitchell and Singh (1974)	1)Noise 2)Quiet	5 adults	ABX	CV in a sentence	2^4	INDSCAL	X	X	X	X	X	NA

Study							Na	Vo	Sib	Cont	Pla	Son
Weiner and Singh (1974)	Quiet	20 adults	CRT for diads	CV	$2^{3.125}$	INDSCAL	NA	X	X	NA	X	NA
Danhauer and Singh (submitted for publication)	Filtering at 1)0.5 kHz 2)2 kHz 3)4 kHz and broadband	1)4 adults with loss at 0.5 kHz 2)4 with loss at 2 kHz 3)4 with loss at 4 kHz	SF, ME, and ABX	CV in a phrase	2^{4}	INDSCAL	NA	X	X	X	X	NA
Danhauer and Singh (in press)	Production/perception	1)12 English 2)12 French 3)12 Serbo-Croation, deaf and hard of hearing	Verbal reporting	CVCV	$2^{4.25}$	INDSCAL	X	X	X	X		X
Danhauer and Appel (in preparation)	1)Visual 2)Tactile 3)Visual and tactile	24 adults	Open choice	CV	$2^{4.5125}$	INDSCAL	X	X	X	X	Labial	

[a]Na., nasality; Vo., voicing; Sib., sibilancy; Cont., continuancy; Pla., place; and Son., sonorancy. The presence of a feature is indicated by X; NA, not applicable. [b]Our interpretation.

retrieved in each of these analyses were tallied before the table was compiled. These tallies indicate that, with a few exceptions, six binary features of the consonants were found to exist (where possible) in these experiments with remarkable consistency. These features were: nasality, voicing, sibilancy, continuancy, place of articulation (front/back), and sonorancy. The table shows how these experiments utilized: 1) different experimental conditions; 2) subjects of different ages, backgrounds, and degrees of hearing disorders; 3) different data collection methods involving different perceptual strategies of the listeners and the different modes of eliciting responses; 4) different phonetic and linguistic contexts; and 5) different stimulus sets. In spite of these differences, which may have affected the emergence of features in their own ways, it can be seen in Table 2 that the above six features have been retrieved when the stimulus sets included the consonants bearing them.

Wilson (1963)   The first three studies in Table 2 involve reanalyses of the Miller and Nicely (1955) data by different multidimensional procedures other than INDSCAL. Wilson (1963) used an earlier version of Shepard's (1962) MDS technique and his own adaption of that technique. He reported clear interpretation of two features in the Miller and Nicely data: voicing and nasality. There are some less clear interpretations possible of Wilson's reported factors or dimensions: sibilancy and continuancy. The feature place of articulation did not show any strength on any dimension, and the feature sonorancy could not have been obtained because sonorants were not included in the stimuli.

Johnson (1967)   Johnson developed a hierarchical clustering scheme and tested the applicability of his model against the Miller and Nicely data. This method utilizes perceived distances between stimuli and converts them into a series of rank-ordered diameters. These diameters are based on both the maximal similarity and the maximal dissimilarity of the objects. The stimuli with maximal similarity, for example, cluster at the top of the hierarchy, and the stimuli with relatively less similarity cluster toward the bottom of the hierarchy. In this method, the diameter values along the vertical dimension can be used to provide certain well bifurcated clusters that are arbitrarily used to define the number of important groupings in the data. The important clusters reported by Johnson from the Miller and Nicely data were related to nasality, voicing, and sibilancy distinctions.

Shepard (1972)   Shepard reanalyzed the Miller and Nicely data by the Shepard technique of scaling and reported the features voicing and nasality in a two dimensional solution. This solution accounted for 99.4% of the variance in the data. The two dimensional solution presented by Shepard actually can be reinterpreted by an additional feature sibilancy, which separated /s, ʃ, z, 3/ from all other consonants.

The next five experiments in Table 2 involve the utilization of the multidimensional analysis techniques of 1) Torgerson (1958) used by Peters (1963); 2) Shepard used by Shepard (1972) in the reanalysis of Peters' data;

and 3) Shepard-Kruskal used by a) Graham and House (1971), b) a reanalysis of Graham and House data by Singh, Woods, and Tishman (1972), and c) analysis of visual and auditory judgment by Jeter and Singh (1972).

Peters (1963) Peters primarily focused on the spatial representation of the 16 English consonants whose interpoint distances were obtained by feeding the psychologically obtained proximities among consonants to an earlier multidimensional analysis technique (Torgerson, 1958). The method used for collecting perceptual judgments was seven-point scaling. Although Peters reported the recovery of the gross perceptual features, voicing, manner, and place, a reexamination of the spatial representations of his stimuli reveals that the feature manner could be elaborated in terms of nasality, sibilancy, and continuancy.

Shepard (1972) Shepard reanalyzed Peters' data using his own multidimensional scaling analysis technique and reported the recovery of the perceptual features, voicing and nasality. A reexamination of Shepard's reanalysis reveals, again, that besides the two reported features, nasality and voicing, sibilancy also can be shown to exist on one of the two dimensions reported.

Graham and House (1971) Graham and House had 4.5-year-old children making same/different judgments of pairs of consonants presented at the word-medial positions. They used the Shepard-Kruskal method of nonmetric multidimensional scaling to determine the dimensionality and the features of consonant perception. Although their attempt to retrieve perceptual attributes of consonants of the young children was praiseworthy, because of their utilization of an arbitrary metric, they failed to obtain significantly relevant perceptual correlates to the expected phonetic features for the 4.5-year-old children. Although they reported the tendency of these children to utilize the features nasality, continuancy, and sonorancy, there was a lack of clear interpretation of the results for all these features.

Singh, Woods, and Tishman (1972) Singh, Woods, and Tishman reanalyzed the Graham and House data with an underlying metric assumption for describing judgments of either Euclidean or City-Block phonemic pairs (see Singh, Woods, and Becker, 1972). The perceptual judgments of children analyzed with these underlying assumptions yielded results compatible with the phonological competence of 4.5-year-old children and were very much consistent with the adult model. The 16 consonants were found to have been perceived by these children in a two dimensional space with nasals, sibilants, continuants, and sonorants each forming distinct perceptual groups.

Jeter and Singh (1972) Jeter and Singh constructed 336 triads from eight prevocalic English consonants and presented them to 60 judges, 30 of whom compared them for auditory similarities and 30 of whom made judgments of visual similarities. All of these judgments were made in an ABX paradigm. The Shepard-Kruskal method was used to analyze these judgments. A plotting of Kruskal's (1964a, 1964b) measure of stress for both auditory and visual perception indicated that these triadic judgments regarding the eight consonants were made in a three dimensional space. The visual data have a lower stress, hence a better fit, than the auditory data. The spatial representation of the graphemes in a three dimensional space revealed that the subjects used vertical-rounded, vertical-crossed, and angular categories exclusively when making visual judgments. The spatial representation of the phonemes in a three dimensional space revealed that the features voicing and sibilancy were used exclusively when making auditory judgments. It was striking however, to note that the features place of articulation and stop/continuant manner were commonly recovered in both visual and auditory modalities. On the basis of the above findings two sets of overlapping feature systems, one for the eight graphemes and another for the eight phonemes, were proposed. When these features were used to predict the MDS dimensions, the multiple R for the visual space was 0.809 and for the auditory space it was 0.677.

Retrieval of Distinctive Features by INDSCAL

The remaining 10 studies included in Table 2 utilized INDSCAL for the analysis of their data. Like other multidimensional scaling analysis, one primary objective of the INDSCAL model is to convert psychological proximity of stimulus X response (δjk) obtained from symmetric or half matrix, to a set of stimulus X dimension coordinates (Xjk). In addition, this method also provides the weightings of individual subjects (or other data sources) (Wik) of the dimensions. As a result the INDSCAL output consists of two matrices, "an $n \times r$ matrix of coordinates of the n objects on the r dimension (group stimulus space) and an $m \times r$ matrix of weights of m subjects on the r dimension (subject space)" (Carroll, 1972). The plottings of both of these spaces can be seen in Figures 22–25. It may be noted that Shepard, in his description of the application of geometric space models to analyze speech perception data, has called this "a powerful new method." The application of this method in speech perception is uniquely suited since: 1) the output of this program is in fixed space and therefore no theoretical targets are required for rotation, and 2) this program also provides subject space along with the stimulus space. A problem with this method is its inability to provide an explicit measure for selecting dimensionality. It may be fruitful to utilize Kruskal's MDS in conjunction with INDSCAL to gain greater insight into the question of dimensionality (Singh, Woods, and Becker, 1972).

Regarding the question of dimensionality, it may be noted that the INDSCAL solution, in general, at the lower dimensionality seems to group the stimuli in broad phonetic categories. With the increase of dimensionality, the grouping becomes more and more subdivided. For example, a two dimensional solution may yield voicing and nasality features. If extended to three, four, and five dimensions, voicing may show a narrower grouping of voiced versus voiceless stops, voiced continuants, and so on (Danhauer and Singh, submitted for publication). Thus, the output of INDSCAL solution seems to indicate that the question of unique dimensional space in phoneme perception may not be relevant.

Wish (1970) Wish reanalyzed the Miller and Nicely (1955) data and reported a solution in a much higher dimensionality than reported earlier by Shepard. Wish found the features nasality, voicing, sibilancy, continuancy, and the second-formant transition. A comparison of INDSCAL analysis of these data via Wish's results with those of the MDS analyses (of the same data) via Wilson's, Shepard's, and Johnson's results shows that a higher and more elaborate structure can be obtained by the INDSCAL analysis. This was not feasible by earlier multidimensional analysis procedures.

Pruzansky (1970) Pruzansky used 16 consonants, the same ones used by Miller and Nicely, and obtained similarity judgments via a sorting device. She

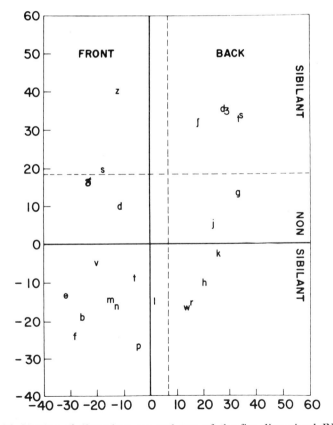

Figure 26. Plotting of dimensions one and two of the five dimensional INDSCAL configurations. Dimension one separates sibilants from nonsibilants, and dimension two separates front place from back. (From Singh, Woods, and Becker, 1972.)

subjected the psychological judgments to INDSCAL analysis and obtained the features, nasality, sibilancy, continuancy, and place of articulation.

Singh, Woods, and Becker (1972) Using three different methods, a large number of subjects, and 22 initial English consonants, Singh, Woods, and Becker (1972) utilized both the Shepard-Kruskal MDS (see under "Phoneme in perceptual space," p. 122) and the INDSCAL procedures to find answers to the questions of appropriate perceptual dimensionality for diadic and triadic comparisons, the weights of the perceptual dimensions under various data collection methods, and the comparison of the features obtained under the a posteriori method of analysis (INDSCAL) with that of a priori feature systems. Figures 26 and 27 show the spatial representations of four of the five dimensions. The fifth dimension was nasality. These figures show front/back, sibilant/nonsibilant, plosive/nonplosive, and voiced/voiceless divisions. The voiced nonplosive consonants can be further subdivided into sonorant

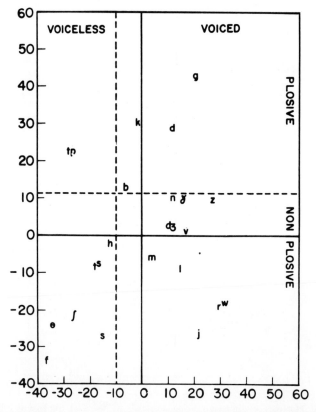

Figure 27. Plotting of dimensions three and four of the five dimensional INDSCAL configurations. Dimension three separates the plosives from the nonplosives, and dimension four separates voiceless from voiced. (From Singh, Woods, and Becker, 1972.)

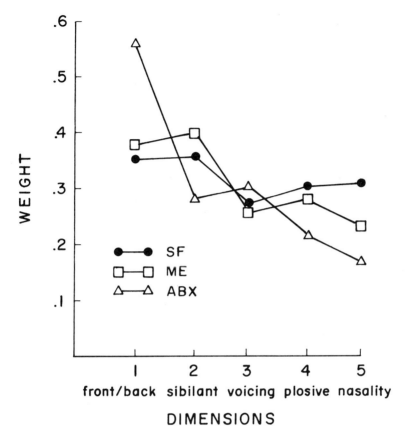

Figure 28. Weighting of dimensions and their feature interpretations by three different methods treated as three individual subjects in the INDSCAL analysis. (From Singh, Woods, and Becker, 1972.)

/m,l,w,r,j/ and nonsonorant /v,ð,z,dʒ/. The phoneme /n/ is an exception to this classification.

The manner in which the three data collection methods, namely SF, ME, and ABX, weigh the five dimensions commonly found is shown in Figure 28. The abscissa represents the five dimensions, each representing a perceptual feature, and the ordinate represents the weighting or contribution of each of these dimensions toward the total explained variance. The diadic methods in the figure show similar weighting tendencies. The triadic method weights place of articulation considerably more than any other feature. The features sibilancy and place are strong for all the three conditions, and nasality is a weak feature. It may be noted that the weakness of nasality and the strength of place as an outcome of psychological judgments directly contradicts the rank order of features in the Miller and Nicely experiment. These reversals may be attributed to the methods of collecting responses and the experimental conditions.

This discrepancy—regarding the weighting of the feature nasality when the results of the multivariate analyses performed by Miller and Nicely (1955), Singh and Black (1966), and Wang and Bilger (1973) are compared with the results of the multidimensional scaling analysis by Singh, Woods, and Becker (1972)—may also be explained by the following argument. Nasality was weighted as the strongest feature when the confusions of consonants were analyzed by the multivariate procedure and was weighted as the weakest feature when the psychological judgments of similarity were analyzed by the multidimensional analysis method. It may be pointed out that the features in the INDSCAL analysis are weighted in terms of their contributions toward the total explained variance in the data. Since there were only two nasal consonants used in the above data sources, their contribution was minimal. To the contrary, in the multivariate analysis the information content of each feature is compared with the maximum possible information pertaining to *that* feature. Thus, this feature may transmit information with high rate.

Singh and Singh (1972) Three sets of perceptual responses to Hindi consonants by the Hindi speakers and listeners were analyzed in this study: one set of responses was obtained for 28 initial consonants at five S/N ratio conditions from 10 Hindi listeners by Singh and Singh (1972). The other two sets of responses were obtained for 29 initial and final consonants in the peak-clipped (Gupta, Agrawal, and Ahmed, 1969) and in the undistorted listening (Ahmed and Agrawal, 1969) conditions.

Initial Hindi consonants in noise Subjects' confusions for these consonants were obtained in five S/N ratio conditions (6 dB, 3 dB, 0 dB, −3 dB, and −6 dB). For the purpose of obtaining common perceptual space across these conditions, in one of the analyses the data for the 10 judges were pooled for each of the five conditions separately, and the conditions themselves were treated as individual subjects. Before the subjects' perceptual confusions were analyzed by INDSCAL, they were analyzed by MDS (Kruskal, 1964) in one to six dimensional spaces. Such a two-step multidimensional scaling strategy facilitates the INDSCAL analysis by reducing the number of iterations it may require for meeting the criterion for solution. Three features—voicing, aspiration, and sibilancy—were obtained on three of the four dimensions of the INDSCAL analysis, while the results in the higher dimensions (five to seven) indicated the presence of some interacting features. Figure 29 shows the plotting of two of the four INDSCAL dimensions. These dimensions were interpreted by the features voicing (/h/ in Hindi is voiced) and aspiration. It may be noted that recovery of the INDSCAL dimensions are constrained by the assumption of the orthogonality or the independence of the coordinate systems. The phonologically distinctive features, voicing and aspiration, therefore, were perceptually utilized independently by the listeners of the Hindi language.

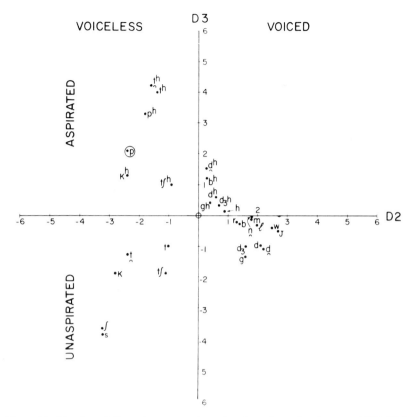

Figure 29. Plotting of dimensions one and two in a four dimensional space of INDSCAL analysis of 29 Hindi consonants. (Based on Singh and Singh, 1972.)

Initial and final Hindi consonants in undistorted and clipped conditions   Four confusion matrices, two involving the initial and final consonants in the undistorted condition and two involving the initial and final consonants in the clipped conditions, were, again, first analyzed by MDS in one to six dimensional spaces. The MDS distances in the six dimensional spaces were analyzed by INDSCAL, treating as individual subjects each of the following four conditions: 1) initial undistorted, 2) final undistorted, 3) initial clipped, and 4) final clipped. Plotting of the measure of "stress" as a function of dimensions in the MDS analysis shows a much lower stress value along the dimensions for the unclipped conditions than for the clipped conditions (Figure 30). The lower stress value is an indication of better fit between the observed and expected distances in the Kruskal method of scaling. It may be noted that the effect of clipping on the magnitude of fit (indicated by "stress") was substantially greater for the postvocalic consonants than it was for the prevocalic consonants. In the undistorted condition, however, the

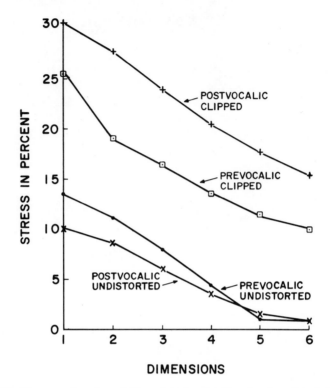

Figure 30. Stress as a function of dimensions for the clipped and undistorted listening conditions in pre- and postvocalic contexts. (Reanalysis of data from Gupta, Agrawal, and Ahmed, 1969, and Ahmed and Agrawal, 1969, by Singh and Singh, 1972.)

position of consonants did not seem to influence stress differently. Figures 31 and 32 show the recovery of the features voicing, aspiration, and sibilancy as common perceptual parameters utilized by the Hindi listeners across the two positions and for the peak-clipped and undistorted listening conditions. The recovery of the feature voicing and aspiration in the four dimensional space, again, showed their independence in the Hindi language. In dimensions higher than four, no clear indication of any other features was apparent. Some indications of interaction of the sonorancy, nasality, and the place features were found.

Walden and Montgomery (1973) Walden and Montgomery obtained similarity judgments for diads of 20 English consonants by 18 subjects, six with normal hearing, six with mild hearing losses, and six with severe hearing losses. Using INDSCAL they found four dimensional space for these groups with the features, voicing, sibilancy, continuancy, and sonorancy.

Mitchell and Singh (1974) Mitchell and Singh collected perceptual judgments via ABX on 16 English consonants embedded in a declarative sentence. These sentences were presented triadically in one condition of quiet and two conditions of noise. The INDSCAL solutions were considered optimal in a four dimensional space for the extreme noise condition and in a five dimensional space for the less noisy and quiet conditions. The features obtained in the five dimensional space were nasality, voicing, sibilancy, continuancy, and place. Since no sonorant consonants other than the nasals were included in the stimuli, there was no provision for the feature sonorancy to be retrieved. The conclusion drawn in this experiment was that the perceptual features obtained in isolated syllables of earlier studies were confirmed to exist also in words embedded in a sentence. For some of the main findings of this experiment, refer also to Figures 22–25.

Weiner and Singh (1974) Weiner and Singh analyzed the cues in same/ different choice reaction time (CRT) judgments of nine continuant consonants. The CRT values entailing each pair of the different consonants were analyzed by INDSCAL analysis. A four dimensional space was considered

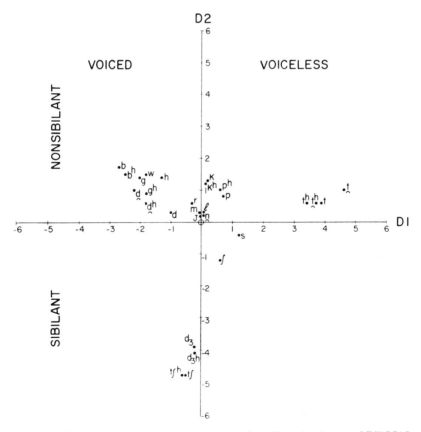

Figure 31. Plotting of dimensions one and two in a four dimensional space of INDSCAL analysis of 28 Hindi consonants. (Reanalysis of data from Gupta, Agrawal, and Ahmed, 1969, and Ahmed and Agrawal, 1969, by Singh and Singh, 1972.)

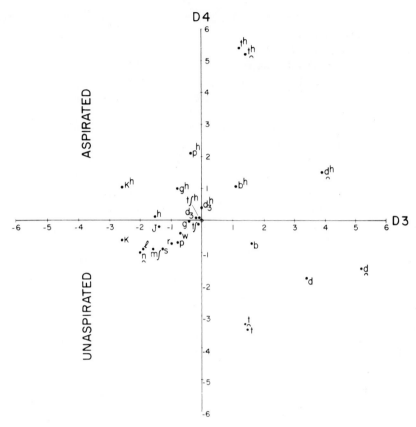

Figure 32. Plotting of dimensions three and four in a four dimensional space of INDSCAL analysis of 28 Hindi consonants. (Reanalysis of data from Gupta, Agrawal, and Ahmed, 1969, and Ahmed and Agrawal, 1969, by Singh and Singh, 1972.)

uniquely appropriate for the judgments of differences by the measure of CRT. These dimensions were interpreted by the features, voicing, sibilancy, and the two places of articulation. The four dimensional solution accounted for 72% of the variance in the subjects' judgments. Of the 72%, D1 (voicing) accounted for 24%; D2 (sibilancy) for 19%; D3 (front/back) for 15%; and D4 (palatal) for 14%. An examination of the individual subject's weighting of these dimensions revealed three different trends. These three trends are reported in Figures 33–35. Figure 33 shows that subjects 4, 7, and 8 weighted sibilancy (D2) as the highest dimension. In contrast, subjects 2, 6, 9, and 10 weighted voicing (D1) as the highest dimension and sibilancy (D2) the lowest (Figure 34). The weightings of the third group of subjects are shown in Figure 35 where subjects 1, 3, and 5 seem to confirm the overall trend of the general stimulus space. It may be noted that all of these 10 subjects had normal speech and hearing and all were college-age students of similar dialectal backgrounds.

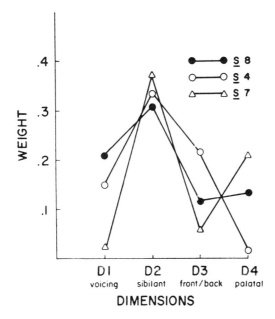

Figure 33. Plotting of weightings of distinctive features made by subjects 4, 7, and 8. (From Weiner and Singh, 1974; copyright 1974 by the American Psychological Association; reprinted by permission.)

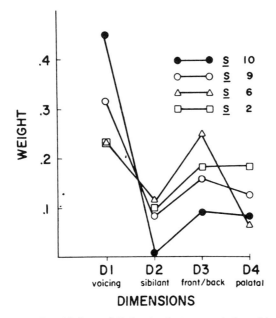

Figure 34. Plotting of weightings of distinctive features made by subjects 2, 6, 9, and 10. (From Weiner and Singh, 1974; copyright 1974 by the American Psychological Association; reprinted by permission.)

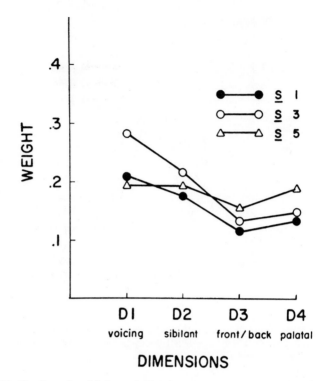

Figure 35. Plotting of weightings of distinctive features made by subjects 1, 3, and 5. (From Weiner and Singh, 1974; copyright 1974 by the American Psychological Association; reprinted by permission.)

These results show that although it is possible to determine a feature system for a group, it is difficult to draw conclusions about the relative weightings of features for that group.

On the basis of the four dimensions recovered in this study, it is assumed that CRT judgments can be used as a criterion for determining phonemic similarity. Figure 36 shows CRT as a function of zero-, one-, two-, three-, and four-feature differences. The top curve in Figure 36, taken from Chananie and Tikofsky (1969), clearly shows a lack of relationship between CRT and distinctive feature differences. The curve labeled "Weiner and Singh GI" represents the mean CRT's for pairs of consonants representing zero-, one-, two-, three-, and four-feature differences obtained for the same 10 subjects whose judgments were utilized for obtaining the perceptual features. The curve labeled "Weiner and Singh GII" is the outcome of a replication experiment conducted to cross validate the trend obtained for the first group of subjects. To determine whether these functions showed similar relationships, a comparison of slopes procedure (Dixon and Massey, 1969) was performed. The result was that the two beta coefficients were not different from each other.

A test of the significance of difference of the mean CRT scores associated with the feature differences by a single factor, repeated measures analysis of variance yielded significant F ratio $(4, 36) = 16.08$, $P < 0.05$. A Tukey (a) comparison of means (Winer, 1971) showed that CRT values for zero-feature differences were significantly greater than values associated with any other feature difference. In addition, the CRT value associated with one-feature difference was significantly greater than differences of three and four features.

The curves labeled "Miller and Nicely GI" and "Miller and Nicely GII" are a result of applying Miller and Nicely features, rather than the features obtained from the INDSCAL analysis, to the Weiner and Singh data. The results attributed to the two sets of features were compatible. The difference between the results of the present investigation and those of Chananie and Tikofsky (1969) may be attributed to their level of reaction time, which was considerably higher than the reaction time obtained in the Weiner and Singh (1974) study. Figure 36 suggests that the number of features distinguishing one phoneme from another becomes more crucial when the overall magnitude

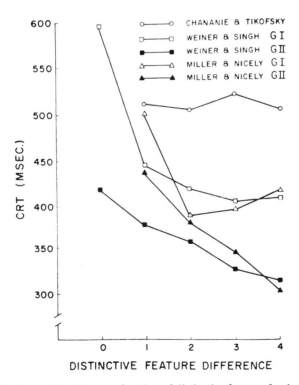

Figure 36. Choice reaction time as a function of distinctive features for data collected from groups 1 (GI) and 2 (GII) in the Weiner and Singh (1974) study as compared with a previous study of Chananie and Tikofsky (1969). (From Weiner and Singh, 1974; copyright 1974 by the American Psychological Association; reprinted by permission.)

of reaction time is lowered. The magnitude was highest in the Chananie and Tikofsky study and the number of features played no role. The magnitude was lower in the Weiner and Singh GI, and the slope was not steep. The magnitude was lower in Weiner and Singh GII and Miller and Nicely GII and the slopes were steepest. Thus, it seems that when extraneous factors contributing to reaction time are minimized, the difference in the number of features begins to play a role.

Danhauer and Singh (**Submitted for Publication**) This research included three experiments dealing with speech perception by hearing-impaired subjects. The overall goal of these experiments was to determine what features were used by these subjects in their perception of consonantal stimuli. Sixteen English consonants, all voiced/voiceless cognates in English, were judged in the context of a phrase. Three psychological methods, SF, ME, and ABX, were employed for obtaining similarity judgments (Danhauer, 1974). The subjects were three different groups of bilateral sensorineural hearing-impaired individuals. One group of four subjects had a loss of 30 dB or greater at and above 4,000 Hz, the other group had a loss of 30 dB or greater at and above 2,000 Hz, and the third group had a loss of 30 dB or greater at and above 500 Hz. The experimental variables consisted of two conditions, one consistent with the slope of the hearing loss for the particular group and the other a nonfiltered condition.

The similarity judgments made by four subjects in each of the three hearing-impaired groups using the three data collection methods under the filtered and nonfiltered conditions were analyzed by INDSCAL. Within each of the three experiments, this analysis was performed for each of the three data collection methods separately. A common perceptual space was then obtained by combining the three data collection methods.

Features for the 4,000-Hz Group The results of INDSCAL analysis in two to seven dimensional spaces revealed that these subjects consistently utilized sibilancy, continuancy, front/back place, and voicing features. In some instances the place feature showed further distinctions of palatal, labial, and dental places.

Features for the 2,000-Hz Group A two to seven dimensional INDSCAL analysis showed that while the feature sibilancy was recovered for the 4,000-Hz group, it was almost never found to exist for the 2,000 Hz. The features retrieved with consistency were plosive, stop/continuant, front/back, and voiceless/voiced.

Features for the 500-Hz Group The commonly retrieved features across the three methods and two conditions for this group were, again, voicing, sibilancy, stop/continuant, and front/back place. The most persistent feature for this group was voicing. For this group one of the strongly weighted dimensions most frequently was interpreted as sibilancy, continuancy, and plosive on one dimension without violating the assumption of orthogonality in INDSCAL. This is an extremely economic and neat perceptual strategy rarely seen in data obtained from normally hearing subjects in undistorted conditions. The fact that subjects with losses above 500 Hz processed consonants utilizing such high frequency features implies that the phoneme perception by these subjects supercedes the concept of critical frequencies.

Conclusions Three conclusions can be drawn from these three experiments. First, the filtering did not affect either the recovery or the weighting of features in any of the experiments in a predictable fashion. Second, the perceptual features of consonants were recovered by invoking "cues" not directly related to acoustic thresholds, thus making it possible for the subjects with sharp slopes in pure tone sensitivity beyond 500 Hz to be able to utilize features of high frequency characteristics. Third, the perceptual features obtained for these three groups of subjects were similar to the ones reported earlier under conditions of noise (Mitchell and Singh, 1974) and quiet (Singh, Woods, and Becker, 1972).

Danhauer and Singh (in Press) Cross linguistic responses were obtained to CVCV stimuli by severely hard of hearing and profoundly deaf French, American, and Yugoslavian subjects with average pure tone thresholds poorer than 90 dB ISO for frequencies above 1,000 Hz. The responses were analyzed by the INDSCAL procedure. The perceptual features obtained from these subjects were nasality, voicing, sonorancy, sibilancy, and continuancy. Although these are aggregated features for all subjects, the extent of hearing disorders in the above subjects (12 for each language—six hard of hearing and six deaf) was such that on the basis of pure tone audiograms, it would not be possible to explain the retrieval of some of these features. It is concluded in this study that the perceptual features of phonemes do not depend directly on the decoding of acoustic cues. These features seemed to be entities unto themselves without direct correlations with the acoustic properties of the stimuli and the auditory capacity of the perceiver.

Danhauer and Appel (in Preparation) The last consonantal study reported in Table 2 involves a cross modality comparison of the perception of consonants. Responses from 24 subjects to the initial consonants of English in visual, tactile, and visual-tactile modalities were obtained to investigate the retrieval of the perceptual features of the consonants from cues other than those supplied directly by the auditory modality. An INDSCAL analysis of the subjects' confusions revealed that these subjects utilized voicing, sibilancy, continuancy, and labial place features.

Conclusions In Table 2, although it has been shown that the features nasality, voicing, sibilancy, continuancy, sonorancy, and place seem to have been retrieved consistently, there are still some cases where they have failed to be recovered. Three reasons for such a lack are being posited here. First, the earlier multidimensional studies did not examine high enough dimensionality to obtain all features (Shepard, 1972). Second, a given perceptual feature was too sensitive to a given experimental condition and assumed zero weight because of that condition. Place of articulation, in noise, was such a feature (Mitchell and Singh, 1974; Singh, 1971). Since the majority of the experiments reported here involved noise, either experimentally induced or because of hearing losses, place feature showed extreme weakness. The third reason is that the weakness in the initial structure of the data, attributable to lack of sufficient observations to warrant involvement of all features (in a confusion matrix), was felt to be another reason for the lack of recovery of certain features (Danhauer and Appel, in preparation).

CONCLUSIONS

Independence of Perceptual Features

The perceptual features appearing persistently in the studies reported in this chapter were voicing, nasality, sibilancy, continuancy, sonorancy, and front/back place. Listener's performance in utilizing these features in various experimental and listening conditions show predictable patterns. These features have potentials of being described simultaneously by the selected articulatory and acoustic features. However, while the perceptual features may utilize the articulatory and acoustic properties in manifesting themselves, they are entities unto themselves, thereby *superceding* man's possibilities in both the auditory and productive domains. The recovery of features like place of articulation and sibilancy, which is perceived by normal subjects in the high frequency regions, for severely hearing-impaired young adults of several languages (Danhauer and Singh, in press), demonstrates the independence of features from close auditory ties. The hearing-impaired subjects, whose audiograms show appreciable hearing losses at and above 500 Hz, have the ability to utilize these features in a complex perceptual task (Danhauer and Singh, submitted for publication). These results cannot be explained by a theory of audition.

Similar to the findings that phonemic perception may defy auditory principles, phonemic perception also defies articulatory principles. In a cross linguistic experiment (Singh and Black, 1966) it has been shown that listeners from Hindi, English, Arabic, and Japanese languages made perceptual errors with sophistication that was not a part of their phonetic repertoire. The perceptual processing of aspiration by the English listeners, liquid/retroflexion by the Japanese listeners, and of a much larger group of fricatives by Hindi listeners, cannot be explained by the phonetic ability of the subjects in these languages. It is concluded, therefore, that like the acoustic parameters, the articulatory parameters provide only a manifesting medium to the perceptual processes.

Satisfaction of Certain General Criteria for a Theory

The six perceptual features of consonants found in the a posteriori analyses are essentially similar in nature to the important features in the a priori experiments. The manner in which these features have been recovered seems to satisfy certain broadly accepted criteria for a theory. These criteria may include: 1) simplicity and economy, 2) unambiguity, and 3) potential to explain data. For simplicity, the only classification system of the perceptual features obtained in the a posteriori studies involved was a clear binary division of the phonemic distinctions, disregarding all other details. For economy, in spite of the inherent redundancy in the phonemic system, the obtained dimensionality in these studies was closely tied with the exponents of the binary base (see Table 2). An examination of several independently conducted research studies involving phoneme perception, with varying subjects, conditions, stimuli, speakers, listeners, modalities, deviances, etc., consistently reveal these perceptual features.

REFERENCES

Ahmed, R., and S. Agrawal. 1969. Significant features in the perception of (Hindi) consonants. J. Acoust. Soc. Amer. 45: 758–763.

Black, J. W. 1957. Multiple-choice intelligibility tests. J. Speech Hear. Disord. 22: 213–235.

Black, J. W. 1970. Interconsonantal differences. In A. J. Bronstein, C. L. Shaver, and C. Stevens (eds.), Essays in Honor of Claude M. Wise, pp 74–96. Standard Printing Co., Hannibal, Mo.

Blumstein, S., and W. Cooper. 1972. Identification versus discrimination of features in speech perception. Q. J. Exp. Psychol. 24: 207–214.

Carroll, J. D. 1972. Introduction to INDSCAL. Handout for Bell-Penn MDS Workshop. Philadelphia.

Carroll, J. D., and J. J. Chang. 1970. Analysis of individual differences in a multidimensional scaling via an n-way generalization of 'Eckart-Young' decomposition. Psychometrika 35: 283–319.

Chananie, J. D., and R. S. Tokofsky. 1969. Choice response time and distinctive features in speech discrimination. J. Exp. Psychol. 81: 161–163.

Chomsky, N., and M. Halle. 1968. The Sound Pattern of English, pp. 176–177 and 303–305. Harper and Row, New York.

Cole, R. A., and B. Scott. 1972. Distinctive feature control of decision time: Same-different judgments of simultaneously heard phonemes. Percept. Psychophys. 12: 91–94.

Crystal, T. H., and A. S. House. Local signal levels and differential performance in dichotic listening. In Proceedings of Speech Communication Seminars, Stockholm. Vol. III, Speech Perception and Automatic Recognition. Almquist and Wiksell International, Stockholm, and John Wiley & Sons, New York. In press.

Danhauer, J. L. 1974. A multidimensional analysis of hearing impaired subjects' responses to sixteen consonants. Unpublished doctoral dissertation, Ohio University, Athens.

Danhauer, J. L., and S. Singh. A multidimensional scaling analysis of phonemic responses from hard of hearing and deaf subjects of three languages. Lang. Speech. In press.

Day, R. S., and J. M. Vigorito. 1972. A parallel between degree of encodedness and the ear advantage: Evidence form a temporal order judgment task. Status Report on Speech Research, SR-31/32, pp. 41–47. Haskins Laboratories, New Haven, Conn.

154   Sadanand Singh

Dixon, W. J., and F. J. Massey. 1969. Introduction to Statistical Analysis. McGraw-Hill, New York. 638p.

Graham, L., and A. House. 1971. Phonological oppositions in children: A perceptual study. J. Acoust. Soc. Amer. 49: 559–566.

Gupta, J. P., S. Agrawal, and R. Ahmed. 1969. Perception of (Hindi) consonants in clipped speech. J. Acoust. Soc. Amer. 45: 770–773.

Halle, M. 1964. On the basis of phonology. In J. A. Fodor and J. J. Katz (eds.), The Structure of Language: Readings in the Philosophy of Language, pp. 324–333. Prentice-Hall, Englewood Cliffs, N.J.

Jakobson, R., G. Fant, and M. Halle. 1951. Preliminaries to Speech Analysis: The Distinctive Features and their Correlates. MIT Press, Cambridge. 58p.

Jeter, I., and S. Singh. 1972. A comparison of phonemic and graphemic features of eight English consonants in auditory and visual modes. J. Speech Hear. Res. 15: 201–210.

Johnson, S. C. 1967. Hierarchical clustering schemes. Psychometrika 32: 241–254.

Kile, J. 1966. Predicting consonantal responses to filtered syllables. Unpublished doctoral dissertation, Ohio State University, Columbus.

Klatt, D. 1968. Structure of confusions in short-term memory between English consonants. J. Acoust. Soc. Amer. 44: 401–407.

Kruskal, J. B. 1964a. Multidimensional scaling by optimizing goodness of fit to a nonmetric hypothesis. Psychometrika 29: 1–27.

Kruskal, J. B. 1964b. Nonmetric multidimensional scaling: A numerical method. Psychometrika 29: 115–129.

McGregor, L. 1972. An investigation of the perceptual structure of sixteen prevocalic English consonants embedded in sentential material. Unpublished doctoral dissertation, Ohio University, Athens.

Miller, G., and P. E. Nicely. 1955. An analysis of perceptual confusions among English consonants. J. Acoust. Soc. Amer. 27: 338–352.

Mitchell, L., and S. Singh. 1974. Perceptual structure of sixteen prevocalic English consonants sententially embedded. J. Acoust. Soc. Amer. 55: 1355–1357.

Peters, R. W. 1963. Dimensions of perception for consonants. J. Acoust. Soc. Amer. 35: 1985–1989.

Pruzansky, S. 1970. Judgments of similarities among initial consonants using an auditory sorting apparatus. Presented at the 80th Meeting of the Acoustical Society of America, November 3–6, Houston.

Shannon, C. E., and W. Weaver. 1963. The Mathematical Theory of Communication. University of Illinois Press, Urbana. 117p.

Shepard, R. N. 1962. The analysis of proximities: Multidimensional scaling with an unknown distance function. Psychometrika 27: 125–140, 219–246.

Shepard, R. N. 1972. Psychological representation of speech sounds. In E. E. David, Jr. and P. B. Denes (eds.), Human Communications: A Unified View, pp. 67–113. McGraw-Hill, New York.

Singh, S. 1966. Cross-language study of perceptual confusion of plosive phonemes in two conditions of distortions. J. Acoust. Soc. Amer. 40: 635–656.

Singh, S. 1968. A distinctive feature analysis of responses to a multiple choice intelligibility test. Int. Rev. Appl. Linguist. 6: 37–53.

Singh, S. 1970a. Initially and transitionally truncated prevocalic English consonants spoken and recognized by native Hindi and English speakers. In A. Rosetti (ed.), Actes Du X Congres international des Linguistes, pp. 245–255. Edition of the Socialist Republic of Rumania, Bucarest.

Singh, S. 1970b. Interrelationship of English consonants. *In* B. Hala, M. Romportl, and P. Janota (eds.), Proceedings of the Sixth International Congress of Phonetic Sciences, pp. 825—828. Publishing House of the Czechoslavak Academy of Sciences, Prague.

Singh, S. 1971. Perceptual similarities and minimal phonemic differences. J. Speech Hear. Res. 14: 113—124.

Singh, S. 1973. A unified theory of speech perception. Presented at the 1973 Annual Convention of American Speech and Hearing Association, October 10—15, Detroit.

Singh, S. A step toward a theory of speech perception. *In* Proceedings of Speech Communication Seminars, Stockholm. Vol. III, Speech Perception and Automatic Recognition. Almquist and Wiksell International, Stockholm, and John Wiley & Sons, New York. In press (a).

Singh, S. Distinctive Features: Theory and Application. University Park Press, Baltimore. In press (b).

Singh, S., and G. M. Becker. 1972. A comparison of four feature systems using data from three psychophysical methods. J. Speech Hear. Res. 15: 821—830.

Singh, S., and J. W. Black. 1966. Study of twenty-six intervocalic consonants as spoken and recognized by four language groups. J. Acoust. Soc. Amer. 39: 372—387.

Singh, S., and K. Singh. 1972. A search for the perceptual features of 29 prevocalic Hindi consonants. Presented at the 83rd Meeting of the Acoustical Society of America, April 18—21, Buffalo.

Singh, S., D. R. Woods, and G. M. Becker. 1972. Perceptual structure of 22 prevocalic English consonants. J. Acoust. Soc. Amer. 52: 1698—1713.

Singh, S., D. R. Woods, and A. Tishman. 1972. An alternative MD-SCAL analysis of the Graham and House data. J. Acoust. Soc. Amer. 51: 666—668.

Studdert-Kennedy, M., and D. Shankweiler. 1970. Hemispheric specialization for speech perception. J. Acoust. Soc. Amer. 48: 579—594.

Torgerson, W. S. 1958. Theory and Method of Scaling. John Wiley & Sons, New York. 460p.

Walden, B. E., and A. A. Montgomery. 1973. Dimensions of consonant perception in normal and hearing impaired listeners. Presented at the 1973 Annual Convention of the American Speech and Hearing Association, October 10—15, Detroit.

Wang, M., and R. C. Bilger. 1973. Consonant confusions in noise: A study of perceptual features. J. Acoust. Soc. Amer. 54: 1248—1266.

Weiner, F. F., and S. Singh. 1974. Multidimensional analysis of choice reaction time judgments on pairs of English fricatives. J. Exp. Psychol. 102: 615—620.

Wickelgren, W. A. 1966. Distinctive features and errors in short-term memory for English consonants. J. Acoust. Soc. Amer. 39: 388—398.

Wilson, K. V. 1963. Multidimensional analysis of confusions of English consonants. Amer. J. Psychol. 76: 89—95.

Winer, B. 1971. Statistical Principles in Experimental Design. McGraw-Hill, New York. 907p.

Wish, M. 1970. An INDSCAL analysis of the Miller and Nicely consonant confusion data. Presented at the 80th Meeting of the Acoustical Society of America, November 3—6, Houston.

The Measurement of Temporal Factors in Auditory Perception

Robert Peters, Ph.D.
Professor and Director
Institute of Speech and Hearing Sciences
The University of North Carolina at Chapel Hill

CONTENTS

INTRODUCTION

Although sound pressure changes in time provide the necessary ingredient for auditory perception, there are no systematic, overall bodies of knowledge or theories that treat temporal properties of perception at acoustic, physiological, or behavioral levels. However, all studies in auditory perception, including audition and the perception of speech and music, are studies of temporal factors because the auditory-perceptual process is characterized by temporal change in order for the detection, discrimination, or recognition processes to occur. The fact that the sequential pattern of sound pressure changes are critical for hearing provides insight into the basic character of auditory perception. That is, since the information in the acoustic signal does not remain available, nor can the auditory system respond to features of the signal as they occur, there must be longer perceptual units that are somehow stored and then processed after the arrival of sufficient information from the sensory input. This characteristic of the auditory system leads to questions about the nature of these meaningful units of perception and whether they are fixed or determined by the stimulus input.

Psychological moment theories (Stroud, 1955) would suggest that perceptual sampling is periodic, perhaps controlled by a central timing mechanism or clock. Other theories place the emphasis for the organization of

157

perceptual units on the incoming stimuli. Regardless of whether or not perceptual sampling is discrete or stimulus organized, or a combination of the two, as is probably the case, the understanding of temporal properties that result in detection, discrimination, and the perception of speech and music is necessarily basic to the knowledge of how man organizes meaning from the pattern of sounds in his environment. As Hirsh (1967) suggested, "Auditory perceptual theory requires the concepts of sequence and temporal pattern to play the same role that Gestalt or form or shape has played in visual perception." He also observed that the rules that govern temporal pattern perception in hearing must be combined with, in the case of speech perception, a different set of rules, also concerned with sequence and temporal relationships, that are provided by the structure of language.

The importance of these observations will be increasingly evident in the following discussion because of the difficulties that are inherent in attempting to understand temporal properties apart from the characteristics of the particular input stimuli. Also, these observations serve to emphasize the possibility that man's processing of sequential sound patterns is not independent of his sound-producing capabilities in speech or music. The performance in the auditory system is probably reflective of the limitations and constraints of speech production and other sound-producing capabilities of man. In fact, the link between speech perception and production may be rhythmic action, a concept proposed by Lashley (1951) and more recently treated by Martin (1972).

Basically, the concept of rhythmic action holds that the natural constraints of human movement-produced sounds, like speech and music, are rhythmically patterned. That is, sequences of sounds that are rhythmic possess a hierarchial organization that has a coherent internal structure at the sound level (Martin, 1972). These sequences of accented and unaccented units are temporally organized such that the locus of each sound element on a time dimension is relative to the locus of the other elements in a particular series. This concept of rhythm is termed relative timing, and the connection between sound production and auditory perception is that if sound sequences produced by man are characteristically organized in a rhythmic fashion, it follows that man's perceptual system will function in ways that take advantage of these rhythmic patterns.

An alternative to a rhythmic concept is that the sound units in a sequence are only concatenated, successive, rather than possessing a temporal structure. The implications that result from regarding rhythmic action as a central concept in a serial order behavior such as auditory perception are that investigators need to be concerned with the properties of this possible temporal structure as well as being concerned with temporal order capabilities when attempts are made to explain auditory perception from temporal order judgment studies. That is, more concern should be placed on longer temporal patterns than on adjacent sound units. As was indicated previously, although studies in auditory perception do concern temporal factors, the focus of this chapter is necessarily limited to what are generally termed temporal order studies. Other aspects of auditory perception that are included are not treated in depth, but are used primarily to bring focus on the central problem of measurement of temporal aspects of auditory perception.

Because perceptual systems extract from the environment information that is biologically relevant to the organism, the first step in measuring temporal factors is to specify the hierarchy in auditory perception that reflects biological needs. Mountcastle (1965), in discussing what the brain faces in sensing, stressed the need for studies that treat problems about functional meaning for the organism. He structured six questions that are particularly appropriate to our discussion on auditory perception. The first question, "Has anything happened in the environment?", is the problem of detection. The next question, "What is it?", leads from the problem of detection to that of identification. The third question, "How much of it is there?", leads from detection and discrimination to the problem of quantification. The fourth question, "Is this stronger than that?", is related to the previous one and deals with the problem of differential discrimination. The next question, "Where is it?", is a problem of localization. The final question is "Does the stimulus move in space or change its properties as a function of time?"

These questions suggest that there is a hierarchy of perception that relates to biological needs and that this hierarchy specifies the kinds of behavioral questions we can ask in the study of auditory perception. From these six questions, it may be observed in general that increasingly lengthened time spans are necessary as one goes from detection to the process of extracting information from an event that is changing its properties in time. In man this can be viewed as going from detection to the perception of speech, and it is important to distinguish between these various levels of performance as we examine the temporal properties of auditory perception. For example, the fact that an observer can detect an order difference between two stimuli in a time magnitude of 1 or 2 msec cannot be construed to mean that he can also perform recognition or speech understanding in the same time domain. There is clearly a difference between the detection of speech—something is happening in the environment—and the understanding of what is being said.

Given that detection, recognition, discrimination, localization, and the more complex behaviors of extracting meaning from sequential patterns of signals provide the basic framework within which studies of temporal properties of auditory perception can be conducted, questions then arise as to the role of measurement and what variables could and should be controlled to lead to basic understandings of these temporal properties. Von Békésy (1960), in his comments on the role of question asking relative to hypothesis-testing research in general, stated that a strategic question is the one of greatest value in formulating research, because it gets at the important variables. He also added that the formulation of strategic questions is probably one of the most difficult aspects of research. His comments do point out, however, the importance of asking the right question in order to understand the role of temporal factors in auditory perception.

When one conceptualizes research as the systematic activity by an investigator in relating observations in nature or the protocol field to the concept or theory domain, hypotheses are formulated by the investigator. These hypotheses are verified, rejected, or modified as a consequence of measurements that are performed at the protocol or data field. Measurement is thus the link between data and concept fields. Within this framework, the temporal properties of acoustic signals need to be controlled in ways that seem to relate to auditory perception. Also, the consequences of these systematic controls and variations on behavioral responses need to be measured, and the results need to be related to general theories of temporal auditory perception. In this process, another general aspect of the theory of measurement becomes involved. Numbers are assigned to objects or phenomena and are then manipulated in various ways to provide information about the phenomena. The importance of these number assignments is that there be a relationship between the properties of the number system and the domain that is under study. This is generally referred to as an isomorphic relationship between a numerical system and the particular phenomena that are being investigated.

As Lashley (1951) properly observed, spatial distribution of excitation in the nervous system has been studied much more than temporal aspects of nervous activity. This applies even today to auditory perception, where explanations of auditory behavior are more likely to be based on spectral interpretations than on temporal factors. Yet Nordmark (1970) concludes after his review of time and frequency analysis that the picture of the ear emerging from various considerations is that of a temporal pattern analyzer. He goes on to comment that once this notion is accepted, auditory phenomena will be much easier to understand than they are at the present time. Because the ear is primarily thought of as a spectral rather than a temporal analyzer, except under special circumstances, such as periodicity pitch, studies tend to be designed and measurements tend to be made on spectral rather than temporal factors. As was indicated previously, the concept of rhythm, or as it is called by Martin (1972), relative timing, could form a theoretical base and lead to the kinds of studies that would be particularly fruitful for understanding many aspects of auditory perception. In addition, if rhythm is considered as a basic organizing structure for both perception and speech production, programs of study such as Allen's personal communication, which propose a theoretical model for timing control for speech, become particularly important also for studies in perception.

Many of the studies treating temporal factors of auditory perception have been concerned with resolving power of the auditory system. For a number of reasons, the results have not been clear, in part because of the failure of investigators to differentiate between various methods of stimulus presentations or observers' responses. For example, as Hirsh and Sherrick (1961) have indicated, temporal resolving power must be broken into at least two measures, one a measure of successiveness and the other a measure of order. Recent studies have also demonstrated that judgments of perceived order differ considerably as a result of different modes of stimulus presentation and kind of responses required from listeners. For example, it is much more difficult for an observer to report the order of tones in a tone train that is constantly being recycled than to report a tone train that is discretely presented.

There are also problems in studies of temporal factors in controlling physical aspects of the signal that is different only in temporal properties. This is particularly true when the signals are only a few milliseconds long. The investigator who reviews or initiates studies on temporal factors needs to be aware of some of these problems. He should be especially cognizant of the fact that detection, discrimination, and recognition responses are different tasks for an observer and will yield results reflecting these differences. In the following sections, measurement of temporal factors in auditory perception will be discussed relative to temporal auditory acuity, temporal order for brief sounds, temporal order for speech, and temporal patterns in music.

Temporal order studies are often justified by investigators on the following basis. Since temporal patterns underly the perception of speech and music, knowledge of basic auditory capabilities is necessary in order to understand the processes involved in extracting meaning from auditory sequences, as in the case of speech. There are other reasons for studying temporal order in its own right, rather than regarding it as only basic to more complete understanding of other phenomena. As was stated earlier, knowledge about the temporal structure of rhythm may well provide a unifying concept for speech production and perception. That is, since there is an orderliness to rhythmic patterns, they do probably, apart from other temporal aspects of speech or music, provide an information-carrying structure that is important for perception. Unfortunately, most of the temporal order studies that have been reported to data treat only two or three sequential events and have not yet come to grips with a longer temporal structure such as rhythm.

There are other reasons for considering the merit of temporal order studies. First is the possibility that these studies can provide information about basic auditory processes. In the case of temporal auditory acuity, the necessary and basic nature of the information is obvious: What is the minimal integration time of the auditory system? Second is the question of whether or not temporal factors of perception are controlled by central mechanisms rather than being peripheral sensory phenomena. Some of the evidence, it would seem, provides support for a central timing mechanism. The results from a study by Hirsh and Sherrick (1961), where perceived order was measured across different sense modalities, was interpreted by the authors to favor the central control process rather than sensory process. Also, as was indicated earlier, since the auditory system cannot respond immediately to incoming stimuli, and must in some form store information before perceptual processes can operate, studies of judgments on temporal order, in which comparisons can be made between objective and subjective orders, possibly could be informative about this process of auditory perception. Evidence from several studies (Peters, 1964, 1967), where perceived order was found to be different from sensory input order, does suggest that the perceptual readout can be different from the sensory input.

MEASUREMENT OF TEMPORAL AUDITORY ACUITY

Temporal auditory acuity is discussed first, not because there are a large number of studies in this area, but because it considers basic resolving powers of the auditory system and is probably—from a stimulus-generation point of view—one of the most difficult areas. In this sense, discussion of temporal acuity will exemplify one major measurement problem, that of specifying with some exactitude the effective stimulus at the ear. Temporal auditory acuity is described as the shortest time interval within which the ear can discriminate the order of auditory events (Green, 1971). In a way it is related to temporal integration, which is concerned with the contributions of duration and intensity to the detectability of a signal. However, whereas in temporal integration performance improves with duration, the concern in these studies is on the minimal integration time. Because several of the studies on auditory acuity utilize the same modes of stimulus preparation, some discussion is given to one of the studies in detail, since it does exemplify problems of experimentation and measurement.

Ronken (1970) reported data on two main areas: 1) whether the auditory system can respond to monaural phase cues contained in short transient signals that fall within nominal time constants of the ear, and 2) the importance of such cues relative to power or energy. His data suggested that the ear can discriminate between very short wide-band signals that differ only in phase, and that observers varied considerably more in their ability to detect phase differences than in their ability to detect power differences. The phase cue, however, was found salient enough to mask significantly the detection of power differences. A problem, however, in the study of the role of phase differences was the ease with which relatively sustained periodic stimuli could vary the phase components. However, with very short duration samples of such stimuli, when the phase spectra are varied, differences are also produced in the energy spectra.

These phase studies are described by Green (1971) and Patterson and Green (1970). Green states that while it is true that the studies could be described as the study of phase perception, this does not seem to be an accurate description. He therefore finds it simpler and more concrete to think of the differences in the order of temporal events within the wave form, rather than as phase spectra. For this reason, these studies are considered to be studies of temporal auditory acuity or minimal integration time (Green, 1973a). The study by Patterson and Green (1970) is a particularly good example of measurement in this area of study, because although for sustained periodic sounds phase spectra can be varied, to have two signals differ in temporal, phase, properties where the sounds last only a few milliseconds, is most difficult.

To overcome these difficulties, the authors generated their signals following a procedure as outlined by Huffman (1962), which is a procedure, in essence, to pass a pair of digital impulses through an all-pass digital filter. In the case of this study, the wave forms under investigation were stored in digital form in a laboratory computer and converted to analog signals by a digital-to-analog converter. All stimuli were filtered by two variable band-pass filters, where the sampling rate could be varied. The stimuli were presented to the subject monaurally, in this case by TDH-39 earphones, and in the experiment the observers responded in a two-alternative, temporal, forced-choice procedure, and were required to indicate the order in which the signals were presented. The two wave forms for each trial were presented in random order, and after each trial the subject was given feedback indicating the correct answer. In general, the task in the study of temporal acuity is to establish a temporal order between two stimuli, and then decrease the total duration of the stimuli until the different orders can no longer be perceived. In this study, it was found that listeners could discriminate differences in temporal order when the total duration of the two signals was as small as 2.5 msec. Green (1971) draws the analogy between his study on temporal acuity and the limits on the perception of the pitch of the residue because the temporal properties for both are very similar.

In a subsequent study, Green (1973b) posed the question as to whether or not the previous findings of minimal temporal acuity were verifiable over a range of frequencies. Two procedures were used, one using the Huffman sequences previously described and the second using two segments of a sinusoidal signal that differed in amplitude and were played either forward or backward in time. The ability to discriminate the order in which the signals were presented was essentially the same at 2,000 and 4,000 Hz, but was not as well discriminated at 1,000 Hz. For both procedures, Huffman and segments of sinusoidal signals, the value of the temporal acuity measure was in the 1–2 msec range.

One question on measurement that is raised in dealing with very short transients and was discussed by Patterson and Green (1970), was whether or not the signal at the ear corresponds to voltage wave form. Ringing characteristics of earphones and also of the ear would raise some questions about whether or not the signals as described were actually the signals processed by the ear. Patterson and Green, however, were of the opinion that—at least to the earphones—the system was linear and the changes that the signal may have undergone from the time it was generated by the computer until it entered the inner ear probably were not transformations that would serve as the basis for discriminating the signals other than relative to the temporal differences.

The studies on temporal auditory acuity stress the need for precise measurements and control of the acoustic signal in order to specify the exact proportions of the signal that relate to differences in behavioral responses.

MEASUREMENT OF TEMPORAL ORDER PERCEPTION

Whereas the previous section treated temporal processes that are concerned with minimal temporal auditory integration and subsequent sections deal with longer and more complex signals such as speech, this section primarily deals with temporal order judgments that result from responses to two or three either sequential or overlapping sounds. The signals employed are usually periodic, and they are often pure tones. The kinds of questions that the experimenter usually asks relate to minimal onset time differences between two signals or interval differences between two or more signals, durations of signals, or other configurations of sound that he believes will measure order perception. If the stimuli consist of sequential sounds, the experimenter may shorten the sounds to that point that observers' judgments meet his criterion of correct or incorrect responses.

Although the fact that perceived temporal order of stimuli does not necessarily correspond to actual physical order has been recognized for at least a century, current work in judgments of temporal order can be properly thought of to have begun with the work of Hirsh (1959) and Hirsh and Sherrick (1961). In the latter article, there is a particularly good review that begins with Exner's work in 1875, and discusses the problem of simultaneity versus successiveness. In the earlier study (Hirsh, 1959), various pairs of sounds were manipulated with respect to time of occurrence, and each member of the sound pair was different from the other with respect to frequency. Among the differences employed were frequency for tones, spectrum for bands of noise, and duration for pairs of sounds that consisted of a brief and a prolonged sound. These differences between the members of each pair of sounds were necessary, as Hirsh emphasized, in order for an observer to be able to identify and attach a label to each of the sounds. Two stimuli presented in the same sense modality, identical in quality and intensity, cannot allow for judgments or temporal order because there is no way for the observer to recognize each stimulus separately.

One of the reasons for historical confusion about temporal judgment was that authors, particularly those who did not have firsthand information about studies, failed to differentiate among the various methods that had been employed to obtain measures of perceived temporal order. The literature had not always been clear in differentiating between judgments of simple successiveness (i.e., are there two sounds as opposed to one?) and judgments of actual order of stimuli. Hirsh (1959) clearly differentiated tasks that dealt with judgments of successiveness and judgments of order. His results indicated that a 2-msec separation was sufficient to provide a judgment that the onset time of two signals was not simultaneous, whereas the time separation that was necessary between the onset of two sounds for the judgment of order (i.e., which one of the sounds was first?) required about 20 msec to provide for 75% correct responses.

In the second of the two studies, Hirsh and Sherrick (1961), using methodological procedures similar to those in the previous study, examined temporal order judgments at various modalities, including visual, auditory, and tactile, and combinations of various modality pairs. They again found an approximate value of 20-msec as the amount of time that must intervene between two events in order for observers to report correctly, 75% of the time, which of the two events preceded the other. The authors concluded that whereas the time between successive stimuli that was required for the stimuli to be perceived as successive rather than simultaneous could depend upon the particular sense modality involved, i.e., visual, auditory, or tactile, the temporal separation that is required for a judgment of perceived order is much longer—in fact, by about a factor of 10—and is independent of the input sense modality. As was indicated previously, this can be viewed, as it was interpreted by Hirsh and Sherrick, that the control of temporal order is served primarily by central mechanisms rather than by the separate sensory channels themselves. This also strongly suggests, for future studies where the intent is to examine aspects of central mechanisms, that stimuli from different sense modalities should be employed in order to avoid problems that may occur when the inputs are through a single sense modality.

Broadbent and Ladefoged (1959), employing three signals, examined auditory temporal order using paired sounds that consisted of either a hiss, a pip, or a buzz, and an **ABX** procedure. They found that identifications were only at the 50% level, although 150-msec intervals separated members of the sound pairs. They suggested that the combination of a trained subject and the quality change attributable to the short temporal intervals between the sounds accounted for the temporal resolving times reported by Hirsh (1959).

White and Lichtenstein (1963) performed an experiment that did not deal with differences in onset time as had the Hirsh studies, but did deal with discrete visual and auditory signals of approximately 10 msec. The observers adjusted differences between stimuli pairs until intermittent stimuli seemed to be regularly spaced. The results were reported as estimates of temporal acuity, and it was found that the optimal value of stimulus separation for auditory judgments of regularity was at about 100 msec for audition and at about 140 msec for vision. Again, this study demonstrates, as do a number of studies, past and present, that the responses are critically task dependent. This is particularly true when stimuli pairs are recycled for a period of time, as opposed to discrete stimuli presentations.

Between the time of the initial work by Hirsh (1959) and a current publication by Divenyi and Hirsh (1974), a number of studies have treated the problem of temporal order judgments. However, no general conclusions can be formulated as to basic properties, especially as to time values, for resolving characteristics of the auditory system. Some investigators have postulated at least dual perceptual mechanisms, for example, one that functions with respect to longer, unfamiliar, sequences of sound and another one that allows fine temporal discrimination on a sound pattern of a few milliseconds. When considering what seem to be conflicting results, it is necessary to specify the nature of the response, where on the hierarchy from detection to the processing of complex signals or speech is the task, and also to understand the biases provided by the input stimuli. Discrimination of quality change in two signals does not necessarily depend on an order judgment, and temporal order judgments for speech are different for nonspeech signals by virtue of speech-processing contributions to the response.

Divenyi and Hirsh (1974), in commenting that a minimal duration or minimal time interval as an indicator of temporal resolution has not emerged, stated that the range of values seems to depend on one or several of three important variables. These are listed as: 1) the number of elements in a sequence of sounds, whether or not the series is cyclical or continuous, as opposed to a single presentation of a sequence; 2) whether the observer's task is to discriminate between two sequences or to identify order; and 3) the amount of training the observer receives. There are probably other factors involved in the discrepancies in results found among the various studies. These could include serial order effects in recall, peripheral masking, perceptual interference among successive signals, and contributions of learning and memory variables to the recall task.

Some of these issues have been treated by recent studies. One consistent finding has been that when four sequential sounds are presented in a continuous, recycled manner, the duration of each sound must be increased from 200 to about 700 msec before inexperienced listeners can identify the correct order. Even for experienced listeners the duration of the sound must be increased to about 300 msec (Warren et al., 1969). These findings are in accord with those reported by Broadbent and Ladefoged (1959) and Thomas and Fitzgibbons (1971). When the sequences are not recycled but are only presented once, these values drop to 200 msec for four sounds (Warren, 1972) and to 50 msec for three sounds (Peters and Wood, 1973a, 1973b). For two sounds the value is about 20 msec (Hirsh, 1959). When order, absolute identifications, are compared to discrimination for a four-sound pattern using single sequence presentations, the minimal durations for each sound drop from approximately 200 msec (Warren, 1972) to 90 msec for dichotically presented tones, and 10 msec for diotic presentations (Leshowitz and Hanzi, 1972). In the latter study, discrimination measures were obtained by asking observers to judge whether the order of presentations was the same or different for two sequences. For two brief sounds, as was summarized in the section on temporal acuity, the duration value for discrimination is in the 1−2 msec range.

It is obvious from the above discussion that different modes of measurement are tapping different response variables and that investigations are needed to explore and explain some of these variables. Divenyi and Hirsh (1974) provided a study of this kind because they systematically explored relevant variables using three contiguous pure tones of different frequencies presented in a single sequence. Their study addressed the questions of tonal component duration necessary to identify sequences, the effect of total and relative frequency range on identification, the isolation of perceptual features in a temporal order identification task, and an ordering of temporal orders from easy to difficult. The results of the study, briefly summarized, were that the minimal duration of each component tone necessary for absolute identification of a sequence was between 2 and 7 msec, that a total frequency range narrower than the one third to two thirds octave decreased identification values, and that for relative frequency ranges, harmonic relationships among the tones made identification easier than for complex harmonic relationships. Also, with respect to direction of frequency change of the component tones, unidirectoral changes were easier to identify than the other changes, and final tone identification, particularly for the highest and lowest tone of a series, was better than for other tones in the sequence.

The study by Divenyi and Hirsh (1974) demonstrated that by examining a variety of factors, ties can begin to be made with other auditory data and theory in ways that will advance understanding of the total auditory process. Thus, beginnings at least have been made in understanding the nature of learning tonal patterns, or Gestalts; the role that critical bands may play in complex pattern perception by establishing frequency limits on component sounds; the contributions that recency effects may provide in the identification of sequences; and how melody perception can be explained by experimental data. The areas just reviewed are all worthy of further measurement and exploration because it would seem that the understanding of temporal properties in perception, at least in part, is dependent upon explaining other known observed behavioral phenomena in the area of hearing.

A series of studies on temporal order judgments (Peters, 1964, 1967) yielded data that seemed to be dependent upon the same processes that yield critical band data, that is, when frequency separations between tones of a sequence reach certain values, perceived order changes, sometimes abruptly. The point at which this change occurs corresponds roughly to critical band distances. In these studies, the experimental method normally involved a three-tone sequence with the first and last tone at the same frequency and the center tone variable and under frequency control by the observer. Each tone might be of 20-msec duration with an interval of 50 msec between each tone. Observers used the method of adjustment to change the frequency of the center tone until the tones were no longer heard as low-high-low, assuming that the observer was increasing the frequency of the center tone, but were heard as low-low-high. The observers were never initially instructed to expect this perceived change; rather, they were asked to change the frequency of the center tone and report their experience. After an observer reported that the order had changed, he was then instructed to adjust the center frequency until the experience of order change occurred. These values were plotted for various frequencies, determined by the first and last tones, and for both ascending and descending center frequencies.

In the studies described above, the sequences were repetitive with a short interval between each sequence. In other variations of the study, the method of constant stimuli was employed, and single sequences rather than repetitive ones were presented. The results for these experiments, however, were similar to those reported above in that perceived order seems to be influenced by frequency characteristics of the tones of a series. When the frequency of the center tone differed sufficiently from the first and last tones, its perceived order usually was last. It would seem that there are implications concerning perceptual grouping of like signals that may relate to a perceptual store. However, when the center tone was at a contralateral ear as compared to the first and last tones, the perceived order shift was difficult to achieve. This would seem to implicate peripheral sensory rather than central mechanisms. Similar results were also found when five- and seven-tone sequences were employed as well as three-tone sequences. The finding that temporal order can be influenced by stimulus properties is known, as, for example, when speech is the stimuli, linguistic factors override temporal ones.

The importance of the studies such as the ones above on perceived temporal order is that they treat a simpler and more basic variable than speech. Thus, although one of the basic reasons for studying temporal order judgments is to understand speech processing, sometimes it is necessary to deal with more basic variables in the process.

Another possible way to study perceptual temporal phenomena is to examine the performance of systems in a breakdown state. The aphasic offers such an opportunity for the study of temporal order. Efron (1963) used both auditory and visual temporal ordering tasks to study left brain-damaged aphasics and right brain-damaged nonaphasics. He concluded that the hemisphere dominant for speech is also important for temporal discriminations. Swisher and Hirsh (1972) presented pairs of auditory and visual stimuli to brain-damaged and nonbrain-damaged subjects. The subjects indicated which member of the pair was first. Although the results are somewhat difficult to interpret, it did seem that temporal ordering problems are part of an aphasic's pattern of deficit and that the study of aphasics may be helpful in understanding temporal perception.

There is another study which, while it did not treat temporal order values directly, does have some relevance to the issues involved. Ptacek and Pinheiro (1970) found that for three temporally spaced white noise bursts involving two elements, soft and loud, that observers required a 10-dB intensity difference within a pattern for 50% correct identification. The just noticeable difference for white noise is about 0.5 dB. Also, a large number of the errors were complete pattern reversals or mirror images. The authors rightly concluded that the results seemed to indicate that the pattern recognition task is a higher auditory function than simple discrimination of intensity differences. This study again demonstrates that although information about the resolving power of the auditory system is necessary, the critical measures for auditory perception are also likely to be found by detailed examination of the characteristics of the error responses, as was done in the Ptacek and Pinheiro study, where the errors were found to be systematic and not random.

MEASUREMENT OF TEMPORAL ORDER FOR SPEECH

The range of potential and available studies with respect to temporal factors in speech is tremendous, and for this reason this section is necessarily limited to treatment of studies that are specifically concerned with temporal order judgments for the purpose of examining variables in speech perception. In the study of temporal order measures for speech, the investigator must isolate temporal, linguistic, and other contributing variables if he is to understand the relative contributions of time to perception. As has been suggested earlier, the tie between speech production and perception may be the concept of rhythm and biological central timing mechanisms. Temporal order studies may help to elucidate these issues.

A major issue for temporal perception relates to average phoneme durations in speech which are between 70 and 80 msec for normal speaking rates. Liberman et al. (1967), in discussing the necessary hypothetical sound alphabet if speech were processed as a successive alphabet, indicated that each phoneme segment could last no longer than 50 msec on the average. Average phoneme rates may not be representative because vowels typically average between 200 and 300 msec, and some consonants are much shorter than the average of 70–80 msec. Also, the fact must be considered that the consonants carry a substantial information load in speech and an average phoneme rate is thus not representative.

Thomas et al. (1970), addressing themselves to the question of temporal order in the perception of vowels, required subjects to determine temporal order in recycled sequences of four vowels. The durations were varied from

75 to 300 msec. The results indicated near perfect scores at approximately 125-msec duration and chance levels for durations of about 100 msec. However, Thomas et al. (1970) report previous studies indicating that vowel durations as short as 27 msec can be correctly identified. This suggests that it is not a matter of failing to identify the vowel but rather the result of the temporal pattern that depresses recognition. These authors raise an issue that may be obscured when considering sounds, tones, or vowels that are successive and adjacent, i.e., that the critical issue may relate to time for auditory processing and not necessarily to durations of the sounds. Thus, sounds of 30-msec duration may be sufficient for correct perceptional sequences of sufficient intervals to separate the sounds to allow for auditory processing.

Several investigators have advantageously studied speech processing by relating temporal order judgments of speech to other variables. These other variables include the established observation that certain speech sounds may be categorically perceived, in that there is a tendency for the discrimination of certain speech sounds to be a function of phonetic categories rather than a function of physical differences between stimuli. For example, the right ear has the advantage in dichotic listening in that when speech pairs are presented simultaneously to the two ears, the stimuli to the right ear are more correctly identified than those presented to the left ear; and that for dichotic listening to syllables, the ear where one syllable onset lags behind the other one has the perceptual advantage. Although the lag effect is primarily helpful to right ear inputs, it also applies to the left ear.

Some of the pertinent studies are reviewed here within this framework. Day (1970a) reported a study where the syllable /tæs/ was presented to one ear, while /tæk/ was presented to the other ear. Relative times varied from 0 to 100 msec in both directions. Although subjects often reported /tæsk/ or /tæks/ they were able to report well on whether /s/ or /k/ was heard last. The author concluded that while both linguistic and nonlinguistic processing levels operate in a normal listening situation, the linguistic level seems to be prepotent in that it can effect selective loss of nonlinguistic information, such as temporal order or acoustic shape information. Warren (1970), in support of the above suggestion, reported that listeners believed they heard a deleted speech sound or syllable in a sentence where the missing sound is replaced by noise. In a related study, Day (1970b) presented dichotically to listeners two speech stimuli that differed only in their initial phonemes, /bæŋkət/ and /læŋkət/. The relative onset times had a 100-msec range. Not only did the subjects report /blæŋkət/, but they were not able to judge the temporal order of the initial phonemes. They reported hearing /b/ first regardless of whether /b/ or /l/ actually was first. The study again reflects the control of temporal judgments by linguistic information. As a demonstration of enhancement of the right ear advantage for speech perception, a temporal lag was found to increase the right ear advantage (Studdert-Kennedy and Shankweiler, 1970).

Day and Bartlett (1972) extended the work of previous studies that concerned speech and temporal order judgments by presenting dichotically paired speech and nonspeech stimuli. The judged order errors for speech/ nonspeech were comparable to those that would be expected for speech/ speech pairs dichotically presented when the response required was which ear led. The error rate did not increase when the required response was which stimulus led, as it did for speech/speech tasks when observers were required to judge order by stimuli. The results are consistent with a view that speech and nonspeech analyses are processed by different processors that do not interfere with each other.

The observations that can be drawn from studies of this kind are that temporal order judgments provide a powerful method for the study of auditory perception, particularly when the effects attributable to speech and nonspeech inputs can be separated and analyzed. Cutting (1973), for example, used discrimination and temporal order tasks to study the rate of formant transitions in speech and nonspeech tasks. The temporal order task merely required the subject to indicate the first item of a dichotic pair. The results indicated that, in general, for both identification and temporal order speech tasks there was a right ear advantage. Nonspeech tasks, on the other hand, whether identification or temporal order, usually yielded left ear advantages. The study further indicated that stimuli with transitions were processed differently than stimuli without transitions regardless of whether or not speech or nonspeech stimuli were involved. As was indicated in this section concerning speech, measurements resulting from two ears, different stimuli classes, and kinds of temporal order responses can be informative about auditory processing in general.

MEASUREMENT OF TEMPORAL ORDER FOR MUSIC

Ortmann (1926), in his monograph on the relativity of tones, wrote that "a melody must have duration or extent in time. . . . interwoven with this extent are the psychological problems of immediate memory, recall and anticipation." He continued to discuss and develop a theory on the perception of tonal sequences that was farsighted, and by today's knowledge, very modern. He recognized, for example, that the perceptual status of any tone in a melody is determined by tonal environment and by its absolute position in the pitch and time series, and furthermore, that any succession of tones in music is not reacted to only melodically, but that harmonic and rhythmic relationships are always present to modify the purely melodic effects.

Ward (1970) comments to the effect that while the last few decades have produced important new procedures and results in regard to auditory process, "advances in knowledge about the perception of music during the same period have, by and large, been much less spectacular." This seems to be true, particularly since Ward (1970) in his comprehensive review of musical perception does not include rhythm or report a melody study that involves temporal properties of music.

Subsequent to Ward's (1970) review, Divenyi (1973) published a major experimental monograph entitled "The rhythmic perception of micro-melodies: Detectability by human observers of a time increment between sinusoidal pulses of two different, successive frequencies." Divenyi stressed that rhythm in music means a good correspondence of an intended recurrence for the performer or expected occurrence for the listener with the actual physical recurrence of musical sounds. When the correspondence is satisfactory, it is termed rhythmic regularity, and when imperfect, it is considered irregular. The questions asked by Divenyi concerned what irregularities could be tolerated by performer and listener and still be recognized as a regular rhythm. A number of specific questions were asked about the effects of frequency, temporal discrimination, and subjective parameters related to the perception of rhythm. A series of experiments were then designed and carried out to provide empirical answers to these questions. The results of the study, described properly by Divenyi as one that has been "investigating a hitherto unexplored segment of auditory spatio-temporal interaction," perhaps raises more questions than have been answered.

However, these questions are important for understanding temporal properties of musical perception. One question concerns the fact that temporal discrimination may be strongly influenced by tonal frequency when time intervals are marked by short tones—that is, perceptual processing may continue after cessation of tones in such a way to interact with successive tones. Another question relates to how long or short tones could be made to result in frequency effects on discriminability of time intervals between tones. Other results that apply to discrimination of tones in complex frequency and time patterns obtained from the study concerned those attributes of frequency, tones, range, and change that affect discrimination judgments. Divenyi also concluded from the study that there seem to be two perceptual processes, perhaps overlapping, that handle temporal discrimination, one process for intervals shorter than 600 msec and the other for intervals longer than 600 msec. His results also indicated less variability for discrimination for short time intervals and greater variability for longer time intervals. The judgments on regularity of rhythmic occurrence seemed to be similar to those that apply to duration estimations. The virtue of Divenyi's (1973) study was that musical perception, especially time factors, were rigorously subjected to modern psychophysical study, resulting in a good beginning toward understanding some of the relevant parameters underlying the perception of melody and the factors in music.

Dowling (1972) considered the question of whether or not melodic transformations—inversion, retrograde, and retrograde inversion—could be recognized by listeners. Inversion, retrograde, and retrograde inversion are transformations that operate on a melodic pattern, as a whole turning it upside down, backwards, or upside down-backwards by altering the pitch with respect to pitch and duration properties, respectively. Transformations are of obvious interest with respect to temporal patterns because although transformed, time patterns are still retained. The listener's task was to judge the exactness of the transformation after hearing the original melody. The results indicated increasing difficulty in judging from inversion to retrograde to retrograde inversions. The results seem to indicate that temporal factors take precedence over pitch factors in making these kinds of judgments because the disturbance of temporal factors is more disruptive of melody recognition than are pitch factors.

Considering rhythmic theory, Martin (1972) states that natural rhythm patterns can have a variety of surface forms, but nevertheless do have a simple underlying structure that is characterized by either one or the other of two obligatory rules. These are given as the relative accent level and the relative timing of elements. The accent rule applies to repeating patterns, and the relative timing relates to rhythm and concerns the relative timing between adjacent and near-adjacent elements in a behavior sequence, as opposed to concatenation of elements. Martin (1972) notes that the rhythm rule makes explicit what the musician knows tacitly in the same way that the linguistic rule makes explicit what the speaker of the language knows tacitly. Such studies of temporal factors in the perception of music seem to indicate that a largely untapped area of study, of considerable interest to temporal perception theorists, exists with respect to music.

SUMMARY

In this chapter the measurement of temporal factors in auditory perception was discussed relative to temporal auditory acuity, temporal order for brief sound, temporal order for speech, and temporal patterns in music. Various issues such as preperceptual storage of auditory inputs, meaningful units of perceptual relationships among man's sound-producing capabilities, and the role of biological needs in auditory perception were reviewed prior to and as a basis for summarizing pertinent studies on temporal factors in auditory perception.

On the basis of the data reviewed, measurement of factors that are involved in temporal auditory perception are found to be dependent, not surprisingly, on the nature of the observer's task and on the characteristics of the auditory stimulus. For example, detection of an order difference can occur in a much shorter time span than can identification of sequential signals. Also, the stimulus, such as speech, can have its own order structure which seems to operate independently of other perceptual order properties. Current work on temporal factors, as exemplified by the studies covered in this chapter, suggests that considerable progress is and can be made toward a broader understanding of all aspects of auditory perception by operating from a framework that emphasizes hearing and a temporal process. In this regard, a particularly important area for future study is that of rhythm as it relates to both speech perception and speech production.

REFERENCES

von Békésy, 1960. Experiments in Hearing. McGraw-Hill, New York. 745p.
Broadbent, D. E., and P. N. Ladefoged. 1959. Letter to the editor: Auditory perception of temporal order. J. Acoust. Soc. Amer. 31: 1539.
Cutting, J. A. 1973. Perception of speech and nonspeech with and without transitions. Status Report 33, pp. 39–46. Haskins Laboratories, New Haven, Conn.
Day, R. S. 1970a. Temporal order judgments in speech: Are individuals language-bound or stimulus-bound? Status Report 21/22, pp. 71–78. Haskins Laboratories, New Haven, Conn.
Day, R. S. 1970b. Temporal order perceptions of reversible phoneme cluster. Status Report 24, pp. 47–56. Hoskins Laboratories, New Haven, Conn.
Day, R. S., and J. C. Bartlett. 1972. Separate speech and nonspeech processing in dichotic listening. J. Acoust. Soc. Amer. 51: 79(A).
Divenyi, P. L. 1973. The rhythmic perception of micromelodies: Detectability by human observers of a time increment between sinusoidal pulses of two different, successive frequencies. In E. Gordon (ed.), Experimental Research in the Psychology of Music. pp. 41–130, Vol. 7, University of Iowa Press, Iowa City.
Divenyi, P. L., and I. J. Hirsh. 1974. Identification of temporal order in three-tone sequences. J. Acoust. Soc. Amer. 55: 144–151.
Dowling, W. J. 1972. Recognition of melodic transformations: Inversion, retrograde, and retrograde inversion. Percept. Psychophys. 12: 417–421.
Efron, R. 1963. Temporal perception, aphasia, and déjà vu. Brain 86: 403–424.
Green, D. M. 1971. Temporal auditory acuity. Psychol. Rev. 78: 540–551.
Green, D. M. 1973a. Minimum integration time. In A. R. Møller (ed.), Basic Mechanisms in Hearing, pp. 829–846. Academic Press, New York.
Green, D. M. 1973b. Temporal acuity as a function of frequency. J. Acoust. Soc. Amer. 54: 373–379.
Hirsh, I. J. 1959. Auditory perception of temporal order. J. Acoust. Soc. Amer. 31: 759–767.
Hirsh, I. J. 1967. Information processing in input channels for speech and language: The significance of serial order of stimuli. In C. H. Millikan and F. L. Darley (eds.), Brain Mechanisms Underlying Speech and Language, pp. 21–38. Grune & Stratton, New York.
Hirsh, I. J., and C. E. Sherrick, Jr. 1961. Perceived order in different sense modalities. J. Exp. Psychol. 62: 423–432.
Huffman, D. A. 1962. The generation of impulse-equivalent pulse trains. IEEE Trans. IT 8, S10–S16.
Lashley, K. S. 1951. The problem of serial order in behavior. In L. A. Jeffress (ed.), Cerebral Mechanisms in Behavior, pp. 112–136. John Wiley & Sons, New York.
Leshowitz, B., and R. Hanzi. 1972. Auditory pattern discrimination in the absence of spectral cues. J. Acoust. Soc. Amer. 52: 166.

Liberman, A., F. S. Cooper, D. P. Shankweiler, and M. Studdert-Kennedy. 1967. Perception of the speech code. Psychol. Rev. 74: 431–461.

Martin, J. G. 1972. Rhythmic (hierarchical) versus serial structure in speech and other behavior. Psychol. Rev. 79: 487–509.

Mountcastle, V. B. 1965. The problem of sensing and the neural coding of sensory events. In G. Quarton, I. Melnechuck and F. Schmitt (ed.), The Neurosciences: A Study Program, pp. 393–408. Rockefeller University Press, New York.

Nordmark, J. O. 1970. Time and frequency analysis. In J. V. Tobias (ed.), Foundations of Modern Auditory Theory, pp. 57–83. Vol. 1. Academic Press, New York.

Ortmann, O. 1926. On the melodic relativity of tones. Psychol. Monogr. 35: 1–47.

Patterson, J. H., and D. M. Green. 1970. Discrimination of transient signals having identical energy spectra. J. Acoust. Soc. Amer. 48: 894–905.

Peters, R. 1964. Perceived order of tone pulses. J. Acoust. Soc. Amer. 36: 1042(A).

Peters, R. 1967. Perceived order of tone pulses. J. Acoust. Soc. Amer. 42: 1216(A).

Peters, R., and T. J. Wood. 1973a. Perception of temporal order for tones. J. Acoust. Soc. Amer. 53: 311–312(A).

Peters, R., and T. J. Wood. 1973b. Perceived order of tone pulses. J. Acoust. Soc. Amer. 54: 315(A).

Ptacek, P. H., and M. L. Pinheiro. 1971. Pattern reversal in auditory perception. J. Acoust. Soc. Amer. 49: 493–498.

Ronken, D. A. 1970. Monaural detection of a phase difference between clicks. J. Acoust. Soc. Amer. 47: 1091–1099.

Stroud, J. M. 1955. The fine structure of psychological time. In H. Quastler (ed.), Information Theory in Psychology, pp. 174–205. Free Press, New York.

Studdert-Kennedy, M., and D. Shankweiler. 1970. Hemispheric specialization for speech perception. J. Acoust. Soc. Amer. 48: 579–594.

Swisher, L., and I. J. Hirsh. 1972. Brain damage and the ordering of two temporally successive stimuli. Neuropsychologia 10: 137–152.

Thomas, I. B., and P. J. Fitzgibbons. 1971. Temporal order and perceptual classes. J. Acoust. Soc. Amer. 50: 86–87.

Thomas, I. B., P. B. Hill, F. S. Carroll, and B. Garcia. 1970. Temporal order in the perception of vowels. J. Acoust. Soc. Amer. 48: 1010–1013.

Vitz, P. C., and T. C. Todd. 1971. A model of the perception of simple geometric figures. Psychol. Rev. 78: 207–228.

Ward, W. D. 1970. Musical Perception. In J. V. Tobias (ed.), Foundations of Modern Auditory Theory, pp. 405–447. Vol. 1. Academic Press, New York.

Warren, R. M. 1970. Perceptual restoration of missing speech sounds. Science 167: 392–393.

Warren, R. M. 1972. Perception of temporal order: Special rules for the initial and terminal sounds of sequences. J. Acoust. Soc. Amer. 52: 167.

Warren, R. M., C. J. Obusek, R. M. Farmer, and R. P. Warren. 1969. Auditory sequence: Confusion of patterns other than speech or music. Science 164: 586–587.

White, C. T., and M. Lichtenstein. 1963. Some aspects of temporal discrimination. In C. T. White and M. Lichtenstein (eds.), Perceptual and Motor Skills, pp. 471–482. Southern University Press, Birmingham, Ala.

The Measurement of the Dimensions of Visual Communication

Herbert J. Oyer, Ph.D.
Professor, Audiology and Speech Sciences
Dean, College of Communication Arts
Michigan State University

CONTENTS

INTRODUCTION

Speech and hearing specialists have given attention to the visual aspect of the spoken code because of the implications it has had for hearing-impaired persons who need supplemental cues provided through the visual input channel. Our great preoccupation has been with variables associated with lipreading.

In this book, the central theme of which is measurement in speech and audition, it would be less than complete not to include some comments about the fast growing research area of nonverbal communication. This contention is reinforced by the writer's own position that places lipreading, as we have traditionally thought of it in speech and hearing science, as only one of the important nonacoustic means of communication. Another important means is via nonverbal communication not necessarily related to speech production.

Visual Communication

One might ask the question as to why time, effort, and money should be spent to study the area of visual communication. The answer to this is quite clear, because much of what man learns is learned from the stimuli that he receives through the visual channel. The blind, who are deprived of this channel, must receive special attention if they are to learn what sighted individuals learn through viewing the world about them.

Those who are actually involved in the study of visual communication differ widely in backgrounds and interests. They might be psychologists who are interested in relating the process of visual communication to cognition. They might be audiologists who are directing their efforts toward assisting the hearing-handicapped individuals to interrelate with those about them by means of the visual channel. They might be researchers in the area of journalism who are determined to understand the effects of the layout of the printed media, the newspaper, the magazine, etc., on the readability of their product. Or they might be professional advertising specialists who, because of their need to know which visual configurations are most successful in selling a product, will spend time and effort to determine how well they can communicate via pictures to the potential buyer of their product. On the other hand, they might be researchers in the area of television broadcasting who are seeking to determine the effects of televised visual messages on viewers. They might be research specialists in the area of communication theory who wish to define more clearly the basic principles of visual communication, whether in mass situations, small groups, or in interpersonal encounters. Obviously, there are many different persons, coming from different areas of interest, who occupy themselves with the study of visual communication.

Attempts at communicating information occur through various means. One attempt is through the use of pictures. This is an ancient method as evidenced by the graphic illustrations found inside caves. The use of pictures has not diminished, but is increasing as we move toward the 21st century. Probably never in the history of man have so many pictorial illustrations been used in an attempt to communicate ideas.

Another mode of visual communication is orthography. This, too, is ancient and dates back to the times when messages were encoded in hieroglyphics. Today, as never before, modern man is being deluged with printed materials. Most psychologists and reading specialists give serious consideration to the study of the form that orthography takes and the ability of humans to learn to read. Sizes and shapes, as well as frequency of occurence of orthographic characters, have been carefully studied to the end that predictions can be made relative to optimal conditions for normal readers. Also, reading specialists have become deeply involved in research that is directed toward understanding the errors that occur in handling the printed word.

There are also researchers who are interested and involved primarily in the area of communication theory and who are carrying out research in visual nonverbal communication. A basic interest of theirs is to gain greater understanding of human responses to visual nonverbal signals and to relate their findings to the developing body of communication theory. More is said about this later in the chapter.

In speech pathology and audiology the focus of visual communication has been and continues to be on lipreading, sometimes referred to as speechreading, and was developed long before speech pathology and audiology had developed as professional entities. The development of lipreading as a tool for the handicapped can be traced back to the 1600's, when attempts were made to teach deaf children to talk. Pedagogical approaches have not changed greatly between then and now. The parameters important to the study of lipreading and the variables that effect the lipreading process have been identified and explored to some extent. The attempts which have been made and the results which have been achieved through this exploration receive attention in this chapter.

Broadly defined, visual communication involves the sending and receiving of visual stimuli that evoke meaning within the receiver. These stimuli might or might not be accompanied by other types of stimuli such as acoustic, tactile, olfactory, and so forth. They might be linguistic or nonlinguistic stimuli.

Nonverbal Communication

Nonverbal communication is an aspect of visual communication. Linguists, anthropologists, psychologists, and sociologists have contributed heavily to the developing field of nonverbal communication. Scholars in the area of communication theory have also begun to give considerable attention to this area of study. One of the finest resumes of the literature on nonverbal communication systems is presented as a separate issue of *The Journal of Communication,* published in December of 1972. In this issue, writers contribute to a variety of topics on special problems that are involved in understanding nonverbal communication systems. Hand movements, visual behavior and social interaction, factors in conversational behavior, experimental analysis of interpersonal influence processes, and conflicts and directions in proxemic research span the offerings therein. In all, it brings together invited papers by researchers who are deeply involved in the study of nonverbal communication.

Harrison and Knapp (1972) state that "looking to the future we anticipate even better theoretical formulations, a diffusion of research technology and methodology, and a quickening pace of empirical research and an ever-increasing application of findings to man's practical communication problems."

Research Patterns

Although the nonverbal communication systems probably antedate verbal systems of communication by several thousands of years, the scientific exploration in this field has been under way for approximately a century. It was Charles Darwin, who in his work, *The Expression of Emotions in Man and Animals,* in 1872, gave attention to the nonverbal aspect of communication.

Harrison and Knapp (1972) imply that the most obvious contributions have been made by anthropologists and psychologists.

The names of Efron (1941, 1972), Birdwhistell (1970), and Hall (1959, 1966) loom large as contributors from the anthropological arena. Psychologists Ruesch and Kees (1971) as well as Ekman (1972) have contributed to the psychological understanding of nonverbal language.

In their review of contributions that researchers have made to the nonverbal communication literature, Harrison et al. (1972) suggest that the pioneers in the area of nonverbal communication, such as Efron (1941) and Ruesch and Kees (1971), are well worth studying. The Ruesch and Kees approach is broad and involves examination of art, biology, electronics, philosophy, and psychiatry. They attempted to organize a nonverbal communication code by differentiating among sign language, action language, and object language. They state that the results of Efron suggest that culture can explain emergent gestural patterns.

Two general texts that introduce the reader to nonverbal communication have been recently published. One is by Mark Knapp (1972) and deals with problems in nonverbal communication and human interaction. Within this work there is integration of findings from several fields to include sociology, psychology, psychiatry, education, anthropology, and speech communication. Yet another book which has been just recently published is by Randall Harrison (1974). The book by Harrison is a comprehensive introduction to the entire field of nonverbal communication and provides the reader with a basic framework with which to understand the total process in humans.

Any sensitive clinician would be quick to see the importance of nonverbal visual cues in relation to the rehabilitation of hearing-handicapped persons, for whom visual expressions and head movements provide information beyond the verbal message. The literature of speech pathology and audiology, however, fails to reveal any research data detailing the extent to which these cues are utilized by those who are hearing handicapped. It has been found through research carried out by Ellsworth and Carlsmith (1968) that the interaction of verbal content and eye contact during an interview bear relation to a subject's reaction to the interview situation. Their findings reveal that the interviewer prefers eye contact and favorable content. Interesting findings by Mehrabian (1968) were that distance from the person being addressed, amount of eye contact, backward lean, and shoulder orientation related in a positive way to the degree to which the speaker was positively or negatively viewed.

RESEARCH IN VISUAL COMMUNICATION FOR THE HARD OF HEARING

Attempts to Test Lipreading

The earliest attempts to view quantitatively the visual aspects of the verbal code were made by researchers who attempted to construct tests of lipreading. It is not the intent to review in detail these early efforts, but merely to refer to the approaches that were utilized in the attempt to measure this aspect of human behavior.

Nitchie (1913) was perhaps the first to measure lipreading skill. Although he made no record of the data he may have gathered, his approach was the use of the silent motion picture film. He constructed three test sentences and photographed them with a camera that moved at 16 frames/sec. Although a crude attempt, it seems to be the point at which some focused attention was directed toward measurement of the visual aspect of the verbal code.

Four years later, in 1917, Conklin developed materials consisting of eight consonants, 52 words, and 20 sentences, and he administered these in a face-to-face arrangement. He presented these materials to subjects at the Oregon State School for the Deaf and scored his items systematically. His analysis showed a high correlation between the scores that were achieved by his subjects and the rankings that were made of the subjects by their teachers.

Eleven years later, in 1928, Day and Fusfeld set about to build two lipreading tests which they administered in a face-to-face situation to over 8,000 deaf pupils. Materials used in this test were four sets of 10 sentences. One interesting finding was that the pupils performed considerably better when their teachers read the lists than when they were read by persons unfamiliar to them.

The Heiders, in 1940, developed several tests of lipreading. One test contained 1,500 unrelated nouns, 15 meaningless phonetic units, 15 names of animals, 15 unrelated sentences, and 10 related sentences. The second test they developed contained names of animals, unrelated sentences and nouns, and stories. The third test was the same as the second except for the elimination of the names of animals. They found through their research that vowels were easier to recognize than consonants and that there was no correlation between the ability to lipread nonsense syllables and general lipreading ability.

Mason (1942) constructed for children filmed lipreading tests that she could score in an objective manner. She was quite rigorous in setting criteria to follow in the development of her tests. In the final development of her third test, she found high correlation among the forms of the tests.

In 1946, Utley constructed a motion picture achievement test of lipreading and standardized the procedures. Her analyses show an interrelationship among the skills involved in lipreading words, sentences, and stories.

In the early years of lipreading research, there were still others interested in measuring lipreading abilities, such as Reid (1947), Kelly (1955), Morkovin (1947), and Pauls (1947).

From the John Tracy Clinic (Los Angeles, Cal.) comes the test entitled Film Test of Lip Reading. Lowell (1957) fabricated an unrelated sentence test of 60 items. The sentences are reasonably simple in content and frequently used in everyday conversation. There are two forms to the test that have been analyzed and found to be similar in difficulty. The test is a reliable one.

Attempts have continued to be made through the years to test lipreading ability. Moser et al. (1960b) developed a film test of visual recognition of one-syllable words. The words were selected from most frequently spoken words, and the test is a reliable one.

There are still others who have attempted to develop tests, including Postove (1962), Nielsen (1970), and Mykelbust and Neyhus (1970).

There remains a great need for the development of a valid and reliable test of lipreading for measuring the ability of subjects to perceive the nonacoustic visual aspect of the verbal code. It is true that there are reliable tests; however, the most that can be said for the validity is that they might have face validity.

Fingerspelling and Sign Language

Disagreement still exists among those who advocate the manual approach as a means of communication for the deaf and those who advocate the use of the oral approach. Of late, there has been a new thrust in this whole area by those recommending total communication as the answer.

Manual language has existed for hundreds of years, but little research has been done to determine whether it is more or less effective than the oral approach. In 1960, Moser et al. (1960a) discussed the manual communication from a historical point of view. It was pointed out that manual alphabets existed for hundreds of years although their usefulness to the education of the deaf has been more recent. Moser et al. (1961) carried out an experiment to determine the feasibility of fingerspelling as a means of communication. One of the variables viewed carefully was that of distance and its effect upon the intelligibility of fingerspelling. It was determined that there was quite good intelligibility up to 175 feet, but that it fell off rapidly thereafter.

A blend of lipreading and manual communication called cued speech was brought about by Cornett (1967). He combined speechreading with a system of manual cues which help the viewer to discriminate between similar visual configurations. This seems to be a reasonable approach, but there is little research evidence that indicates its usefulness.

As with tests of lipreading, there should be developed tests of fingerspelling and signing. Only serious, well controlled investigations will shed light upon the efficacy of the manual approach.

Lipreading Research

This section of the chapter is not meant to be exhaustive of the research that has been accomplished in the area of lipreading; however, the principal purpose is to draw attention to selected speaker, code, channel, and receiver variables that have been investigated.

Selected Speaker Variables The selected speaker variables to be considered in this section are facial expression, lip movement, facial exposure, sex of speaker, whispered versus voiced speech, rate of speech, and amount of information the speaker provides.

Stone (1957) and Vos (1965) have indicated through research that normal mouth movements are preferable to exaggerated movements of the lips. O'Neill (1951) has found that persons who are most intelligible visually as speakers are also most intelligible under nonvisual conditions. In Finland, Pesonen (1968) supported O'Neill's findings through similar study of Finnish speakers. Generally, the findings suggest that normal speaking style is best for optimal lipreadability.

The question arises as to how much of the face is necessary for viewing for good lipreading. Stone (1957) and Greenberg and Bode (1968) have found that, for lipreading success, exposure to the full face is preferable to exposure of lips only.

Research results show that there really is no difference in sex of speakers as regards their lipreadability. Aylesworth (1964) failed to find any significant differences among lipreading scores as related to difference of sex of speakers. Sahlstrom (1967), in a study in the physiology laboratory, used rubber strain gauge instrumentation to determine facial movements of selected areas of the faces of speakers. He found that male speakers were speaking with greater intensity of facial movement over the duration of the words than were female speakers. Leonard (1968), in a follow-up of the strain gage study of Sahlstrom, determined there was no difference in facial movement associated with voice or whispered speech. This might have implications for training.

Question has been raised as to whether or not changing the rate of speech might facilitate lipreading performance. Measurement has been accomplished to attempt to answer the question in a study by Byers and Lieberman (1959) and Black, O'Reilly, and Peck (1963). Rate of speech was not found to have significant effect on lipreading performance by either of these groups of investigators.

Must a viewer be able to see every movement of the face and lips of the speaker in order to lipread successfully? The answer to the question as found by Subar (1963) would indicate that much of the signal can be lost and yet the viewer can be successful in the lipreading task. She randomly blocked out frames of filmed speakers uttering words in order to deprive the viewer of specified amounts of information. Up to 45% deletion caused no significant deterioration in lipreading performance.

Selected Code Variables In 1961, Roback tested the ability of college students to identify homophenous words through the use of visual cues as they were presented on a silent film. The results of her testing showed that homophenous words really should not be considered the same but, in effect, are somewhat different one from another. Her subjects were able to identify in a multiple choice test more correct words than would have been possible through chance occurrence alone. In a follow-up study Joergenson (1962) made physical measurements of the words most frequently identified correctly by the Roback subjects. She found that the sizes and shapes of the mouth opening might have given beneficial cues to the subjects of Roback. Words that were supposedly homophenous, upon analysis of the stimuli as they appeared on the film, were shown to vary considerably through time as they were produced by the same speaker.

In a study designed to investigate the influence of the stem of monosyllabic words on the identification of the initial consonants by lipreaders, Franks and Oyer (1967) determined that the influence of the stem on the identification of the initial consonant was prominent. The same consonant united with different vowel-consonant word stems, was identified with different degrees of accuracy.

As shown by Greenberg and Bode (1968), the position of consonants within words does relate to their lipreadability. They employed the Modified Rhyme Lists as stimuli. Their subjects attained scores that were higher for consonants when the consonants were in the initial position of the word.

Pesonen (1968) took a look at Finnish phonemes and concluded that the main reason for confusion in visual confusion of vowels was dissimilarity in size and shape of the lip openings. He stated that consonants were most easily discriminated by his subjects because of the place of their articulation.

Upon viewing familiarity as a code factor in lipreading sentences, Lloyd and Price (1971) found that in their investigation of both normal hearing subjects and hearing-impaired subjects, there was significant agreement between the two types of subjects in their ability to rate familiarity of sentences along a five-point scale.

Greene (1964) took a look at the ability of viewer subjects to determine where the accents fall in three-syllable words. She found that her viewers were able to determine the accented syllable 70% of the time, well above chance level.

Nielsen (1966) found through experimental investigation that it does no particular good to repeat words if the subject does not lipread them successfully the first time. Her subjects viewed filmed presentations of the stimuli and were not helped by additional repetition of the words.

Schwartz and Black (1967) studied the influence of grammatical form in sentence intelligibility by lipreaders. They used six kernel sentences, each of which contained a noun phrase and a verb phrase. These were subjected to seven grammatical transformations including the negative, interrogative, and passive, and combinations of these. They found that subjects were able to identify the kernel sentences most readily. Low intelligibility scores were evident on the negative form. Their scores ranged from 86.8% for the kernel sentences to 62.0% for the negative-interrogative transformation.

Selected Channel Variables Too few measurements have been made relative to the effects of channel for the transmission of the visual stimulus to the lipreader. In 1961, Oyer determined through an experiment that the medium of television can provide successful teaching of lipreading. Following the training of his subjects on the monosyllabic word list, errors in subjects' responses were substantially reduced.

Thomas (1962) studied the amount of light in which lipreading takes place; her subjects were highly trained on the vocabulary. She found that the illumination can be reduced from normal classroom lighting to virtual darkness before scores change noticeably.

One would think that distractions of a visual type might have highly deleterious effects upon lipreading. However, several studies seem to indicate that auditory distractions have far greater deteriorating effects upon lipreading performance than do visual distractions.

There has long been the question concerning optimal distance and angle between speaker and receiver. Research measurements made in this area yield results which are not necessarily corroborative or conflicting. Mulligan (1954), Erber (1971), and Quigley (1966) have been concerned with this area of inquiry, and it is probably safe to say that as a result of their investigations a distance of 10 feet between speaker and viewer does not have harmful effects upon visual reception. In terms of angle of incidence, it would seem that the best angle for presentation of lipreading stimuli ranges from 0 to 45 degrees.

Selected Receiver Variables Researchers who have focused their attention on receiver variables have invariably asked the question as to the differentiating characteristics of good and poor lipreaders. One of the problems in this type of research has been the lack of a lipreading test that can be considered valid. With the tools at hand, however, studies have been made of a number of subvariables. O'Neill and Davidson (1956) and Simmons (1959) studied a number of variables, such as concept formation, level of aspiration, reading comprehension, and intelligence as related to visual perception. Unfortunately, their results are not mutually supportive. O'Neill and Davidson found, however, that concept formation scores significantly correlated with lipreading scores of their subjects. Subject and method differences obviously contributed to lack of agreement in results.

Some researchers hypothesized that the ability to synthesize and analyze really might bear some relationship to lipreading performance. Tatoul and Davidson (1961) compared lipreading performance and letter prediction but found no significant results on the letter prediction test.

Kitchen (1968) probably has done the most comprehensive evaluation relative to visual perception of both the spoken code and visual synthesis as measured by several tasks. He looked at recognition speed for geometric forms, speed of organizing geometric form patterns, speed of organizing words from letters, recognition speed of common words, speed of organizing sentences from scattered words, and several other tasks. He found some relationship between the speed of forming words from scattered letters, lipreading scores, and a total synthesis score for each subject over all subtests that were positively related to lipreading.

Only a very low correlations has been found by Bode, Nerbonne, and Sahlstrom (1970) between lipreading performance and skill in the filling in of missing letters in sentences. The whole area of analysis and synthesis and the relationship to lipreading is in need of much more research.

There is some evidence that visual acuity is a factor in lipreading performance. Hardick, Oyer, and Irion (1970) found that good lipreaders were of the normal vision group whereas poor lipreaders sustained some diminution of visual acuity. These findings do not agree with those of Goetzinger (1964), who found that minor variations in acuity and in the phorias had no significant effect on lipreading performance.

NEEDS FOR FURTHER RESEARCH

There is still need for the development of a valid and reliable test of lipreading. This is not to say that the criteria that have been employed for the development of the various items within existing tests are not reasonable. However, in order to develop the items that really reflect the task of lipreading as it takes place in society at large and not within a restricted laboratory environment, test items must be selected from various situations in which hard-of-hearing persons find themselves as they go about their daily routines.

Still another need is to determine the amount of information that is available in the visual component of the spoken code. This has been worked out rather carefully for the acoustic aspect of the code, but one cannot generalize those results to the visual aspect. Homopheneity of words certainly makes the determination of the visual information quite a different task.

Yet another need is for researchers in the area of lipreading to acquaint themselves much more fully with the general, fast developing field of nonverbal communication. It would seem that this area gives promise of valuable information for those who would hope to understand the lipreading process completely.

REFERENCES

Aylesworth, D. L. 1964. The talker and the lipreader in face to face testing of lipreading ability. Unpublished masters thesis. Michigan State University, East Lansing.

Birdwhistell, R. L. 1970. Kinesics and Context. University of Philadelphia Press, Philadelphia. 338p.

Black, J. W., P. P. O'Reilly, and L. Peck. 1963. Self-administered training in lipreading. J. Speech Hear. Disord. 28: 183–186.

Bode, D. L., G. P. Nerbonne, and L. J. Sahlstrom. 1970. Speechreading and the synthesis of distorted printed sentences. J. Speech Hear. Res. 13: 115–121.

Byers, V. W., and L. Lieberman. 1959. Lipreading performance and the rate of the speaker. J. Speech Hear. Res. 2: 271–276.

Conklin, E. S. 1917. A method for the determination of relative skill in lip-reading. Volta Rev. 19: 216–220.

Cornett, R. O. 1967. Cued speech. Amer. Ann. Deaf. 112: 3–13.

Darwin, C. 1872. The Expression of Emotions in Man and Animals. John Murray, London (Republished. 1966. The University of Chicago Press, Chicago.)

Day, H. E., I. S. Fusfeld, and R. Pintner. 1928. A Survey of American Schools for the Deaf: 1924–1925. National Research Council, Washington, D.C.

Efron, D. 1941. Gesture and Environment. King's Crown, New York. (Republished 1972. Gesture, Race and Culture. Mouton, The Hague. 266p.)

Ekman, P. 1972. Universal cultural differences in facial expressions of emotions Symposium on Motivation, 1971. University of Nebraska Press, Lincoln.

Ellsworth, P. C., and J. M. Carlsmith. 1968. Effects of eye contact and verbal content on affective response to a dyadic interaction. J. Person. Soc. Psychol. 10: 15–20.

Erber, N. P. 1971. Effects of distance on the visual reception of speech. J. Speech Hear. Res. 14: 848–857.

Franks, J. R., and H. J. Oyer. 1967. Factors influencing the identification of English sounds in lipreading. J. Speech Hear. Res. 10: 757–767.

Goetzinger, C. P. 1964. A study of monocular versus binocular vision in lipreading. Report of the Proceedings of the International Congress on Education of the Deaf. Gallaudet College, June 22–28. U.S. Government Printing Office, Washington, D.C. pp. 326–333.

Greenberg, H. J., and D. L. Bode. 1968. Visual discrimination of consonants. J. Speech Hear. Res. 11: 869–874.

Greene, J. D. 1964. An investigation of the ability of unskilled lipreaders to determine the accented syllable of polysyllabic words. Unpublished masters thesis. Michigan State University, East Lansing.

Hall E. 1959. The Silent Language. Doubleday, Garden City, N.Y. 240p.

Hall, E. T. 1966. The Hidden Dimension. Doubleday, Garden City, N.Y. 201p.

Hardick, E. J., H. J. Oyer, and P. E. Irion. 1970. Lipreading performance as related to measurements of vision. J. Speech Hear. Res. 13: 92–100.

Harrison, R. P. 1974. Beyond Words: An Introduction to Nonverbal Communication. Prentice-Hall, Englewood-Cliffs, N.J. 210p.

Harrison, R. P., A. A. Cohen, W. W. Crouch, B. K. L. Genova, and M. Steinberg. 1972. Special Book Review Section: The Nonverbal Communication Literature. J. Commun. 22: 460–476.

Harrison, R. P., and M. L. Knapp. 1972. Toward an understanding of nonverbal communication systems. J. Commun. 22: 339–352.

Heider, F. K., and G. M. Heider. 1940. Studies in the Psychology of the Deaf. Psychol. Monogr. 52: 124–133.

Joergenson, A. 1962. The measurement of homophonous words. Unpublished masters thesis. Michigan State University, East Lansing.

Kelly, J. C. 1955. Audio-visual speech reading. University of Illinois. Monograph. 39p.

Kitchen, D. H. 1968. The relationship of visual synthesis to lipreading performance. Unpublished doctoral dissertation. Michigan State University, East Lansing.

Knapp, M. L. 1972. Nonverbal Communication in Human Interaction. Holt, Rinehart and Winston, New York. 213p.

Leonard, R. 1968. Facial movements of males and females while producing common expressions and sentences by voice and by whisper. Unpublished doctoral dissertation. Michigan State University, East Lansing.

Lloyd, L. L., and Price, J. G. 1971. Sentence familiarity as a factor in visual speech reception (lipreading) of deaf college students. J. Speech Hear. Res. 14: 291–294.

Lowell E. L. 1957. A film test of lip reading. John Tracy Research Papers II. John Tracy Clinic. Los Angeles, California.

Mason, M. K. 1942. A cinematographic technique for testing more objectively the visual speech comprehension of young deaf and hard of hearing children. Unpublished doctoral dissertation. The Ohio State University Department of Speech, Columbus.

Mehrabian, A. 1968. Relationship of attitude to seated posture, orientation, and distance. J. Pers. Soc. Psychol. 10: 26–30.

Morkovin, B. V. 1947. Rehabilitation of the aurally handicapped through the study of speech reading in life situations. J. Speech Hear. Disord. 12: 363–368.

Moser, H. M., J. J. O'Neill, H. J. Oyer, S. M. Wolfe, E. A. Abernathy, and B. M. Showe, Jr. 1960a. Historical aspects of manual communication. J. Speech Hear. Disord. 25: 145–151.

Moser, H. M., J. J. O'Neill, H. J. Oyer, E. A. Abernathy, and B. M. Showe, Jr. 1961. Distance and fingerspelling. J. Speech Hear. Res. 4: 61–71.

Moser, H. M., H. J. Oyer, J. J. O'Neill, and H. J. Gardner. 1960b. Selection of items for testing skill in visual recognition of one-syllable words. The Ohio State University Development Fund Project Number 5818, Columbus.

Mulligan, M. 1954. Variables in the reception of visual speech from motion pictures. Unpublished masters thesis. Ohio State University, Columbus.

Mykelbust, H. R., and A. I. Neyhus. 1970. Diagnostic test of speechreading. Grune & Stratton, New York.

Nielsen, H. B. 1970. Measurement of visual speech comprehension. J. Speech Hear. Res. 13: 856–860.

Nielsen, K. M. 1966. The effect of redundacy on the visual recognition of frequency employed spoken words. Unpublished doctoral dissertation. Michigan State University, East Lansing.

Nitchie, E. G. 1913. Moving pictures applied to lipreading. Volta Rev. 15: 117–125.

O'Neill J. J. 1951. Contributions of the visual components of oral symbols to the speech comprehension of listeners with normal hearing. Unpublished doctoral dissertation. Ohio State University, Columbus.

O'Neill J. J., and J. L. Davidson. 1956. Relationship between lipreading ability and five psychological factors. J. Speech Hear. Disord. 21: 478–481.

Oyer, H. J. 1961. Teaching lipreading by television. Volta Rev. 63: 131–132, 141.

Pauls, M. 1947. Speech reading. *In* H. Davis (ed.), Hearing and Deafness. Murray Hill Books, New York. p. 269.

Pesonen, J. 1968. Phoneme communication of the deaf. Ann. Acad. Sci. Fenn. Series B: 151–152.

Postove, M. J. 1962. Selection of items for a speechreading test by means of scaleogram analysis. J. Speech Hear. Disord. 27: 71–75.

Quigley, S. P. 1966. Language research in countries other than the United States. Volta Rev. 68: 68–83.

Reid, G. 1947. A preliminary investigation in the testing of lipreading achievement. J. Speech Hear. Disord. 12: 77–82.

Roback, I. M. 1961. Homophonous words. Unpublished masters thesis. Michigan State University, East Lansing.

Ruesch, J., and W. Kees, 1971. Nonverbal Communication: Notes on the Visual Perception of Human Relations. 2nd Ed. University of California Press, Berkeley, 205p.

Sahlstrom, L. J. 1967. Objective measurement of certain facial movements during production of homophonous words. Unpublished doctoral dissertation. Michigan State University, East Lansing.

Schwartz, J. R., and J. W. Black, 1967. Some effects of sentence structure on speechreading. Cent. States Speech J. 18: 86–90.

Simmons, A. A. 1959. Factors related to lipreading. J. Speech Hear. Res. 2: 340–352.

Stone, L. 1957. Facial cues of context in lipreading. Los Angeles School of Education, University of Southern California. John Tracy Clinic, Los Angeles.

Subar, B. E. 1963. The effects of visual deprivation on lipreading performance. Unpublished masters thesis. Michigan State University, East Lansing.

Tatoul, C. M., and G. D. Davidson. 1961. Lipreading and letter prediction. J. Speech Hear. Res. 4: 178–181.

The Journal of Communication. 1972. 22: 4.

Thomas, S. 1962. Lipreading performance as a function of light levels. Unpublished masters thesis. Michigan State University, East Lansing.

Utley, J. 1946. Factors involved in the teaching and testing of lipreading ability through the use of motion pictures. Volta Rev. 48: 657–659.

Vos, L. J. 1965. The effects of exaggerated and non-exaggerated stimuli on lipreading ability. Unpublished masters thesis. Michigan State University, East Lansing.

Measurement of Aural Speech Perception and Oral Speech Production of the Hearing Impaired

Carl W. Asp, Ph.D.
Professor and Director
Aural Habilitation and Rehabilitation
Department of Audiology and Speech Pathology
University of Tennessee

CONTENTS

INTRODUCTION

This chapter discusses some procedures for measuring the speech perception and production of hearing-impaired children and adults. It emphasizes techniques that have been developed in our laboratory. These techniques, such as a similarity scale, are used to quantify the results of an ongoing auditory training program for hearing-impaired children and adults. The training procedures for our program are modeled after the Verbo-tonal method (Guberina, 1964). References to other studies and techniques are used only to clarify points and to obtain a perspective.

Clinical research should not weaken or distract from the service that is provided, especially for young children who are in their formative years. The researcher should be accountable, and keep the well-being of the child and family in perspective at all times. The measurement techniques need to be brief, simple, and practical. Even with these constraints, this type of research can be very productive.

I became aware of the importance of measurement as a graduate student under Professor John W. Black. He stressed measurement as the key to understanding the speech and hearing process. It is not enough to see changes in behavior; one needs to measure them in order to understand the factors that contributed to these changes. Generally, it is easier to measure the perception and production of normal hearing people. However, studies with normal hearers may not be directly applicable to the perception of the hearing impaired (Rosen, 1962). For example, persons with high frequency losses probably use acoustic clues that are not recognized by normal hearers (Rhodes, 1966), or at least are not the primary clues.

The measurement techniques that are needed for the young deaf child are quite different than those that are needed for the adult with an acquired hearing loss. The deaf child has a problem with speech perception which affects his speech production; the lack of normal development of both limit the language competence and performance of the child. On the other hand, the hearing-impaired adult has normal speech production that makes it easier to evaluate the deficiency in speech perception. The adult can describe what he perceives. This type of measurement is more difficult with young deaf children.

This chapter emphasizes the perception and production of the speech signal. Although perception can be achieved from auditory, visual, tactile, or any combination of these sensory inputs, this discussion concentrates on auditory perception because this modality has been affected most by the hearing impairment. The greatest gains can be realized through the measurement and training of the impaired modality.

Highlighting the procedures in our laboratory risks the preliminary consideration of different techniques that have not withstood the scrutiny of time and usability. These procedures and the discussion that follows reflect the ideas, questions, and biases of this writer. Many of these procedures and ideas have been developed through contact with others, but this writer takes full responsibility for what is expressed in this chapter. Hopefully, these procedures provide a different reference point for evaluating the perceptual problems of the hearing impaired. We think some improvement has been made with these procedures, but we are not completely satisfied. Additional research is continually needed in this area.

This chapter is divided into: 1) oral speech production, 2) aural speech perception, 3) measurement of the effects of training, and 4) a summary. Each section is divided into testing procedures for deaf children and for hearing-impaired adults.

ORAL SPEECH PRODUCTION

Deaf Children

Deafness Deafness is one of the most severe handicaps. The factors that affect it are the time of onset, the degree, and the etiology of the hearing loss. If it is a prelingual hearing loss, it restricts the development of oral communication, and language competence and performance. In the case of early onset, the deaf child has both a perceptual and a linguistic problem. Measurement procedures need to take this into account.

The degree of the hearing loss is directly related to the severity of the communication problem. Audiometric criteria are usually used to classify the child as hard of hearing or deaf, or as having a mild, moderate, severe, or profound hearing loss.

The common etiologies are heredity, rubella, meningitis, high fever, and premature birth. There is also a large category of unknown etiologies. The severity and type of etiology is a major factor in determining the degree of success in habilitating the deaf child. More research is needed to determine the specific problems that result from each type of etiology.

Deafness is seldom, if ever, total. Huizing (1959) reported that 95–97% of the children in residential schools for the deaf have some measurable hearing, usually below 500 Hz. The task of auditory training is to develop perceptual skills with the use of measurable hearing. If a deaf child receives the proper training, he can function more like a hard-of-hearing child and possibly be integrated into a regular public school classroom. Figure 1 shows this integration model. On the other hand, if the proper training is not provided, a hard-of-hearing child may regress and function like a deaf child. It is not uncommon to find hard-of-hearing children in programs that emphasize manual communication. In these cases, the aural speech perception was not developed, causing these children to regress in oral communication skills and to have difficulty integrating with normal hearing children.

If the deaf child has a normal central nervous system, we hypothesize that he can be trained to compensate for the hearing loss by using the portion of the acoustic energy that is transmitted through the residuum of hearing to the brain. For example, by selecting auditory training stimuli which are pertinent to the frequency, intensity, and temporal discrimination deficits of the

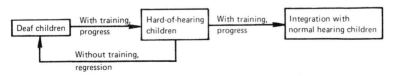

Figure 1. An integration model for training deaf and hard-of-hearing children for integration with normal hearing children.

individual it should be possible to improve significantly the hearing-impaired person's use of auditory information in communication (Danaher, Osberger, and Pickett, 1973).

Proper training during the early years is crucial to the child's development. The "normal" development of speech production seems to facilitate the perception of speech when both are trained together. If the child can develop adequate aural and oral communication skills, he should achieve normal educational, social, and vocational levels. Thus, the potential is great for the habilitation of deaf children. This potential can be achieved if sophisticated tools are available for the measurement and training of speech production and perception.

Intelligibility A multiple choice intelligibility test was developed that derives an intelligibility score for each speaker and a score for each listener (Black, 1957, 1963a, 1963b, 1968). The speaker score is determined by computing the mean score from the panel of listeners. The listener score is the mean score that a listener achieves from judging a series of speakers. This test has been used to evaluate the progress of students who are learning a foreign language. These students usually vary in speakers and listener intelligibility. A student may be a better speaker than a listener, and vice versa.

As speakers, some deaf children are very unintelligible, while other children become intelligible speakers after many hours of auditory training. The lack of speaker intelligibility makes it difficult to administer a standard test that uses the oral response (speech) of the child to determine a speech discrimination score. The listening experience of the tester is a factor in scoring this test.

Realizing this problem, a major study used as listeners teachers and college students who had experience in listening to the speech of deaf children (Hudgins and Numbers, 1942). The authors reported that persons totally naive with regard to speech of deaf pupils are of little value as auditors because they are often distracted by the peculiar voice qualities common to deaf pupils and thus lose much of the content. That is to say, the naive auditors would assign a poorer speaker score for the deaf pupils than would be assigned by the experienced teachers.

If listeners vary in ability to understand deaf speakers, the threshold of intelligibility must be unique for each listener, and this threshold must be affected by the listening experience of the listener. Relative to this threshold is a subintelligible region and an intelligible region. For example, a classroom teacher of deaf children may boast about the great improvement a deaf child has achieved and may provide an example of it for a naive classroom observer. The observer may be puzzled because the speech of the child is unintelligible and the observer cannot understand the point the teacher is attempting to make. What is intelligible for the teacher is not intelligible for the observer.

Thus, in order to evaluate the distorted speech patterns of deaf speakers, a procedure is needed that can measure both the subintelligible and intelligible levels. The procedure should be capable of quantifying and supporting the classroom teacher's example of the improvement in a deaf child. In addition, it should be usable for naive listeners to make valid judgments of deaf speakers. The most reasonable threshold of intelligibility is the one established by the naive listener because it determines if the deaf speaker will be intelligible to the majority of citizens in our society.

Several measures of the quality of deaf speech were developed by this author and are reported in an interim report (Asp, 1972) and a final report (Asp, 1973a). These measures are described and compared in the following sections. The author hopes they can be used successfully in other types of studies.

A Similarity Scale A similarity scale was developed that could be used by naive listeners to evaluate deaf speakers who varied in intelligibility (Asp and Alison, 1968). The tester spoke a word and a deaf speaker attempted to imitate it by speaking the same word. These pairs of speech samples (stimulus-response) were recorded, randomized, and judged by a panel of normal hearing college students, naive about the speech patterns of deaf speakers. A nine-point similarity scale of equal appearing intervals was used. The listeners assigned a number 1 if the response was totally similar to the tester's stimulus, and a number 9 if it was totally dissimilar. If neither was appropriate, the numbers between one and nine could be used to represent the degree of similarity. The tester had intelligible speech patterns. If the deaf speakers responses were judged to be totally similar, it was assumed that he was as intelligible as the tester.

We adapted this testing procedure to evaluate the progress of young deaf children (Asp, 1969, 1970). Fifteen one- and two-syllable words were selected that were familiar to young deaf children and represented a wide range of perceptual difficulty. These test words were spoken by the tester under four test conditions. These conditions evaluated the auditory perception of the children with and without visual clues, and with and without amplification. The similarity scores were better when both visual clues and amplification were available (Asp, 1969; Asp, 1973a; Asp, French, and Lawson, 1970a, 1970b). In fact, some children improved (a decrease in similarity score) even though their speech was not intelligible. Thus, changes in the subintelligible region were measured by this procedure even though they are not measurable by most other tests.

The next section establishes the threshold of intelligibility for the similarity scale and relates the similarity scores to other measures that could identify and explain the factors that are responsible for the changes in the children's performance.

Relationship of Intelligibility and Similarity Scores In order to identify the portion of the similarity scale that contributed to intelligible speech, the children's responses from the pairs of speech samples were separated from the tester's stimuli, randomized, dubbed on a separate tape, and judged by

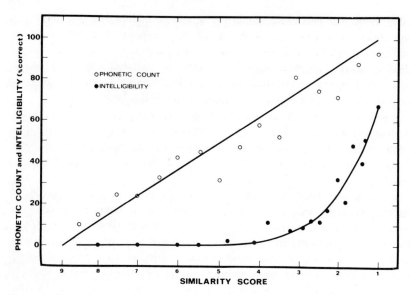

Figure 2. Phonetic count and intelligibility of deaf children in percentage of correct answers as a function of the similarity scores.

normal hearing college students (Asp, 1973a). The listeners wrote a word for each child's response. The mean intelligibility score in percentage of correct answers was computed for each interval of the similarity scale; these means are represented by the solid circles in Figure 2. The exponential line seems to be the best approximation of these data points.

Between 9 and 5 on the similarity scale, the scores were 0% correct in intelligibility. From 5 to 1 on the scale, the scores increased to approximately 70% correct for a scale value of 1. As a result, the midpoint on the scale (a value of 5) was considered the threshold or the beginning of intelligibility. It divided the scale into two distinct parts: the subintelligible region from 9 to 5, and the intelligible region from 5 to 1.

A comparison of these two measures revealed that children can achieve a significant improvement in similarity scores between 9 and 5 on the scale, and not be intelligible. The similarity scale is sensitive to changes in both the subintelligible and intelligible regions, making it useful for evaluating the progress of deaf speakers. On the other hand, the nonlinear growth of the intelligibility scores limits the usefulness of this measure for evaluating progress. Intelligibility tests should be used only with deaf speakers whose speech is intelligible because it is insensitive to changes in the subintelligible region.

The results of this comparison indicated that other measures were needed to determine the parameters that are responsible for the changes in the children's performance, especially in the subintelligible region. Some of th~~

changes, which may be considered as improvements, are necessary for establishing the normal patterns of rhythm and intonation.

Segmental Measures To further analyze these data, a phonetic transcription of each sample (stimulus and response) was written by a person highly trained in listening to the speech of the deaf. For each speech sample, the transcriptions were compared to determine the number of phonemes that were correctly imitated by the child's response. Next, a representative number of responses were selected at every half point (0.5) on the similarity scale. The mean percentage of correct phonemes for each interval are plotted as open circles in Figure 2. A Pearson correlation coefficient was computed between the phonetic count and similarity score. The coefficient was −0.96.

This indicated that a similarity score and a phonetic count were linearly related to each other. The diagonal line in Figure 2 approximated the linear relationship. Fifty percent of the phonemes are correct when the scale value is 5. Both of these correspond to the threshold of intelligibility for 0% correct. In other words, when the deaf child had 50% of the phonemes correct and a similarity score of 5, he was at the threshold of intelligibility for single word response.

Because of the linear relationship, the phonetic count can be used for evaluating the entire range from the subintelligible to the intelligible regions. It is less time consuming than obtaining similarity scores and therefore should be more feasible for evaluating progress in a clinical setting.

Suprasegmental Measures The similarity scale and the phonetic count are useful in evaluating progress in speech production from the subintelligible to the intelligible level. To estimate the contribution of the suprasegmental features to the correctness of the produced word, narrow- and wide-band spectrograms (Kay Elemetrics (Pine Brook, N.J.), model 6061A) were made for the speech samples (stimulus and response) for one testing condition. This reduced the amount of data for the analysis.

The following measurements were obtained from spectrograms: 1) mean fundamental frequency (F_o) in hertz, 2) intonational contour in percentage of correct contours, 3) syllable match in percentage of correct syllables, 4) voice duration in milliseconds and reported as a response/stimulus ratio, and 5) the latency in milliseconds for the time between the termination of the tester's stimulus and the onset of the child's response. Most of these measures were taken from the narrow-band display, with the wide-band display used to confirm the judgments. A description of the measurement procedures is provided in a final report of a research project (Asp, 1973a). The choice of the parameters was based on several studies (Lehiste, 1970; Eguchi and Hirsch, 1969) and on the experience of the writer.

Speech samples were grouped in equal intervals of 0.5 based on the similarity score that had been previously assigned to each sample. The mean and standard deviations were computed for each interval on the scale and are displayed graphically in Figure 3 as X's and open circles, respectively. The

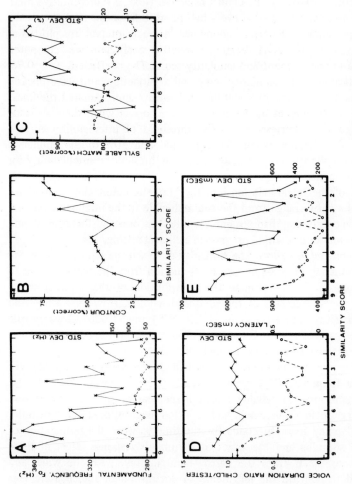

Figure 3. Acoustic measures of deaf children as a function of similarity scores: fundamental frequency (F_0) in hertz, intonational contour in percentage of correct contours, syllable match in percentage of correct matches, voice duration as a ratio, and latency in milliseconds. The X's represent the means, and the open circles represent the standard deviations. In addition, the means for normal hearing children are identified in the left ordinate by ← N.

units for the means are on the left ordinate of each graph, and the units for the standard deviations are on the right ordinate. (The standard deviations for Figure 3B could not be calculated.) For example, the interval 1.0–1.4 in Figure 3A had a mean F_0 of 285 Hz and a standard deviation of 51 Hz. In Figure 3C, the interval 8.5–9.0 had a mean syllable match of 74% and a standard deviation of 26%.

To estimate equivalent acoustic measures for normal hearing children, four normal hearing children of similar ages were evaluated by the same tester and the test procedure described earlier for the condition without amplification. These speech samples were analyzed spectrographically with the same procedure. The mean values for this group are identified by arrows ($\leftarrow$ N) on the left ordinate of each graph in Figure 3. These mean values for the normal hearing children are used as reference points in discussing the following measurements on the deaf children.

As the speech production improved from 9 to 1 in similarity score, the mean F_0 of the hearing-impaired children decreased to a value that was similar to mean F_0 for normal hearing children (see Figure 3A). It seems that training, maturation, and other factors contribute to this improvement. We believe that training is the most significant of these factors.

Intonational contour displayed a 51% improvement from 9 to 1 on the scale (see Figure 3B), and was slightly below the mean for normal hearing children.

Syllable match (see Figure 3C) improved 24%, and the final score exceeded the mean for normal hearing children. When deaf children achieved a similarity score of 1, their ability for syllable match received a higher score than the one for intonational contour.

The mean ratio for the voice duration (see Figure 3D) showed a gradual decrease as similarity score decreased. It approximated the mean value for normal hearing children. This implies that the child's voice duration changed from a duration that was longer than the tester's stimuli to a duration that was either equal to or less than the duration of the tester's stimuli.

The mean latency (see Figure 3E) tended to decrease but displayed great variability for adjacent intervals on the scale. The shortest latency for a similarity score of 1 was longer than the mean latency for normal hearing children. The deaf children showed some decrease, but seemed to take longer to respond to the stimuli than did normal hearing children.

A Pearson product moment correlation coefficient was computed between each of the above measures and the similarity scores (N = 16 subjects). (See Table 1.) Mean F_0, intonation, and syllable match had a higher correlation with the similarity scores than was detected for voice duration and latency, and may contribute more than the latter two measures to an improved similarity score.

Interaction among Intelligibility, Segmental, and Suprasegmental Features The similarity scale provides a separate measure and a unique way of

Table 1. Pearson product moment correlation coefficients between the similarity scores and the
measurements related to the suprasegmental aspects of children's responses

Measurements	Correlation coefficient
Fundamental frequency	+0.72
Intonational contour	−0.84
Syllable match	−0.87
Voice duration	+0.45
Latency	+0.48

comparing intelligibility, segmental, and suprasegmental features. The contribution of intelligibility and the segmental feature (phonetic count) are
easier to ascertain than the contribution of suprasegmental features of speech.
When the deaf child's speech is judged as totally dissimilar to the tester's
stimulus (a scale value of 9), both the intelligibility and phonetic feature are
0% correct, and the suprasegmental features are quite different than those for
normal hearing children. At the threshold of intelligibility (similarity score of
5), the segmental feature has improved to 50% correct, and the suprasegmental features have changed and are closer to those for normal hearing children.
The pitch of the deaf child's voice has decreased approximately 50 Hz, while
the intonation and the syllable match have improved approximately 25%.

One could assume that the 50% improvement in the segmental feature
was responsible for reaching the threshold of intelligibility, especially if
measures of the suprasegmental features were not available. The improvement
in intonation and rhythm (syllable match) probably is necessary for the
correct identification of segmental phonemes. These changes are occurring in
the subintelligible region and probably are essential for achieving a higher
level of intelligible speech.

Possibly some insights can be obtained by considering the speech development of normal hearing children. The young child who is 1.5 or 2 years old is
usually intelligible to the mother, but mostly unintelligible to a naive observer. Most children of this age have developed normal rhythm and intonation and are very capable of imitating the rhythm and intonation of others if
it is within their auditory memory span. Their suprasegmental patterns are
probably developed further than those of the hearing-impaired children when
both are at the threshold of intelligibility.

The habilitation of speech production and perception of young deaf
children should parallel the development for normal hearing children. This
suggests that the early stages of training should emphasize the development of
the suprasegmental aspects of speech rather than the segmental features. The
former seems to be more difficult to train and measure than the latter.

Measurement of Vocalizations Most young deaf children produce speech
with prolonged duration (Hudgins and Numbers, 1942). It seems that their

timing mechanism for the temporal aspects of speech is not functioning properly. These excessive prolongations affect the syllable rate, which in turn affects the intelligibility of their speech. It is necessary to have a measurement technique for quantifying this aspect of production.

A procedure was developed for measuring and controlling the vocalizations of young deaf children (Asp and Lawerence, 1970). This study showed that normal hearing children produce significantly more vocalizations (25/min) than did deaf children (8/min). The second part of the study demonstrated a significant increase in the rate of vocalization of the deaf children by using an operant conditioning technique with visual feedback. This increased rate of 25/min was comparable with that of normal hearing children. Thus, deaf children are capable of producing an adequate rate if the proper learning conditions are used.

As a follow-up, a wireless FM system was designed to measure the vocalizations from a remote location while the child was free to move in a natural environment (Asp, Wood, and Keller, 1971). Deaf and normal hearing children from 5 to 17 years of age were sampled. As before, the normal hearing children vocalized at a similar rate (23/min) regardless of age. However, the rate for deaf children was significantly different as a function of age. The rate was highest (8/min) for younger deaf children (5 and 7 years) and lowest (1/min) for older children (11, 13, 17 years). Regardless of the reason, the lower rate after 11 years of age reduces the chances of these children developing intelligible speech (Asp, Wood, and Keller, 1971).

One investigator reported that young deaf children who had received auditory training on a unit that had an extended low frequency response vocalized significantly more than children who were on a unit with a narrower frequency response. Both groups increased in vocalization rate and decreased in vocalization duration as a function of the training (Berry, 1972).

Distinctive Feature Analysis of Errors Earlier studies (Hudgins and Number, 1942) listed the common errors in the speech of the deaf but did not do a detailed analysis of the type of misarticulations. A recent study (Bradberry, 1970) analyzed the errors with a distinctive feature system (Singh, 1968). The children had fewer errors when both auditory and visual clues were available; however, there was less distinctive feature disparity of the errors when only auditory clues were available. Visual clues are helpful in minimizing errors, but they can be detrimental by increasing the magnitude of the distinctive feature difference.

The earlier section on suprasegmentals identified some acoustic measures that detected changes in the child's speech at the subintelligible level. A distinctive features system is needed to analyze the suprasegmental aspects of the child's speech. One investigator (Takefuta, 1974) used a computer simulation to analyze the intonational signals of listeners. He used a feature extraction by dividing fundamental frequency variations into four levels. This feature extraction seems to be a refinement of an earlier measure on the rate of pitch change (Fairbanks, 1940).

Fundamental frequency is an important parameter in both the intonation and the stress patterns of speech (Lehiste, 1970). Thus, it may be the starting point for developing a distinctive feature system for the suprasegmental aspects of speech.

Vibrotactile Input It has been our experience that the bone vibrator (oscillator) is a very useful transducer for improving the production and perception of young deaf children. At the outset of training, most young deaf children cannot discriminate speech through a headset or a bone vibrator on the head. However, most of them can discriminate speech patterns that are presented through a bone vibrator that is placed in their hand. When the vibrator is used in daily training, there is an improvement in rhythm and intonation. After a period of training, there is usually an improvement in their perception through the headsets.

Other investigators have reported that hearing-impaired children have better detection thresholds when a vibrator is used with the air-conduction signal (Bender, 1973).

We have found that the bone vibrator is also very helpful in improving the perception of adults with sensorineural hearing losses. The vibrator is placed on the head during the training session. Training increases the distance at which the person can perceive speech with the unaided ear. The increased distance probably signifies that the patient has learned to discriminate speech at a poorer speech-to-noise ratio.

Hearing-impaired Adults

If an adult has a postlingual hearing loss and has acquired normal linguistic skills, a standard picture articulation test can be administered to identify possible misarticulations. This is a relatively easy task for a well qualified speech pathologist. After a period of time, the hearing loss may affect the articulation of high frequency consonants such as fricatives and may affect the voice quality. Auditory training to correct the perceptual problem should eliminate the misarticulations and help the adult maintain an intelligible level of speech production.

AURAL SPEECH PERCEPTION

Deaf Children

The direct measurement of aural speech perception in young deaf children is a very difficult if not impossible task. One procedure is to have the child respond manually by pointing or pressing a button to identify the appropriate picture or object. The number and type of objects should be appropriate for the language level of the child. Miniature figures and toys can be used. To test the deaf child, the acoustic signal (speech) should be presented through an amplification system, such as a hearing aid or an auditory training unit, without visual clues. The child responds by identifying the object that corresponds to the spoken word.

If the task is too difficult for the deaf child, the test should begin by presenting the appropriate object and spoken word simultaneously, with visual clues available for both. After the child establishes the correct association, he can be tested without visual clues. The child attempts to identify the object that corresponds to the spoken word. If the child responds correctly, the order of the test should be reversed. The object should be presented and the child attempts to speak the correct word. If the child can both identify the correct object and produce the correct word, he probably is perceiving it correctly. However, if he can identify it and not produce it, he probably is capable of discrimination within a closed set of stimuli, but cannot produce it from auditory memory.

Most young deaf children cannot be evaluated with standard tests of speech discrimination, such as the CID auditory test W-22. The oral response may be unintelligible to the tester, and a written response may be affected by the lack of normal language ability. In these early stages of the child's development, it is necessary to make a detailed analysis of the child's production (e.g. phonetic count) in order to make any inferences of aural speech perception. However, after the child has developed some auditory perception and speech production through training, it is possible to use some standard tests for evaluating speech discrimination.

Hearing-impaired Adults

An adult with an acquired hearing loss is easier to test than a young deaf child because the adult usually has normal speech and language skills. An adult can respond by speaking what was heard or by writing a response. The speech stimuli can be presented live or recorded. For the live presentation, the speech discrimination score may vary for different speakers. The low pitched male voice is usually easier to perceive than a high pitched female voice.

Conventional Audiometric Test Clinical testing usually includes pure tone detection thresholds, a speech reception threshold, and a speech discrimination score for each ear. Although these tests are standardized and accepted in the United States, they do not provide specific information for determining the frequency response that is optimal for auditory training and hearing aid placement. For example, some adults with similar pure tone detection thresholds will perform quite differently on a suprathreshold test of speech discrimination while others will achieve the same discrimination score with different detection thresholds. It seems that the perception of some combinations of speech sounds is not affected by changes in the audiogram. A more appropriate test should consist of words or nonsense syllables that measure errors in speech discrimination that have resulted from a hearing loss at low, medium, or high frequencies. On the other hand, at least one investigator (Lipscomb, in press) questioned whether pure tone thresholds accurately reflect the amount of cell damage. It seems that additional tests are needed to supplement, confirm, or replace some of the audiometric tests currently in use.

Filtered and Nonfiltered Nonsense Syllables In order to develop new tests, recorded vowels were passed through an octave band-pass filter and normal listeners reported what they heard (Guberina, 1964, 1972). The octaves were 50–100, 75–150, 100–200, . . . , and 6,400–12,800 Hz. The responses of the listeners were analyzed to determine the octave band that had the most frequent perception of each vowel. This band was considered the optimal octave of the bands that were used. The following optimal octaves were identified: /u/, 150–300 Hz; /o/, 300–600 Hz; /a/, 600–1,200 Hz; /e/ 1,200–2,400 Hz; and /i/, 2,400–4,800 Hz. A similar experiment was conducted for consonants. Two of the optimal octaves for consonants are /b/ 150–300 Hz and /s/ 6,400–12,800 Hz. A listing of these can be found in an interim report (Asp, 1972).

Based on this concept, nonsense syllables were constructed with consonant and vowel with similar or adjacent optimal octaves (Guberina, 1964). These nonsense syllables (logatomes), /bru, mu, bu, vo, la, ke, ti, ʃi, si/, (Asp, 1972, 1973b; (Black, 1968) served as the basis for Verbo-tonal audiometry (Guberina, 1964). It was hypothesized that these logatomes would differentiate among hearing losses at low, medium, or high frequencies.

The nonsense syllable test includes paired syllables that were prerecorded and presented as either filtered or nonfiltered test stimuli. For the filtered test, for example, the paired nonsense syllables /bu-bu/ was prerecorded through the octave band-pass filter of 150–300 Hz, the nonsense syllable /si-si/ through the filter band 4,800–9,600 Hz, etc. Filtered stimuli are available from the lowest octave band of 50–100 Hz to the highest band of 6,400–12,800 Hz. Each nonsense syllable is recorded twice to provide the rhythm and linguistic redundancy of speech.

Both the filtered and the nonfiltered test stimuli (logatomes) are used to obtain detection thresholds for air conduction and for bone conduction for each ear. These thresholds are recorded as the hearing level in decibels. The filtered stimuli are compared directly with the pure tone stimuli. For example, the detection threshold for /bu-bu/ filtered through the 150–300 Hz band is compared with the threshold of the 250-Hz pure tone. These thresholds can be plotted on the same audiogram for a close visual comparison to identify any discrepancies that might occur.

For testing young deaf children, one study (Asp, 1973a) reported no significant difference between the air conduction detection thresholds for filtered logatomes and pure tone stimuli. In other words, the filtered stimuli confirmed the detection thresholds for the pure tone stimuli. However, our work with hearing-impaired adults suggests that the filtered nonsense syllables provide additional information. For example, the filtered stimuli may give better thresholds above 1,000 Hz than those measured with pure tone stimuli.

The detection thresholds of the nonfiltered logatomes are compared to the thresholds of the filtered logatomes and pure tone stimuli within the same frequency region. For example, the threshold for the nonfiltered logatome /si-si/ would be compared with both the filtered (4,800–9,600 Hz) threshold for /si-si/ and the pure tone threshold (6,000 Hz). The nonfiltered logatome usually has the better threshold because it may be detected by the more sensitive area of hearing, which is usually in the low frequencies. That is to say, the thresholds that have the greatest hearing loss cannot be responsible for the lower detection of the unfiltered logatomes.

Thresholds of intelligibility can be tested with both the filtered and nonfiltered stimuli by having the patient repeat what he hears. The intelligibility threshold is the lowest level where the patient can accurately identify each logatome. For some of the high frequency logatomes (e.g., /si-si/), a threshold of intelligibility may not be possible for the filtered logatome, even at the maximal level of the audiometer. However, it may be possible to establish it for the nonfiltered logatome. Comparisons between the thresholds for filtered and nonfiltered logatomes as well as detection and intelligibility thresholds are made. These thresholds can vary considerably. In some additional tests, logatomes are presented through unoptimal filtered bands. These tests are not discussed in this chapter, but this information is available in an interim report (Asp, 1972).

Tonality Word Test Peterson and Asp (1972) reported a significant correlation between the pitch of prevocalic consonants and the optimal octaves that were reported by Guberina (1972). The results of this study agree with Guberina's hypothesis that the optimal octave and the pitch of each phoneme are related. For the purpose of this discussion, the word tonality will be used to mean the pitch of the speech sounds that is perceived by the listener. This pitch probably includes more than the fundamental frequency (F_0) and probably contributes to the discrimination among the phonemes.

A monosyllabic word test was constructed in our laboratory based on the optimal octaves that were used for the nonsense syllable test described above. For each test word, phonemes (consonant (s) and a vowel) were selected that had the same or similar optimal octave. These stimuli were called tonality test words.

Test words were selected according to five tonality categories: 1) low, 2) low-middle, 3) middle, 4) middle-high, and 5) high. An example of a test word for each category is "moon, bud, cat, hit, see," respectively. Forty test words having the same or similar optimal octave were assigned to each tonality category. These test words are used regularly in our clinic to test hearing-impaired patients to determine the frequency response that would be optimal for auditory training and hearing aid placement.

For the clinical administration of this test, five words are randomly selected from each tonality category and are spoken orally by the tester in an unfiltered form. The test words are spoken naturally at normal conversational

Table 2. Results of a tonality test presented to a hard-of-hearing
patient with a high frequency sensorineural hearing loss[a]

	Low	Low-middle	Middle	Middle-high	High
1	+	+	− − (hot)	− +	− − − (six)
2	+	+	− +	+	− − − (east)
3	+	+	+	− − − (each)	− − − (since)
4	+	+	+	− − − (yeast)	− − − (itch)
5	+	+	+	+	− − − (teeth)
	100%	100%	60%	40%	0%

[a]A plus (+) is a correct response and a minus (−) is an incorrect response.
The words in the parentheses are the perceptual errors. With the first
presentation, 60% of 25 words were correct; with the second presentation,
8% of the words were correct. Therefore, the total percentage of correct
words was 68%.

level. If a test word is not perceived correctly, it is presented a second or a
third time. The percentage of correct responses is computed for each category
based on the response to the first presentation of each test word. Table 2
displays the typical results for testing an adult with an acquired high frequency, sensorineural hearing loss. In this example, the percentage of correct
responses for each category is: low, 100%; low-middle, 100%; middle, 60%;
middle-high, 40%; and high, 0%. For this patient the pure tone audiogram
usually would have a sharp downward slope toward the high frequencies and
no detection thresholds above 2,000 Hz.

This test is also scored in total percentage of correct words for all 25 test
words by adding the percentage of correct words for first (60%) and second
(8%) presentations (see Table 2). If the percentage of correct words for the
second presentation is 20% or greater, the intensity level (loudness) is increased and the patient is retested. The total percentage of correct words is
compared with the speech discrimination score as measured by the CID
auditory test W-22.

Articulation Curve Measured with Tonalities The speech discrimination
score depends on the presentation level in decibels. If the test is administered
at only one presentation level, a valid estimate of the patient's maximal
discrimination score can be obtained only when the score is 100%. If the
score is less than 100%, there is no way of knowing if it represents the
patient's best performance (Carhart, 1965).

Most audiologists use one presentation level at about 30 or 40 dB above
speech reception threshold. If the CID W-22 test list is used, this is referred to
as "PB Max" (Newby, 1964). In order to obtain a valid estimate of the
maximal discrimination score, it is necessary to present the test at several
presentation levels. Therefore, short wordlists are desirable to complete the
test in a reasonable amount of time. Some investigators have presented 10

test words at each presentation level, eliminated the use of a carrier phrase, and used successive presentation levels of 5 or 10 dB to plot the articulation curve (Asp, in press; Boothroyd, 1967). In one case, the same 30 phonemes (10 vowels and 20 consonants) were used for each list of 10 words. These were referred to as isophonemic word lists (Boothroyd, 1967).

In our laboratory, the test results indicate that grouping the speech sounds according to tonalities provides a systematic means of measuring and analyzing the perceptual errors that are attributable to the frequencies with the greatest hearing loss. As a result, the tonality words were used to construct a test to measure the speech articulation curve.

Twenty lists, with 10 words in each list, were tape recorded. Each list has two monosyllabic words from each of the five tonality categories described earlier. That is to say, there are two low, two low-middle, two middle, two middle-high, and two high-tonality words in each list. This test was standardized with normal hearing adults to determine the hearing level in decibels for the articulation curve.

The words are presented at 5-sec intervals without a carrier phrase. The rhythmic occurrence of the test words seems to alert the patient and reduce the need for an introductory phrase. We and other investigators (Boothroyd, 1967) have not detected any problems with this procedure, and it serves to shorten the testing time.

For the hearing-impaired patient, the level for speech detection is established. Then, 10 test words (one list) are presented at successive 10-dB steps above speech detection. These 10-dB increments are continued until the level of discomfort and/or the limit of the audiometer is reached. For more sample points, 5-dB increments can be used.

From these measurements, the articulation curve is plotted, displaying the percentage of correct words at each presentation level. The following information is available from this curve: 1) the patient's detection level for speech (e.g., 50 dB); 2) the hearing loss for speech, measured in decibels as the difference between the patient's detection threshold and that of normals; 3) the maximal percentage of correct words (e.g., 70%); 4) the level needed for the maximal percentage of correct words relative to 0 dB for normal listeners (e.g., 80 dB); 5) the intensity that the patient needed above his detection threshold to achieve maximal discrimination ($80 - 50 = 30$ dB); and 6) whether there was a decrease in the score after the maximal discrimination was achieved.

Optimal Field of Hearing The test results from our laboratory indicate that the frequency response of the amplification system is an important factor in auditory training and hearing aid placement for adults. We find the best test results when the frequency response and level includes the most sensitive area (residuum) of hearing plus any additional frequencies that may be needed. This frequency response will produce the best discrimination score at the lowest level. Guberina (1964, 1972) identified this as the optimal field of hearing (OFH). The identification of the OFH is a complex task that requires an experienced tester to adjust to the unique perceptual problems of each patient. The goal of this section is to discuss the rationale and measurement procedure for identifying the OFH.

One study demonstrated that patients with high frequency hearing losses had discrimination scores (58.8%) significantly better (28%) than those of normal hearing persons while listening to words that were passed through a 1,000-Hz low-pass filter (Rhodes, 1966). The frequency response of the filter was similar to the pure tone detection thresholds of the hearing-impaired patients, thus emphasizing the most sensitive area of hearing. Hearing-impaired patients probably use acoustic cues not recognized by normal hearers, and probably can learn to discriminate speech through existing hearing rather than resurrecting hearing that has not been used (Rhodes, 1966). These results seem to confirm our clinical observations of the importance of the OFH.

Other studies (Shore, Bilger, and Hirsh, 1960) found no difference among hearing aids with different frequency responses. These hearing aids emphasized the frequency region where the patients had the greatest hearing loss. If the measurements are limited to the area of the greatest loss, the chances of finding a difference are probably minimized. Another factor to be considered is that some conventional tests may be insensitive to these differences.

Previously in this section, three tests were discussed: a nonsense syllable test, a tonality word test, and a test to determine the articulation curve. We find that these tests in combination are useful for identifying the OFH. The following is our procedure for identifying OFH.

The detection thresholds for the filtered nonsense syllable test are compared to the thresholds obtained with pure tones. When the results of these two tests agree, the most sensitive area of hearing is identified. If there is some disagreement, it usually occurs in the high frequency region where the thresholds for filtered logatomes are better than those for the pure tones. The wider bandwidth of the filtered logatomes may be a factor in detecting this difference.

Next, the tonality word test is administered under the following conditions: 1) the unaided ear, with no amplification; 2) wide-band amplification, through the auditory training unit; 3) the filtered response of the training unit set to correspond to the OFH; and 4) a wearable hearing aid that corresponds to the OFH.

For the unaided test condition, the patient uses no amplification or acoustic system. With the nontest ear plugged, the tester speaks practice words at different distances in order to determine the distance that produces the most comfortable loudness (MCL) for the test ear. For example, the optimal distance may be 6 inches for one patient but 15 feet for another. The tester always speaks the words at a normal conversational level.

The tonality word test is administered at the distance for MCL. It is scored in percentage of correct words for each of the five tonality categories and also for the total score (see Table 2). For a patient with a high frequency hearing loss, discrimination scores will be poorer for the higher tonalities, as displayed in Table 2. That is to say, the results of the categories of the tonality test usually include the residuum of hearing, which suggests that the patient is perceiving better in frequency regions where there is more sensitivity.

Next, the patient is placed under earphones and tested with the wide-band amplification of the auditory training unit that is set for MCL. The total percentage of correct words for this condition is usually better than the total score for the unaided condition. Although both test conditions use MCL, the wide-band amplification probably produces a better discrimination score because of the better speech-to-noise ratio at the test ear. The relative difference among the five tonality categories in percentage of correct words usually is similar for both test conditions. For example, there may be a 40% difference between the middle-high and high categories for both conditions (see Table 2). For most patients, the use of wide-band amplification does not correct the perceptual errors for the high category.

With the unaided and wide-band test condition producing similar results, the wide-band condition can be eliminated in the test procedure after the tester has developed the skills necessary to obtain reliable results in the unaided condition. The most difficult task for the unaided condition is to establish the distance that produces MCL. There are at least two ways to check this. One is to make sure that the percentage of correct words that were presented a second time does not exceed approximately 20% (see Table 2). Another way is to decrease the distance (increase the intensity) for a test word that was not perceived correctly. If it is not a conductive hearing loss, the patient usually will not perceive the word correctly, even when the distance is reduced.

The test results from the unaided condition and the filtered logatome test usually agree for patients who have severe to profound hearing losses and have not worn a hearing aid. For these patients, the OFH usually corresponds closely to the residuum of hearing, and it is easy to identify. In some cases, however, patients who have worn a hearing aid and/or received auditory training will have an OFH that may be slightly different than would be expected.

The test results from the unaided tonality test and the filtered logatome test are then used to select the frequency response that will improve the speech discrimination scores. First, the auditory training unit (a multifilter system) is set to correspond to the residuum of hearing. For example, for a high frequency hearing loss, the unit might be set for a cutoff frequency of 1,000 Hz, with a slope of 6 dB/octave toward low frequencies and a 65-dB slope toward high frequencies. The patient is asked if the pitch of the testers voice is too high or too low. If this frequency response is near the OFH, the pitch will be normal. At this point, the tester may adjust the slopes, the cutoff frequency, or both to improve the quality of the sound. For some patients, this may include adding a high-pass or high-peaking filter where the patient is less sensitive, but it is kept below the detection threshold for these frequencies.

The patient is tested with the tonality word test for one or more of these frequency responses. The test scores are usually better for the filtered frequency response than for the unaided or the wide-band condition. For example, a patient may improve from 0% to 40% in the high category. The tester selects the filtered frequency response that produces the best test scores and identifies it as the OFH. Usually, the OFH includes the residuum of hearing and possibly some additional frequencies. The tonality test is valuable in determining OFH because it seems to be sensitive to perceptual errors of the patient.

The test results from nonsense syllable and the tonality tests are used to identify the OFH through the auditory training unit. For example, for a high frequency hearing loss, the training unit might be set for a cutoff frequency of 1,000 Hz, with a slope of 6 dB/octave toward low frequencies and a 65-dB slope toward high frequencies. The tonality test is administered through this frequency response and compared to the results for the unaided and wide-band amplification conditions. Usually, the filtered frequency response produces better discrimination scores for the tonality categories with the poorest scores.

Next, testing under earphones in a sound-treated booth determines the articulation curve that was described earlier. The speech level that is needed for the maximal discrimination on the curve is compared with the presentation level of the OFH determined earlier. If there is an agreement, the level and the frequency response are considered to be appropriate. If there is a disagreement, other frequency responses are evaluated with the tonality test to determine OFH.

After the initial diagnostic information is obtained and the OFH is determined, the patient is scheduled for individual auditory training, for two or three sessions per week. The OFH is set on the training unit for each ear separately. The OFH is reevaluated periodically with the tonality test to see if any modifications may improve aural perception of the patient. Training continues until the patient does not show any additional improvement in speech discrimination.

As mentioned earlier, the procedure for identifying the OFH is complex and requires an experienced tester. This procedure needs more research to make it less dependent on the tester's skills and more dependent on the systematic use of the tests. However, we have observed noticeable improvements with the patient's discrimination after the OFH is identified and trained properly. Essentially, we find that most patients can be trained to perceive most speech sounds through the OFH.

Hearing Aid Placement Hearing aids that have a frequency response and gain (in decibels) that is similar to the optimal field of hearing are selected for evaluation. The emphasis is on amplification where the patient is most sensitive. The tonality test is used to compare the aids; the aid with the best score is selected. If the score is less than the score for the OFH through the training unit, the patient receives additional auditory training through the aid. Then, the patient is tested in a sound-treated booth with the CID W-22 lists, and an articulation curve is determined using tonality word lists. If the test results agree, the patient is referred to a hearing aid dealer for purchase of the aid that corresponds to the OFH. This extensive program in measurement, training, and hearing aid placement usually results in a significant increase in the communication ability of the patient, for he is able to function better in both quiet and noisy conditions.

Other Test Conditions The test conditions that are used to evaluate the aural speech perception should similate and/or predict that patient's performance for the everyday listening conditions. Most diagnosticians test in quiet with a short reverberation time. This ideal condition does not similate a typical listening condition for the hearing-impaired patient. It is more realistic to vary the speech-to-noise ratio and reverberation time. The performance of hearing-impaired people is poorer at longer than at shorter reverberation times (T = 0.6 and T = 0.3 sec, respectively) while listening through a hearing aid in the presence of noise and in quiet (Nabelek and Pickett, 1974). The unaided testing conditions that were described earlier simulate a speech-to-noise ratio and reverberation time of everyday listening conditions.

Another factor to consider is the length of the test stimuli. The tonality words are also used to construct sentences that have words with similar tonalities. This is more typical for listening, but is more difficult to score.

Thus far, this chapter has emphasized the measurement and training of each ear separately. Recent research has identified the right ear (left temporal lobe) as predominant for verbal acoustic functions, especially for consonants (Berlin and Lowe, 1972; Kimura, 1961). For a hearing-impaired patient, the right ear may have poorer detection thresholds than the left ear. Therefore, in this case it seems logical to spend more time training the left (better) ear. However, we have encountered some problems when the right ear is less sensitive than the left ear. Possibly both ears should not be trained equally, if one is to serve as the preferred ear. Investigators need to evaluate this potential problem more thoroughly, possibly by testing and comparing with a binaural condition.

The tests that have been described in this chapter used percentage of correct responses as a measure of speech discrimination and failed to emphasize the importance of analyzing the perceptual errors of the patient. We use the tonality criterion for analyzing the direction of the errors. For example, if the error (response) is lower in tonality than the stimulus, then the frequency response needs to be adjusted to compensate for this error. The type and the direction of the error provides important information for diagnosis and training.

MEASUREMENT OF THE EFFECTS OF TRAINING

Deaf Children

The speech production of deaf children is often unintelligible without training and cannot be measured with standard procedures for evaluating speech intelligibility. Thus, a new procedure was developed and identified as the similarity scale. It is described in an earlier section.

Twenty young deaf children received daily auditory training by the Verbo-tonal method (Asp, 1973a) and were tested at 4-month intervals according to the procedures described in the earlier section on the similarity scale. The test conditions were:

1. *Without* visual clues and *without* amplification ($\overline{\mathrm{VA}}$)
2. *Without* visual clues and with amplification ($\overline{\mathrm{V}}\mathrm{A}$)
3. With visual clues and *without* amplification ($\mathrm{V}\overline{\mathrm{A}}$)
4. With visual clues and with amplification (VA)

There was a significant improvement (a decrease in similarity score) ($P <$ 0.0001) over the first three test times (test 1 = 7.6, test 2 = 7.1, and test 3 = 6.8). The testing conditions with amplification (7.1) were slightly better than without amplification (7.2), but the difference was not significant ($P < 0.07$). The testing condition with visual clues (7.0) was significantly better ($P < 0.002$) than without visual clues (7.3). The interactions were not significant. In other words, these deaf children improved significantly in reception/production skills as a function of training and showed better scores when both visual clues and amplification were available. The similarity scale was sensitive enough to detect these differences.

Figure 4 displays the similarity scores for two of these children, one with a 90-dB hearing loss and one with a 78-dB hearing loss. The left ordinate represents the similarity score; the abscissa represents eight tests at 4-month intervals. The child in Figure 4A had a similarity score of 9.0 for all four test conditions at test 1. She improved on all these conditions over the eight tests. The right ordinate shows the scales for phonetic count and intelligibility. She achieved at least 80% correct on the phonetic count at test 8.

Figure 4B displays another child who showed a different pattern of improvement. She also improved on all four test conditions.

With regard to measurement of the suprasegmental features, both children showed a significant decrease in mean fundamental frequency (F_o). In addition, the child in Figure 4B had a significant improvement in syllable match. Both children improved significantly in the latency of their response.

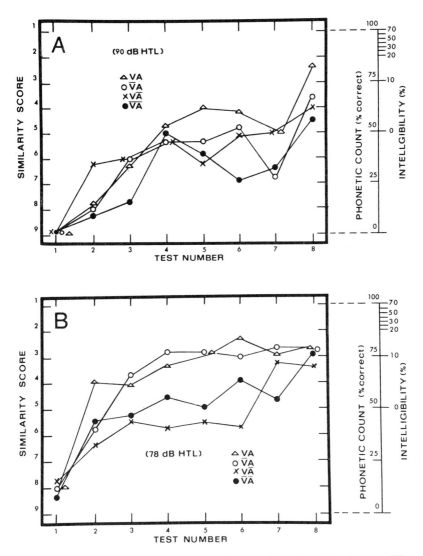

Figure 4. Mean similarity scores for two subjects as a function of four test conditions and the relationships of these scores to phonetic count and intelligibility.

Hearing-impaired Adults

For young deaf children, it takes years of daily training to achieve a level where they can communicate effectively with their normal peers. Most hard-of-hearing adults can be rehabilitated in 1–3 months and achieve a 20% or more improvement in speech discrimination. The following are some examples of typical adult cases that have improved their oral communication

Table 3. Percentage of correct responses for a high frequency and a low frequency hearing aid according to the five tonality categories and the total score for all five categories

Type of hearing aid response	Tonality categories in percentage of correct responses for 1st presentation					Total score for 1st and 2nd presentations
	Low-middle	Low-middle	Middle	Middle-high	High	
High frequency	80	100	80	80	20	80
Low frequency	100	100	100	100	100	100

by receiving auditory training and hearing aid placement that emphasized their most sensitive area of hearing.

Case 1 A 47-year-old counselor has a high frequency sensorineural hearing loss. Earlier, he had been fitted with a conventional hearing aid that amplified mostly high frequencies where he had the greatest hearing loss (see Table 3). He could not understand speech through this aid, especially in noisy situations. He was referred to our program where another aid was selected that emphasized the low frequencies at which he had better hearing; therefore less amplification was needed. The low frequency aid produced a 20% improvement in the total scores, and an 80% improvement in the high tonality category (see Table 3). This improvement was achieved by fitting the aid to the OFH, and using a brief period of training. He has been able to continue his work as a counselor.

Case 2 A 39-year-old veterinarian had a high frequency, sensorineural hearing loss in both ears. He was fitted with a high frequency hearing aid by a local hearing aid dealer but could not adjust to it in noisy situations. He was referred to our program for training and testing. Before training, the tonality score through the auditory training unit with it set on the OFH (96%) was 14% better than the score with a flat frequency response (82%) through the unit. His unaided score was 44%. After auditory training, there was a 48% improvement in the unaided score (44–92%) at the same distance of 7 feet. In addition, he achieved a score of 84% through the hearing aid using only the left ear, and 100% using both ears. This allowed him to improve his ability to function as a veterinarian.

Case 3 A 48-year-old business man had a moderate to severe mixed hearing impairment at the right ear and a profound sensorineural loss at the left ear. Results are presented for the right ear only. His speech reception threshold improved 15 dB, and speech discrimination (W-22) improved 18% at a 5-dB lower presentation level. His tonality score improved 20%. Speech discrimination through a hearing aid improved 16% (from 76% to 92%).

Case 4 A 68-year-old housewife had a mild to moderate presbycusic type of hearing loss. Initial testing indicated speech reception thresholds of 45 dB bilaterally, and a speech discrimination score of 82% at the right ear at normal conversational level (50 dB). At the left ear, speech discrimination ability improved 24% at the same presentation level.

SUMMARY

This chapter offers some unique procedures for measuring aural speech perception and oral speech production of hearing-impaired children and adults. The new testing measures used with the children are for evaluating progress in speech production from the subintelligible to the intelligible level. These measures include: 1) the similarity scale, 2) the phonetic count, and 3) a battery of acoustic measures which include fundamental frequency, intonation contour, syllable match, voice duration, and latency. The similarity scale and the phonetic count measure the entire continuum from the subintelligible to the intelligible level. Both provide a single measure that is easier to interpret than the acoustic measures. Of these two, the phonetic count is the more practical measure, since it is easier and less time consuming to obtain in a clinical situation. Acoustic measures, however, provide more insight into the suprasegmental development of the speech because several parameters can be studied simultaneously.

For the hearing-impaired adult, the tonality word test, the nonsense syllable test, and the articulation curve provide some unique information for diagnosis, training, and hearing aid placement. The optimal field of hearing usually produces better speech discrimination scores than wide-band amplification or a frequency response that amplifies the frequencies that have the greatest hearing loss. With training, some patients achieve a high discrimination score through the OFH, even though the frequency response does not include most of the energy for the second formant. For example, some patients can achieve a high score through a 600-Hz low-pass filter.

The intent of this chapter is to spur a greater interest in developing and evaluating measurement procedures for hearing-impaired people. Measurement is the key to isolating and understanding the perceptual problems of the hearing impaired, and finding solutions to these problems. Although this chapter does not review all possible procedures, hopefully it does identify new areas that need more research so that the appropriate measurement techniques can be developed.

ACKNOWLEDGMENT

Professor John W. Black was the person who stimulated me to stress measurement techniques for gaining more knowledge of the speech and hearing process. His tireless efforts as a teacher, researcher, colleague, and a friend have been outstanding. I would like to thank him for providing this stimulation for me and others.

I would also like to thank A. K. Nabelek, P. J. Carney, J. S. Berry, and A. P. Stewart for making suggestions for this chapter.

REFERENCES

Asp, C. W. 1969. Some results of aural habilitation of preschool deaf children. Presented at the Tennessee Speech and Hearing Association, Nashville.

Asp, C. W. 1970. A design to evaluate low-frequency amplification for habilitating preschool deaf children. J. Acoust. Soc. Amer. 48: 87(A).

Asp, C. W. 1972. The effectiveness of low-frequency amplification and filtered-speech testing for preschool deaf children. An Interim Report for the Bureau for Education of the Handicapped, HEW. Project 522113. ERIC Document Reproduction Service (Report ED-065-977), Bethesda, Md.

Asp, C. W. 1973a. The effectiveness of low-frequency amplification and filtered-speech testing for preschool deaf children. A Final Report for the Bureau of Education for the Handicapped, HEW. Project 522113. ERIC Document Reproduction Service, Bethesda, Md.

Asp, C. W. 1973b. The Verbo-tonal method as a alternative to present auditory training techniques. In J. W. Wingo and G. F. Holloway (eds.), An Appraisal of Speech Pathology and Audiology: A Symposium, pp. 134–145. Charles C Thomas, Springfield, Ill.

Asp, C. W. The Verbo-tonal method; Innovative aural rehabilitation for the adult deaf person. Deafness. Professional Workers with Adult Deaf, Inc. Silver Spring, Md. In press.

Asp, C. W., and C. Alison. 1968. A procedure for evaluating the aural habilitation of hearing-impaired children. Presented at the American Speech and Hearing Association, Denver.

Asp, C. W., E. French, and G. Lawson. 1970a. A preliminary evaluation of some aspects of the Verbo-tonal method as utilized at the University of Tennessee. Presented at the 10th International Audiological Convention, Dallas.

Asp, C. W., E. French, and G. Lawson. 1970b. Visual and/or auditory clues as a function of therapy time, familiarity, and phonetic content in a preschool deaf population. Presented at the American Speech and Hearing Association, New York.

Asp, C. W., and C. Lawerence. 1970. Measurement and operant conditioning of the vocalizations of preschool deaf children. J. Acoust. Soc. Amer. 47: 129(A).

Asp, C. W., W. S. Wood, and J. Keller. 1971. Vocalization rate of deaf and normal-hearing children. J. Acoust. Soc. Amer. 50: 140(A).

Bender, R. 1973. Thresholds of hearing of normal and hard of hearing children with and without a supplementary tactile vibrator. Volta Rev. 75: 47–53.

Berlin, C. I., and S. S. Lowe. 1972. Differential diagnostic evaluation: Central auditory function. In J. Katz (ed.), Handbook of Clinical Audiology, pp. 280–312. Williams & Wilkins, Baltimore.

Berry, J. 1972. The rate and duration of the vocalizations of preschool deaf children receiving two types of amplification and the Verbo-tonal method. Unpublished thesis. University of Tennessee, Knoxville.

Black, J. W. 1957. Multiple-choice intelligibility tests. J. Speech Hear. Disord. 22: 213–235.

Black, J. W. 1963a. Multiple-choice intelligibility tests, forms A and B. J. Speech Hear. Disord. 28: 77–186.

Black, J. W. 1963b. Multiple-Choice Intelligibility Tests. Interstate Printers and Publishers, Danville, Ill.

Black, J. W. 1968. Perception of altered acoustic stimuli by the deaf. A study for Social and Rehabilitation Services, HEW. Grant RD-1226-5-68-C4.

Boothroyd, 1967. Developments in speech audiometry. Presented at the Inaugural Meeting of the British Society of Audiology.

Bradberry, M. E. 1970. A distinctive feature analysis of initial consonants of preschool deaf children who received Verbo-tonal therapy. Unpublished thesis. University of Tennessee, Knoxville.

Carhart, R. 1965. Problems in the measurements of speech discrimination. Arch. Otolaryngol. 82: 253–260.

Danaher, E. M., J. J. Osberger, and J. M. Pickett. 1973. Discrimination of format frequency transitions in synthetic vowels. J. Speech Hear. Res. 16: 439–451.

Eguchi, S., and I. G. Hirsch. 1969. Development of speech sounds in children. Acta Otolaryngol. (suppl.): 257.

Fairbanks, G. 1940. Recent experimental investigations of vocal pitch in speech. J. Acoust. Soc. Amer. 11: 457–466.

Guberina, P. 1964. Verbo-tonal method: Its application to rehabilitation of the deaf. Proceedings of the International Congress in Education of the Deaf. U.S. Government Printing Office, Washington, D.C.

Guberina, P. 1972. Case studies in the use of restricted bands of frequencies in auditory rehabilitation of deaf. Office of Vocational Rehabilitation, HEW. Contract OVR-YUGO-2-63.

Hudgins, C. V., and F. D. Numbers. 1942. An investigation of the intelligibility of the speech of the deaf. Genet. Psychol. Monogr. 25: 289–392.

Huizing, H. C. 1959. Deaf mutism: Modern trends in treatment and prevention. Ann. Otol. Rhinol. Laryngol. 5: 74–106.

Kimura, D. 1961. Some effects of temporal-lobe damage on auditory perception. Can. J. Psychol. 15: 156–165.

Lehiste, I. 1970. Suprasegmentals. MIT Press, Cambridge, Mass. 194 p.

Lipscomb, D. What is the audiogram really telling us. Parts 1 and 2. Maico Audiol. Lib. Ser. In press.

Nabelek, A. K., and J. W. Pickett. 1974. Monaural and binaural speech perception through hearing aids under noise and reverberation with normal and hearing-impaired listeners. J. Speech Hear. Res. 17: 724–739.

Newby, H. 1964. Audiology. Appleton-Century-Crofts, New York. 400 p.

Peterson, H., and C. W. Asp. 1972. The perceived pitch of 23 prevocalic consonants. J. Acoust. Soc. Amer. 52: 146(A).

Rhodes, R. 1966. Discrimination of filtered CNC Lists by normals and hypacusics. J. Aud. Res. 6: 219–133.

Rosen, J. 1962. Phoneme identification in sensorineural deafness. Unpublished doctoral dissertation. Stanford University, Stanford, Cal.

Shore, I., R. C. Bilger, and I. J. Hirsh. 1960. Hearing aid evaluation: Reliability of repeated measurement. J. Speech Hear. Disord. 25: 152–170.

Singh, S. 1968. A distinctive feature analysis of responses to a multiple-choice intelligence test. Int. Rev. Appl. Linguist. 6–1: 37–53.

Takefuta, Y. 1974. Analysis of intonational signals by computer simulation of pitch-perception behavior in human listeners. A study for the Department of the Navy. Contract N00014-67-A-0232-0003, Office of Naval Research, Arlington, Virginia.

Measurement of Hearing by Tests of Speech and Language

John J. O'Neill, Ph.D.
Professor and Head
Department of Speech and
Hearing Science
University of Illinois

CONTENTS

Speech has been used to evaluate hearing since the early days of otological practice. Voice and whisper tests were used, and are still being used, to determine hearing acuity as well as to assist in the determination of the anatomic location of the hearing problem. Present day testing practices have moved to the use of controlled speech samples to assist in the determination of the "site of lesion" as well as to determine communicative efficiency. The latter approach has great appeal because it assists in determining how a loss of hearing may have affected developing and existing language ability and how reductions in hearing acuity have affected academic and vocational performance. In essence, the major reason for using speech to evaluate hearing capacity is that individuals usually request such an evaluation because they have not been hearing the speech of others as well as they should or as well as they would like to.

Speech samples also have been used to evaluate the transmission qualities of telephone systems and other voice communication systems where the major concern in such instances is how well the speech of others is understood when transmitted through such systems.

INTRODUCTION

Interest in the use of speech and language samples as measures of hearing has been centered around two orientations, a philosophic-research orientation and a practical-clinical orientation. The first orientation has resulted in research in areas such as experimental phonetics, intelligibility, the appraisal of voice transmission systems, the effects of various types of distortion upon the reception of speech, listening ability, speaker identification, and areas of linguistics such as learning of language, language barriers, and the effects of context. The second orientation has led to research in areas such as the effects of hearing loss upon the reception of speech, auditory processing, the effects of amplification, and modifications in the range of reception of speech. The second area of interest grew out of the research in the first area. Once there was some understanding of how the normal auditory mechanism received and processed speech, it was only natural that there would be an interest in evaluating how a faulty auditory system (faulty because of pathology or interference in the system) would receive and process speech. The first area, in a sense, provided a yardstick that could be used to measure the effects of various types of interference upon auditory transmission.

In this chapter attention is directed toward describing how speech stimuli, other than isolated phonetic units, have been used to evaluate hearing or listening ability. Attention is focused on a review of approaches that have used words and other, longer connected units of speech to evaluate normal and disordered hearing acuity. The aim is not to explain how certain sounds or the spectra of individual speech units contribute to the recognition of speech or how such discrete elements explain the process of speech. Rather, efforts are directed toward explaining how certain forms of meaningful speech stimuli have been used to evaluate the function of the ear. What follows is not intended to be an exhaustive survey of the research literature.

Rather, it will reflect an effort to cite representative studies that have contributed to the basic concepts of the areas under discussion.

Philosophic Orientation

Under this heading attention is directed to an area that has been labeled by Curtis (1954) as psychophysical phonetics and by Black and Singh (1968) as the psychological basis of phonetics.

Malmberg (1966) indicated that the knowledge we can have of speech sounds depends entirely but not exclusively on the acoustic characteristics of the ear. In a further elaboration of this viewpoint Flanagan (1965) indicated that speech is a multidimensional signal that elicits a linguistic association. He warned that theorizing about speech perception with its linguistic and over-learned functions abounds with pitfalls. He further indicated that while intelligibility and articulation tests can help to identify factors upon which perception depends, they cannot supply a description of the process itself.

An excellent orientation to this chapter can be developed in terms of part of Black's (1968) comprehensive definition of speech perception: "Speech perception is the identification of phonemes, that is, the vowels and conso-nants of language, largely from acoustic cues, and the recognition of pho-nemes in combination as a word." Also, he listed other clues such as rules of syntax, linguistic probabilities, precision of utterance, interfering noise, and familiarity with the language. Attention in this chapter is not directed toward the items (vowels and consonants) listed in the first part of Black's definition.

The study of the acoustic characteristics of speech has mainly involved research in the identification of various identifiable parts of audible speech by the ear of a listener. Thus, if we are to discuss the identification of words or the confusability of speech, we will need to depend upon the auditory preception of these elements. For example, if we are to evaluate intelligibility and articulation, we will need the ear or ears of listeners to identify or sort out such phenomena before any instrumental evaluations can be made. Furthermore, if judgments of vocabulary, grammar, and other linguistic aspects are to be made, a listener must make the initial judgments. Thus, it should be obvious that if we are to have any understanding of the perception of speech or language, there will always be the need to start from an auditory perception of what was uttered.

Initial research in speech processing involved the study of factors that contributed to the successful transmission of speech. The earliest work in this area is exemplified by tests developed at the Bell Telephone Laboratories in the 1920's for the evaluation of telephone systems. Later, other tests of speech perception were developed to test the adequacy of voice transmission systems used in the military services. These studies were undertaken at the Harvard Psychoacoustic Laboratory, Waco Air Force Base (Waco, Tex.), and the United States Naval School of Aviation Medicine (Pensacola, Fla.). Along with the studies of voice transmission systems went the need to understand the factors that make for successful transmission of speech by a variety of users of the systems.

More recently, research focusing on topics such as the distinctiveness of speech (dialect, stress, etc.) has received considerable attention along with studies of the contributions that linguistic elements such as vocabulary and grammar have upon the transmission of information. The direction of the research has followed a basic "philosophic itch" brought on by the desire to have a better understanding of how the various elements of human speech contribute to the transmission of information.

A final area of interest involves the study of the contributions that various linguistic elements provide in the above mentioned transmission of information. Examples of such an approach are exemplified in reports by Black (1963) and recent interests in speech perception and auditory processing in articles by Aten (1972) and Weener (1972).

Practical Reasons

As previously stated, the emphasis of this chapter is on the applied aspects of speech perception as they relate to the evaluation of normal hearing and faulty hearing.

Interestingly enough, the first printed statement concerning the use of speech to evaluate hearing dealt with its use in a clinical vein. In 1874, Wolf indicated that he felt the human voice was the "most perfect conceivable measure of hearing." In 1890, he recorded on an Edison wax cylinder words which were then used in the testing of the hearing of his patients.

BASIC RESEARCH ON WORD TESTS

Normal Hearing

The Bell Telephone Laboratories were responsible for the development of the first test lists to be used in the evaluation of telephone systems. Individuals such as Campbell and Crandall and Fletcher were identified with the development of these lists. Fletcher utilized the results obtained from such tests to develop measures of the frequency and intensity characteristics of the various sounds in the English language. Also, he developed a series of word lists and vowel and consonant lists. The lists were developed so that listeners not familiar with phonetic transcription could be used in the studies of telephone systems. A few years later Nussbaum (1927) developed a word test which was to be used in spoken voice tests. The words were selected on the basis of having sounds that were of uniform acoustic value.

With the advent of World War II, considerable research effort went into the development of speech tests to be used in the evaluation of military communication systems and equipment. A major share of the research was carried out at the Harvard Psychoacoustic Laboratory. This research, initiated in 1941, led to the development of the Harvard spondee, phonetically balanced (PB), and sentence tests. The first two tests were based on several assumptions that were to stay with the area of speech testing up until the present time. The construction of the spondee tests was based on the concept of threshold for speech being defined as the intensity level at which a group of listeners was able to discriminate 50% of the items. Also, certain basic criteria were employed in the development of the spondee lists: 1) the words used should be a normal representation of English speech sounds; 2) the words should be familiar to the listener; 3) the test items should be dissimilar in phonetic construction; and 4) the test items should have similar audibility values. In the instance of the PB word lists, 20 lists of 50 words each were constructed. The words that were grouped on the basis of phonetic similarity to the first part of each word were selected to conform to the following criteria: monosyllabic structure, equal average difficulty, equal range of difficulty, equal phonetic composition, a composition that was representative of English speech, and words that were in common usage. These two tests received extensive use in clinical situations by Hallowell Davis and his colleagues at the Central Institute for the Deaf. The PB word lists were officially adopted in 1960 by the American Standards Institute as part of its standards for measurement of monosyllabic word intelligibility.

Concurrent with the research being done at Harvard, a voice communication training program was being established at the Voice Communication Laboratory (VCL) at Waco Air Force Base. Haagen (1944) developed 24 write-down tests. The words used in the tests were selected from the most frequently used words listed in Thorndike's book of 20,000 words. The lists were equated on the basis of the reception scores obtained by a panel of listeners while they listened over an airplane intercommunication system in the presence of simulated aircraft noise. Also, while the Harvard approach required the repeating of the words that were heard, the Haagen method required listeners to write down their responses. Because of difficulties associated with write-down tests, Haagen (1945) developed a second test of 24 equated lists which were cast into a multiple choice format. The words which were used in the multiple choice test were selected from error responses to the test words in the original write-down test, and they were grouped with the selected test word. The resulting multiple choice tests were judged to be satisfactory in terms of three criteria. First, each of the lists of 24 words was not significantly dissimilar in terms of mean difficulty. Second, the tests distinguished between trained and untrained listeners. Third, the items were internally consistent.

The multiple choice lists were used in research at Purdue University (Lafayette, Ind.) and the Acoustic Laboratory of the United States Naval School of Aviation Medicine. The latter program was later expanded as a joint program with the Ohio State University (Columbus, Ohio) and involved over 10 years of research which was concentrated on several areas of interest: problems of voice intelligibility, the effects of voice level upon intelligibility, listening behavior, the effects of side tone, and the language of voice communication. Also, two more forms (C and D) of the multiple choice test were developed.

In 1952 another project under the sponsorship of the United States Air Force was initiated at Ohio State University. This project, under the direction of Henry Moser, was concerned with research on the language of voice procedures used in Air Force Operations. Also, the project was involved in the development of an international voice radio language for air operations. The two Ohio State projects were terminated in the early 1960's. Some of the major findings from these projects are discussed in the sections that follow.

Defective Hearing

Tillman and Olsen (1973) have provided a comprehensive review of the development and clinical applications of the Harvard tests as well as similar discussions of the CID auditory tests W-1, W-2, and W-22, the CNC lists, and such multiple choice tests as the Fairbanks' Rhyme Test, the Modified Rhyme Test, and a multiple choice form of the CID W-22 test. Rather than repeat that review, attention is directed toward the reporting of a few, representative clinical studies. Oyer and Doudna (1959) evaluated the test results obtained by 400 defective ears for the W-22 auditory test and found that the most common type of error response was the substitution of some word other than the correct word. Ears with nonconductive hearing losses gave results which indicated more confusions for both vowels and consonants than did ears with a conductive loss. In a later study Oyer and Doudna (1960) found that 38 of the 200 PB words accounted for 50% of the total errors made by their hard-of-hearing subjects. One hundred eighty-one hearing-impaired subjects were administered W-22 tests by Schultz (1964). The results indicated that there was a clustering of responses in terms of highly familiar words and that words not included in the 10,000 most familiar made up 14% of the incorrect responses. The possibility of using the VCL word lists developed by Haagen in the testing of hearing was investigated by Doyne and Steer (1951). They found that the test could be used in clinical evaluation. The threshold for the VCL test was 26 dB as compared to 15 dB for Auditory Test 9.

Other Tests

Irwin (1947) developed a test that would assess the acuity for speech as well as the semantic skills of the listener. This test was not developed for commercial use. Experimental word lists consisting of paired series which differed only in voicing, pressure pattern, or influence, as determined from analysis with the visible speech unit of the Bell Telephone Laboratories, were developed by Siegenthaler (1949). One hundred twelve words were used in the test. They differed on the basis of differences between voiced and unvoiced consonants. When the test was used with hard-of-hearing subjects the results indicated that persons with different types of hearing losses gave different responses to the test words. A new set of test words was developed with the words being placed in three groupings of 45 words. One group contained only voicing differences, a second group contained only pressure pattern differences, and the final set contained only individual differences. Experimental results indicated that the test did not differentiate between types of hearing loss.

Sentence Tests

Some researchers have felt that single word tests do not provide a true picture of a listener's ability to receive everyday speech. They indicate that tests utilizing longer units, such as phrases or sentences, might provide a better indication of everyday listening ability. The earliest sentence tests were developed at the Bell Telephone Laboratories by Fletcher and Steinberg (1929). The lists consisted of interrogative sentences that were to be answered by listeners. A correct answer was taken as an indication that the sentence material was correctly understood. The format posed problems in that the sentences were parochial (required knowledge of events and places in New York) and required listeners to have a certain degree of knowledge.

During World War II two types of sentences lists were developed at the Harvard Psychoacoustic Laboratory. The first test, Auditory Test 12, consisted of simple questions which could be answered with one word. The tests which were described by Hudgins et al. (1947) were attenuated so that a threshold for speech could be obtained. The second test required that the listener write down or repeat the sentence. Each sentence contained five key words, four monosyllabic and one dissyllabic. A set of sentences developed at the Central Institute for the Deaf was evaluated in 1953 by a working group of the Armed Forces-National Research Council's Committee on Hearing and Bioacoustics to determine if the sentences represented a reasonable sample of everyday speech. The group approved a revised list of 200 sentences as representing a sample of everyday speech. A scoring system, which was based on the correct recognition of 50 key words in each list of 10 sentences, was developed. Recordings of the sentences have been made but no formal test has been developed.

The development of a test of intelligibility based on units larger than a word, the synthetic sentences identification test was developed by Speaks and Jerger (1965). Sets of 10 sentences were developed from a pool of 1,000 familiar words taken from the Thorndike and Lorge Wordbook. Each successive word in a sentence was selected on the basis of the probabilities or approximations of word sequences. Three different sets of sentences were developed in terms of the degree of approximation of the words (first order, second order, and third order approximations). Approximation involved giving each word a chance to occur proportional to its relative frequency of occurrence after the word that preceded it, in terms of the statistics of normal English. Subjects responded by selecting the correct sentence from a closed set of 10 sentences. Speaks, Jerger, and Jerger (1966) reported that performance for the tests, which were filtered, was related to the contextual constraints of the message sets. Also, the performance-intensity functions for the three sets of sentences were quite similar. Jerger (1970) indicated that the synthetic sentence approach provided for a more realistic appraisal of speech understanding than is gained from tests utilizing word lists. Also, with the use of synthetic sentences it is possible to have control of sentence length and semantic content, a condition that is not too easily realized with real or everyday sentences.

FACTORS AFFECTING THE PERCEPTION OF SPEECH

In considering factors that can affect the perception of speech, there are several major factors or primary areas that need to be considered. These areas are listeners, speakers, mode of listening, and effects of noise. Research which has been undertaken in each of these areas is described, followed by a discussion of subareas of these primary areas.

Listeners

Of major importance to the study of speech perception is the listener or receiver of the basic speech signal. Several important characteristics of the listener are obvious: basic hearing ability, training in listening, language background, previous experience in listening to speech, and set and motivation.

Basic Hearing Ability

It seems quite logical to assume that acuity of hearing should be related to the ability to perceive speech. Also, that listening with both ears rather than with one ear should lead to better reception of speech. Measures of normal hearing acuity for speech are based on measures of speech reception and speech discrimination.

Very little detailed research has been reported in regard to the effects of hearing acuity upon intelligibility. The basic assumption is made that persons with normal hearing are selected for nonclinical studies. Also, the majority of the research has involved the presentation of materials at intensity levels which ensure that the materials can be heard. Most of the interest has been directed toward the effects of other factors. Many studies have supported the assumption that hearing levels for the three frequencies of 500, 1,000, and 2,000 Hz relate quite closely to acuity for speech reception. Also, the Committee on the Conservation of Hearing of the American Academy of Opthalmology and Otolaryngology has recommended that the hearing level for these three frequencies should be used as a measure of a person's ability to hear everyday speech under everyday conditions. Kryter, Williams, and Green (1962) reported that when speech intelligibility (discrimination) scores were compared with pure tone results, the most significant frequencies were 2,000 and 3,000 Hz while pure tone losses at only 500 and 1,000 Hz were important for spondee thresholds. When performance on the PB tests was considered in terms of speech thresholds, the results for 500, 1,000, and 2,000 Hz were the most important frequencies. Kryter (1963) reported that an average hearing level of 15 dB at 1,000, 2,000, and 3,000 Hz would not produce too great a reduction in the understanding of sentences.

Training in Listening

Providing listeners with training prior to the actual listening task should improve their listening performance. The results of several studies bear out that such is the case. Egan (1948) found that 10–15 hr of listening practice produced stable listening scores. Moser and Dreher (1953) found that 8–10 hr of training resulted in stable test scores if no more than 1 week's extinction was involved. In a later study Moser and Dreher (1955) found that training over three test sessions resulted in a significant improvement in intelligibility scores. Also, they suggested that subjects who were to be used in laboratory listening experiments should be either completely new to the lists they were to be tested on or they should be completely trained. Stuckey (1963) reported that after 20 hr of training, a team of listeners was fully trained, in terms of an established criterion.

Several other investigators have hinted at or indicated in general terms that listening practice improved the performance of their listeners. For example, Denes (1964) utilized 15 training periods to evaluate the efficacy of the motor theory of speech perception. While he found that there was close to a 30% improvement in speech recognition scores, he did not find a significant difference between listeners who merely listened and listeners who listened and repeated the words as they heard them. Also, other investigators, such as Pollack, Rubenstein, and Decker (1959), Miller and Isard (1963), Licklider and Pollack (1948), Farrimond (1962), Epstein, Giolas, and Owens (1968), and Jerger et al. (1969), reported that improvement in listener's performance occurred as the experiment progressed. Speaks, Karmen, and Benitez (1967) reported that naive listeners did not perform as well as did trained listeners while listening to synthetic sentences. Licklider, Bindra, and Pollack (1948) found that when two listeners were trained over 10 successive days, they improved considerably more in their understanding of infinitely clipped speech than they did in understanding normal speech. Peters (1956) reported that with increased exposure to training messages (12 as compared to four sessions) and with a decreased speech-to-noise ratio, there was a significant increase in terms of selecting error response words which were correct responses for the training words.

Black, Lang, and Singh (1967) reported on the use of a self-administered procedure for the improvement of intelligibility. The results of the study indicated that subjects could teach themselves to recognize an increasing number of words that they had spoken in quiet and had heard in noise. Gillespie and Black (1967), utilizing another self-administered approach, found that its use led to significantly improved intelligibility scores.

Another training approach involved familiarizing listeners with the voice of speakers, especially foreign speakers whose dialect when they were speaking English words produced listening problems. Studies by Chaiklin (1955) and Hauptmann (1952), which allowed for a brief 3–5 min familiarization with speaker's voices did not produce significant improvements in intelligibility scores. Black and Tolhurst (1955) evaluated the effects of 2 hr of listening practice for a group of British, French, and American naval officers. They found that such practice led to significant improvements in intelligibility scores for English words spoken in the two dialects.

Speakers

It has been fairly well documented that individual speakers vary in terms of their intelligibility. O'Neill (1954) found that speakers from the Midwest and East Central areas of the United States were rated as being the most intelligible. Also, Tolhurst (1954) reported that verbal instructions to a speaker resulted in improvements in intelligibility. Stuntz (1963) indicated that intelligibility was influenced, not only by the individual characteristics of each speaker, but also by the characteristics of other talkers with whom the individual is being compared. Also, Silverstein et al. (1953) found that male speakers were significantly more intelligible than female speakers. Brandy (1966) studied speaker's time-to-time variation in live and recorded presentations. He found that the recorded presentations were more reliable than live presentations. In other words, a speaker may show significant variability on successive days of testing with identical test materials. These results seem to indicate that speaker variability should be recognized as an important factor in intelligibility or discrimination testing. It should be controlled through approaches such as recorded rather than live presentation, and a sufficient number of speakers should be employed, especially when distortion is introduced into the testing situation.

Mode of Listening

Published research has indicated that listening to speech with two ears results in better intelligibility scores than does listening with one ear. The binaural threshold for speech was found by Shaw, Newman, and Hirsh (1947) to be approximately 3 dB lower than the threshold for either ear alone. Also, Chappell, Kavangh, and Zerlin (1963) and Heffler and Schultz (1964) found that binaural listening led to better intelligibility scores than monaural listening did. Carhart (1967) indicates that the 3-dB difference holds for hearing of filtered monosyllables (high-pass and low-pass filtering), and it produces an increase of 16% for the discrimination of unfiltered material and 11–12% for the filtered materials. Tolhurst and Peters (1956) reported that if two messages were presented binaurally with no instructions as to which message was to be selected that the louder message was always better reported. Also, MacKeith and Coles (1971) found that discrimination was superior for binaural listening than for various conditions of monaural listening.

Effects of Noise

Egan (1948) published a series of studies that dealt with the effects of noise on speech communication. In his study of listening in aircraft noise and a white noise background, he found that high intensities of speech plus noise were detrimental to intelligibility and that white noise interfered with speech more than other noises did. Miller (1947) reported that as the level of a masking noise increased that the following occurred. At low intensity levels, low frequency noise bands did not mask speech as well as high frequency bands of noise did, but at high intensities the effectiveness of the masking was reversed, i.e., low frequency bands masked speech much more effectively than high frequency bands of noise. Similar results were reported by Pickett and Kryter (1958) when sloped broad-band noises were used to mask speech. Webster and Thompson (1953), in an investigation of the effects of noise on speech intelligibility in aircraft control towers, found that the most objectionable noise in such a situation was the noise that accompanied messages received through loudspeakers. Also, the best reception occurred when the ambient noise level was kept below 70 dB. In one of the more frequently quoted studies, Hawkins and Stevens (1950) reported that when white noise was above a level of 40 dB, speech thresholds increased linearly with increases in noise level. Mason (1946) reported that listeners trained in noise showed improvement in listening scores. Three hours of training, which included familiarization with half of the test vocabulary, produced a 21.7-point improvement in intelligibility.

Kryter (1970) and Webster (1969) have brought the record of research in this area up to date as of the 1960's. Keith and Talis (1972) investigated the effects of white noise upon lists 1 and 2 of the CID auditory test W-22. For their normal listeners, speech discrimination scores of the following order were obtained with the indicated speech-to-noise (S/N) ratios: +8-dB S/N ratio, 92.2%; 0-dB S/N ratio, 81.6%; and −8-dB S/N ratio, 47.2% for an overall deterioration of 52%. They further reported that as the noise level increased, there was an increase in the variability of scores among listeners.

Recently Carhart (1970) has expanded on the concept of release from masking during binaural listening in a noise background. In essence, speech intelligibility in the presence of background noise will be better under some conditions of listening. He plotted function curves of masking level differences for spondee words and monosyllabic words with phase differences between the signals. On the basis of the obtained results, he concluded that when speech had to be understood, binaural escape from masking over monaural efficiency was between 3 and 7 dB. Masking level difference was computed on the basis of the masking level differences for the frequencies important in the understanding of speech (500–2,000 Hz).

Earlier work in this area has been reported by Licklider (1948) and later research was undertaken by Weston, Miller, and Hirsh (1965). Licklider (1948) conducted experiments which indicated that speech intelligibility was the greatest for binaural noise and speech when they were of opposite phase, and was minimal when monaural noise and speech was in the same ear. Feldmann (1965) reported that intelligibility was significantly improved for binaural hearing when the opposite ear was presented with the same noise but not the speech signal. He further indicated that an intraaural time difference that occurred when either the noise or signal was delayed for one ear led to improved intelligibility. Gerber (1967) did not find the type of performance reported by Feldmann. In fact, he reported that intelligibility was not significantly better for phase differences of 90 or 180 degrees. When filtered versions of Northwestern University Auditory Test 4 were presented to normal hearing subjects under monaural and binaural conditions, the slope of the binaural function for filtered materials (high-pass filtered material presented to one ear and low-pass filtered material to the other ear) was superior to the slope for monaural function for either type of signal (Tillman and Carhart, 1965). Zelnick (1970) utilized a dummy head fitted either with microphones at the position of the ear drums or with two commercial hearing aids. The output from the microphone was led to subjects who listened under monotic or dichotic conditions to revised CNC lists. The results indicated that binaural listening always resulted in better performance than monaural listening did.

PROBLEMS IN LISTENING

The term listening is used to signify that the individual may be required to receive and understand speech materials under conditions different from those previously described in this chapter. In other words, interest is centered on the effects that factors other than noise or mode of listening will have on intelligibility. Five basic areas are reviewed in the discussion to follow. All of these areas could be fitted under the heading of selective listening to speech which was proposed by Broadbent (1952).

Competing Messages

The first area of interest is competing messages, which can be subdivided into two areas. First is the physical masking of one message or speech sample by another speech sample. This phenomenon, which has been labeled as the "cocktail party" effect, has been utilized in the study of intelligibility. This form of noise causes a greater amount of masking than white noise does because it contains components similar to those in the speech stimuli. The second subdivision, and the one emphasized here, is the interference effects of the competing signal. The earliest research in the listening of simultaneous messages was undertaken, among others, by Broadbent (1958), who concluded that different speech tasks interfere with one another. He reported that when pairs of messages are presented simultaneously with a slight time difference provided between the messages that the listener could, after repeated presentations, separate the messages. Cherry (1953) reported that a listener could, after repeated presentations, separate out two different speech passages recorded by the same voice. Such results led Broadbent to conclude that a central rather than a sensory factor was involved when two messages were presented at the same time. Also, he further indicated that the rate at which the information was being transmitted affected the correct recognition of speech materials.

Peters (1954b) reported that unwanted speech which was similar in content to the basic or wanted message produced decreases in intelligibility. Extraneous messages which immediately followed a primary message were found by Peters (1954a) to be ususally more damaging to reception than were extraneous messages which immediately preceded the primary message. Also, he indicated that a greater amount of interference occurred when the extraneous messages were similar in phonetic content and temporal pattern to the primary message. Dirks and Bower (1969), as the result of a series of studies with synthetic sentences, reported that distractional factors attributable to the semantic content of a competing message had no measurable effect on the performance-intensity functions of synthetic sentences. This finding was based on the comparison of results obtained with the masking message played backwards or with the masking message recorded in Latin, thus voiding the semantic effects of the message. Because synthetic sentences do not have any "true" semantic meaning, the results of the study seem to support the notion that semantic masking does not interfere with the reception of individual speech elements that do not have a semantic nature.

In an effort to increase the sensitivity of conventional intelligibility tests, several investigators have examined reaction time to test items as a possible additional measure that might improve the sensitivity of the tests. Pollack and Rubinstein (1963) examined response times to test words presented in noise and found a close relationship between response time and intelligibility.

Reaction times for the Modified Rhyme Test were investigated by Hecker, Stevens, and Williams (1966). They reported that measures of intelligibility and reaction time were independent to some degree and that reaction time to a test item seemed to be dependent on the speech-to-noise ratio at which the item was presented but was largely independent of whether the item was correctly identified. Holloway (1972) reported the results of a study which used alphabet letters and a speed score (the time between the first and last response for each set of letters). The results indicated that it may be difficult to improve on the intelligibility test score as the most appropriate index for the evaluation of intelligibility.

Effect of Distortion

Another approach that can be used to introduce more difficulty in the test situation is to produce distortions in the basic test materials. In other words, known, controllable changes are introduced with the intent of investigating how such changes have influenced intelligibility. The most frequently used methods of producing such distortions involve changes in the temporal pattern of the signal or changes in the amplitude of the signal.

Amplitude Licklider (1946) investigated the effects that several types of amplitude distortion had upon the intelligibility of speech. In his study he utilized symmetrical and asymetrical peak clipping, center clipping, and linear amplification of words presented in quiet and in 110 dB of ambient noise. The peak clipping did not have too great an effect on intelligibility in quiet or in noise. On the other hand, amplitude distortion (center clipping) was more deleterious for intelligibility performance in noise. "Square speech," which was produced when upward and downward peaks of normal speech were clipped off, reamplified, and clipped, was found by Licklider, Bindra, and Pollack (1948) to be surprisingly intelligible.

Temporal Changes It is possible to speed up or slow down speech. The most popular approach involves the speeding up of speech. One of the most frequently used methods involves the removal of portions of the speech pattern through the use of a chopping technique, which can be accomplished with an electronic switch, with actual removal of sections of a magnetic tape containing a recording of the speech signal, or with a speech compressor.

In 1950, Miller and Licklider removed portions of a speech pattern by means of an electronic switch that periodically turned off the speech. They found that if the interruption occurred more than 10 times/sec that there was very little effect on the intelligibility of monosyllabic words. In fact, intelligibility scores remained at levels of 90% or higher until 50% of the speech signal had been discarded. Garvey (1953) removed portions of a magnetic tape which contained recordings of spondaic words; 3 cm of tape were removed and 1 cm was left. The 1-cm portions that were left were spliced together. The resulting tape provided intelligibility scores of 40%. This type of procedure allowed for a 300% speeding up of the speech signal. An electromechanical device that was developed by Fairbanks, Everitt, and Jaeger (1954) was used for the compression of recorded tape materials. The device utilized a rotating arrangement of equally spaced playback heads to sample portions of the recorded tape. In this fashion the portions of the tape that passed across the playback head were transferred to another tape while the portion of the tape not in contact with the playback heads was discarded. Fairbanks, Guttman, and Miron (1957), Fairbanks and Kodman (1957), and Kurtzrock (1956) reported that with a compression rate of 85–87% an intelligibility score of 50% was obtained. Also, they found very little difference in the comprehension of materials presented at rates of 141, 201, and 282 words/min.

Foulke and Sticht (1969) found a loss of 6% in comprehension when the rate was changed from 225 to 325 words/min and a loss of 14% when the rate was changed from 325 to 425 words/min. DeQuiros (1964) reported that when words were presented at rates of 140, 250, and 350 words/min that there were no significant changes in the threshold of detectability for the words. However, there was a difference of 10 dB between the various rates in terms of the presentation level required to obtain a maximal intelligibility score. Compression rates of 36, 46, and 59% were used by Sticht and Gray (1969) in a study of the effects age had upon reception of compressed speech. They reported that with increasing age there was a decrease in the ability to discriminate time-compressed words. Similar results were found by Schon (1970), in terms of 30 and 50% compression rates. Beasley, Forman, and Rintelmann (1972), using the Northwestern Auditory Test 6 and compression rates of 30, 40, 50, 60, and 70%, found that intelligibility decreased to about 80% as the compression rate increased to 70%.

The intelligibility of slow played speech (speech played at a speed slower than which it was recorded) was studied by Tiffany and Bennett (1961). They found that intelligibility was markedly reduced with a downward shift in the speed of playback. They attributed their results to a downward shift in frequency produced by the slow up of playback.

A comprehensive review of the area of compressed speech has been provided by Foulke and Sticht (1969).

Effect of Training

Several investigators have been interested in determining if intelligibility scores that have been depressed because of certain modifications in the speech signal could be improved through training. Licklider, Bindra, and Pollack (1948) trained two listeners in listening to squared speech in five speech-to-noise ratios for 10 days. The results indicated that the listeners improved considerably in their ability to understand the squared speech. Garvey and Henneman (1950) reported that while they did not conduct any systematic investigation of the effects of practice, some preliminary investigation indicated that with three or four practice trials there was a considerable increase in intelligibility for their versions of speeded speech. Several investigators reported that training can produce an improvement in the comprehension of accelerated speech. Voor and Miller (1965) found that 17.5 min of training with speech presented at 380 words/min resulted in an improvement in comprehension scores. A 29.3% increase in the comprehension of materials presented at 475 words/min resulted from several weeks of training with materials that varied in rate from 25 to 325 to 475 words/min was reported by Orr, Friedman, and Williams (1965). Foulke (1964) found that 25 hr of training with blind subjects led to significant differences in intelligibility. Training with slow played speech also resulted in significant improvement in intelligibility scores, according to the results reported by Tiffany and Bennett (1961) and Eakins (1969). Thus, it seems that a period of training enables listeners to improve their intelligibility in terms of listening to distorted speech.

Filtering

The frequency of the speech signal can also be modified through the use of filters. Various types of filters can be used, such as high pass, low pass and band pass. Fletcher and Steinberg (1929) indicated that the frequencies above and below 1,900 Hz contributed equally to intelligibility. Hirsh, Reynolds, and Joseph (1954) reported that when frequencies above or below 1,600 Hz were eliminated, the intelligibility of words was not seriously impaired. Also, Black (1959) found that the important frequencies for the intelligibility of speech were comparable to those reported by Fletcher and Steinberg. Egan and Weiner (1946) indicated that the band from 340 to 3,900 Hz, which includes the first three formants, passed nearly all of the information that was necessary for accurate speech discrimination. Also, the band from 870 to 2,500 Hz carried the bulk of the information in speech. Thomas (1966) reported that this particular band included most of the second formant, which the results of his study indicated was the major contributor to speech intelligibility. However, Hirsh, Reynolds, and Joseph (1954) indicated that, in the instance of polysyllabic words, when all frequencies above 1,800 Hz were removed, intelligibility scores for the words was 97%. When all frequencies above 800 Hz were removed a score of about 95% was obtained.

Sergeant (1964) used three bandwidths—500, 1,000, and 1,500 Hz—with center frequencies for each of the bandwidths of 800, 1,200, 1,600, 1,900, and 2,200 Hz. He reported that when the center frequency was 1,600 Hz, the bandwidth could be as narrow as 500 Hz and intelligibility was not decreased more than 5–10%. Also, there was a greater spread of intelligibility scores across bandwidths for the low frequencies than for the middle or higher frequencies, and if the bandwidth was as broad as 1,500, the center frequency could be as low as 800 Hz and as high as 1,900 Hz without producing appreciable changes in intelligibility. However, when the center frequency was at 2,200 Hz there was a pronounced decrease in intelligibility.

Effect of Hearing Loss

Several of the areas described above have been involved in studies of persons with hearing impairment. Carhart and Tillman (1970) found that subjects with sensorineural hearing losses experienced considerable difficulty in listening when competing messages were presented. The subjects experienced a shift of about 14 dB in masking as a result of the competing messages. Schon (1970) reported that young males with sensorineural hearing losses showed significantly reduced discrimination for time-compressed words. Earlier, De-Quiros (1964) had indicated that time compression had no significant effects upon intelligibility scores for subjects with sensorineural hearing losses, except for compression rates of 350 words/min. Sticht and Gray (1969) also indicated that sensorineural hearing losses did not produce significant effects upon the intelligibility of time-compressed PB words. Bennett and Byers (1967) found that for individuals with sensorineural hearing loss, slow playback of Rhyme Test words led to decreased intelligibility scores for 60 and 70% slow down and increased intelligibility at 80% of normal speed. Rhodes (1966) utilized CNC lists with hearing-impaired subjects. The filter was set at either 1,000 or 2,000 Hz low pass. The results indicated that the hearing-impaired subjects achieved better discrimination scores for the 1,000-Hz low-pass condition than normal hearing subjects did and that their performance was similar to that of a normal hearing group for the 2,000-Hz low-pass condition.

Low-pass filtering has been used to "sensitize" speech tests for the evaluation of central auditory problems. Bocca, Calearo, and Cassinari (1954) presented dysyllabic words with low-pass (500 Hz) filtering at progressively increasing intensities, first to one ear and then to the other ear of a subject with a right temporal lobe tumor. They found reduced scores for the ear contralateral to the lesion. Similar results were obtained by Bocca et al. (1955) with low-pass filtering of 1,000 Hz for 18 subjects with unilateral temporal lobe tumors. While normal subjects obtained scores of 70–80%, subjects with temporal lobe tumors obtained scores of 50% for the ear contralateral to the tumor and 65–75% for the ipsilateral ear. A similar type of performance for subjects with brainstem lesions was reported by Antonelli and Calearo (1968).

Jerger (1960) used PB words that had been subjected to filtering (500 Hz) in the study of two subjects with temporal lobe disorders. He found reduced scores for the ear contralateral to the lesion. In a later study Jerger (1964) found, for a group of subjects with brainstem lesions affecting the central nervous system and Heschel's gyrus, that there was marked reduction in the speech score for the ear contralateral to the lesion. Several investigators have utilized a procedure where words are presented through one type of filtering to one ear and another type of filtering to the other ear. Matzker (1959) presented two-syllable words in a dichotic mode. One ear received the words through a 500–800 Hz band-pass filter while the other ear received the words through a 1,815–2,500 Hz band-pass filter. Normal hearing subjects had very few errors for such a procedure while patients with brainstem lesions made many errors. Smith and Resnick (1972) utilized a somewhat similar approach. However, they utilized words from the CNC lists and utilized band-pass filters from 360–890 Hz for one ear and band-pass filters from 1,750–2,200 Hz for the other ear. They found that the test performance for subjects with brainstem lesions was quite different from the performance of subjects with normal hearing or temporal lobe lesions.

Katz (1962) utilized spondee words in the development of a dichotic test procedure that he labeled the staggered spondaic word test (SSW). A different spondaic word is presented to each ear. The first part of the word appears at the right ear; there is an overlapping of the second part of the first word and the first part of the second word; and the last part of the second word is heard at the left ear. Scoring is done in terms of incorrect responses. In several later studies Katz (1968) and Katz, Basil, and Smith (1963) obtained results that indicated that the SSW was capable of differentiating normal subjects from patients with central auditory disorders. These results were supported by Balas (1971), who found that 60% of his temporal lobe patients were identified on the basis of SSW scores.

LINGUISTIC ASPECTS OF SPEECH PERCEPTION

Within the past few years, research in speech perception has moved into the realm of linguistics, where attention is directed to the code of speech and especially to the encoding aspects of perception. Various areas are considered here: vocabulary, word predictability, effect of context, and phonetic factors.

Vocabulary

Early studies by Howes (1957), Rosenzweig and Postman (1957), and Black (1952) indicated that word intelligibility increased directly as word familiarity increased. Also, Black indicated that words with more sounds were more intelligible than words with fewer sounds. In 1961 Owens, utilizing PB-50 and W-22 lists, found a significant relationship between familiarity and intelligibility. Epstein, Giolas, and Owens (1968) found a significant relationship between intelligibility and familiarity of words from PB-50 and W-22 lists presented under conditions of distortion. The W-22 lists were used in the study of a school-aged population by Hutton and Weaver (1959), who found a significant relationship between familiarity and intelligibility in terms of the 15 least familiar and the 15 most familiar words.

Word Predictability

In 1951 Shannon developed a technique for predicting the occurrence of letters in English. The technique was applied by Black (1955) to a study of the predictability of five-syllable phrases. Also, Black and Morrison (1957) studied the prediction of missing words in sentences. From one to six words were omitted from each of 130 sentences. Subjects were to reconstruct the sentences. For single word deletions responses were approximately 50% correct. The proportion of correct responses decreased as additional words were deleted and as randomization was introduced, in terms of the order of the words. Rubenstein and Pollack (1963) investigated predictability and the intelligibility of monosyllabic words in noise. They found that intelligibility was a simple power function of the probability of occurrence of the words. Also, they proposed an equation which related intelligibility, probability, and speech-to-noise ratio.

Giolas, Cooker, and Duffy (1970) evaluated the predictability of several sentence lists (CID sentence lists, B and D, revised sentence list C, and synthetic sentences). The results indicated that the revised list C was considerably less predictable than lists B and D, which were highly predictable. On the other hand, the synthetic sentences had a negligible predictability. The materials used in this study were re-recorded with low-pass filtering at 420 and 360 Hz by Duffy, Giolas, and Sergeant (1971). They found that easy-to-predict words yielded the highest scores and the difficult-to-predict words received the lowest scores. These results led the investigators to suggest that in any development of sentence intelligibility tests, the constructors of such tests should carefully consider the relative predictability of key words in the sentences.

Effect of Context

The results of a study by Miller, Heise, and Lichten (1951) provided evidence that words heard in context were more intelligible than when they were heard in isolation. Similar results were obtained by O'Neill (1957). Fifty one- and two-syllable words were presented in five contexts in a study undertaken by Traul and Black (1965). They found that intelligibility was enhanced by higher orders of approximation (more contextual cues). Also, grammatical sentences presented in noise were much more intelligible than anomalous or ungrammatical sentences. Miller and Isard (1963) postulated that the use of sentence context by listeners was based on an intimate knowledge of linguistic rules. In a study which compared responses to spondaic words, PB words, and synthetic sentences, Speaks (1967) found that listeners always identified a higher percentage of sentences than either spondaic or monosyllabic words. In a study which utilized pseudosentences presented in noise, Miller (1962) found that when time was short (pauses between successive sentences were eliminated) and the words did not follow a familiar grammatical pattern, that intelligibility was decreased as opposed to when time was short and the words followed a grammatical context. Miller interpreted the results as indicating the existence of perceptual units larger than a single word.

The effects of sequence on syntactic and nonsyntactic materials was investigated by Moser et al. (1956). Listeners, when aurally presented the first half of a spondee, could reproduce the whole word with more success than when presented with the latter half. Also, when presented with couplets, they could more readily identify the couplets when they were heard in the common order than in the uncommon order. Moreover, the intelligibility of a sequence of three unrelated words, as used in three-unit call signs, was independent of their order of occurrence. The method of extrapolation (forward association) or continuation of a sentence, and interpolation (forward-backward association) or filling of gaps in sentences, was used by Poulton (1954) to determine the contributions that these two approaches made when short gaps were introduced in connected, verbal material. The results indicated that the two procedures did not necessarily give different results. Interpolation was more difficult than extrapolation, and if there was a change of postcontexts, changes could be made in the meanings and first words of the answers. Also, Bruce (1955) reported that words connected with a particular topic were more readily identified when the listener was aware of the subject to which they referred.

Phonetic Factors

Interest in this section is not directed to the recognition of isolated vowels and consonants as sounds of speech but rather to the contributions that certain aspects of phonetic elements make to intelligibility. Black (1952) reported that words with many sounds were more intelligible than words with few sounds. Also, familiar words (low Thorndike ratings) had fewer sounds than the less familiar words (high Thorndike ratings). Black further reported that while it was not possible to predict word intelligibility from phonetic content alone, there were 18 sounds that did tend to enhance the recognition of words and seven that tended to detract from such recognition.

In another vein Moser et al. (1957) studied the role of expectation in the reception of speech. Listening panels of American and foreign airmen were provided with printed lists of monosyllabic words, polysyllabic words, and air traffic instructions. They were required to decide whether these printed messages were in agreement or disagreement with tape-recorded presentations of the same materials. The results indicated that listeners who expected to hear matching messages were less likely to detect contradictory messages while listeners who expected different messages were less likely to identify matching messages. Also, errors of identification and discrimination were more frequent for phrases than for words and were more frequent for polysyllabic than for monosyllabic words. Black (1961) reported that the length of sentences and the amount of environmental noise in which the sentences are heard had definite effects upon auditory reception, in that there was a reduction in score with an increase of the number of words in a sentence and with an increase in the masking noise.

AUDITORY PROCESSING

Auditory processing has been defined in many ways. It has been defined as including the transmission of the signal from the external ear to the auditory cortex and as including the transmission from the cochlea to the cortex. Luria (1966) indicated that the auditory analyzer is a crucial link in the development or disorganization of other systems. It causes neurological processes to become diffuse, and closely related stimuli are no longer clearly differentiated. Teatini (1970) wrote that when a neural channel is disturbed by a pathological process, the neural pattern of the message may be sent on an equivalent, still unimpaired channel. This collateral channel acts as an emergency path. The message will not be lost, but processing is less perfect and refined, and as a result redundancy is lowered and intelligibility is decreased.

Most of the recent interest in auditory processing has been directed toward breakdowns in the process. However, there seem to be several areas that can be considered in terms of normal auditory processing. Included among these areas are the roles of attention, auditory experience, and cognitive aspects.

Attention

Broadbent (1962) has been quite involved in research in the area of attention. He indicated that a major factor is the strategy that the listener adopts. Peters (1967), in discussing the motor theory of perception, indicated that a listener hears what he expects to hear because he has learned what to expect, as much from speaking as from listening. Poulton (1953) described covering type masking (inattention) as it affected two-channel listening. Moser et al. (1957) presented 50 operational phrases to listeners who had a printed list of the same phrases before them. They might or might not hear the phrase that was on the printed list. The results indicated that listeners who expected to hear a matching message were less likely to detect contradictory messages, and listeners who were expecting different messages were less likely to identify matching messages. Moray (1969) discusses a model of speech perception that indicates that a selective operation is performed on the input to the primary channel and that the selection is not completely random. The probability of a particular class of events being selected is increased by certain properties of the events and certain states of the organism.

Auditory Experience

Previous listening experience in listening to speech and familiarity with the language obviously plays an important role in auditory processing. This past experience provides the material for the comparator or dictionary that the listener uses in his evaluation of speech stimuli. Previous sections of this chapter have described the effects that familiarity and the organization of language play upon the perception of speech. The next section deals with cognitive factors, especially the role of memory.

Cognitive Aspects

Consideration in the area of cognitive aspects is devoted to the role that memory plays in speech perception. Research indicates that two different processes need to be considered: short-term and long-term memory. Broadbent (1970) stated that most recent speech events are placed in a sensory type of storage and that there is also a storage system that is restricted to a fixed number of elements. Crowder and Morton (1969) have described a system for precategorical storage of acoustic information, in which short-term storage involves storage of articulatory functions while semantic functions involve long-term processing. Short-term memory will be affected by a similarity in acoustic signals, and long-term memory will be affected by semantic similarities. Bryden (1971), in studies of dichotic listening, reported that pre-perceptual auditory storage is relatively long lasting but can be disrupted by subsequent auditory input. He further reported that when the dichotic listening task involved an unattended and attended ear paradigm, then material presented to the unattended ear was stored and remembered in a fashion quite different from material presented to the unattended ear. Items in short-term memory were more subject to output interference than items in echoic memory. Also, Glucksberg and Cowen (1971) found that verbal material presented auditorily to an unattended channel persisted briefly but was not transferred into long-term storage. Wickelgren (1973), in a review of recent research, favored the use of the terms short and long memory traces. Also, he indicated that retention function was quite different for the two types of traces.

SUGGESTED MODELS

Several models have been developed to relate specific aspects of auditory function to processing, in terms of the recognition of language. Lafon (1969) has presented a very broad, general schematic representation of auditory function and the reception of language as well as possible sites of language pathology (Figure 1). A model that is specific to the process of speech perception has been described by Stevens and House (1972). The model also provides for representation of the mechanisms of speech production. Figure 2 shows the major elements of the model. The signal enters the peripheral auditory analyzer which yields auditory patterns that are placed in the temporary store. The preliminary analyzer develops from the signal the

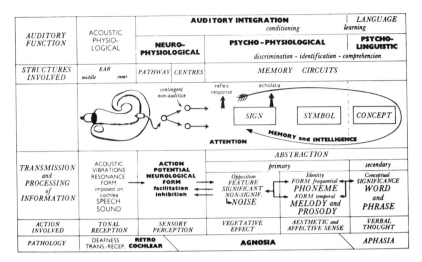

AUDITORY FUNCTION	ACOUSTIC PHYSIO-LOGICAL	AUDITORY INTEGRATION *conditioning*		LANGUAGE *learning*
		NEURO-PHYSIOLOGICAL	PSYCHO-PHYSIOLOGICAL	PSYCHO-LINGUISTIC
			discrimination - identification - comprehension	
STRUCTURES INVOLVED	EAR *middle inner*	PATHWAY CENTRES	MEMORY CIRCUITS	

Figure 1. Lafon's schematic representation of the transmission of verbal information from the reception of acoustic signals to the comprehension of the message received. (Reprinted with permission: Lafon, 1968.)

phonetic features which are then made available for an analysis by the control component. This component develops a hypothesis concerning the representation of the received utterance in terms of phonetic segments and features. This hypothesized representation forms the input to the generative rules component which is then compared in the comparator. The authors describe the principal feature of the model as follows: "It regards speech perception as an active process in which the listener participates equally with the talker." In other words, the listener hypothesizes the message that the speaker is intending to transmit and internalizes the production of the message within the same linguistic framework he would use if he were to produce the message.

Several other models are based on the concept of selective listening as it relates to the concept of attention. The initial model in this area was

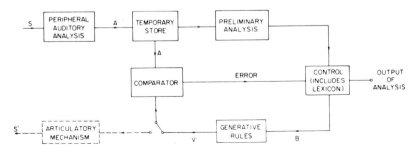

Figure 2. Proposed model by Stevens and House of the speech perception and production processes. (Reprinted with permission: Stevens and House, 1972.)

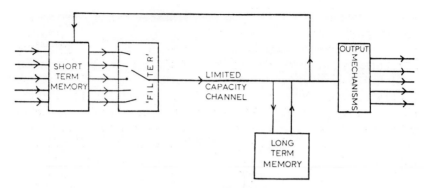

Figure 3. Broadbent's filter theory. (After Broadbent, 1958; reprinted with permission: Moray, 1970.)

proposed by Broadbent (1958), whose model is based on the concept that the speech signal is received by a filter mechanism that selects a stimulus on the basis of certain characteristics and then allows it to enter the central analyzing mechanisms of the brain (Figure 3). A second model (Figure 4) has been proposed by Treisman (1964). Her model is based on the concept of

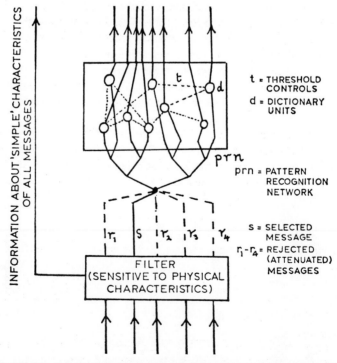

Figure 4. Model of Treisman's input selection. (Reprinted with permission: Moray, 1970.)

selective action by a filter. This filter samples the various input channels and analyzes simple physical characteristics such as pitch, loudness, and temporal characteristics. The resulting information is used by the filter to identify the channel that is to be selected. All other channels are attenuated in a manner not described by Treisman. The signal that has been selected "fires" a single dictionary unit and the word is recognized. The thresholds for the dictionary unit differ and are variable. Deutsch and Deutsch (1963) described a modification of the Treisman model in which the output from the dictionary units become of greater importance, in that it is assumed that the output from the dictionary unit is proportional to the importance of the signal. Thus, the more important the stimulus, the more strongly the dictionary unit fires. Importance is a function of past experience.

Clinical Aspects

Clinical interest in auditory processing has developed because of assumptions that disturbances in auditory processing are related to learning disabilities. Chalfant and Scheffelin (1969) provide a review of the function of auditory processing in the larger context of central processing dysfunctions. Also, Rampp (1972) has provided a discussion of disturbances of auditory perception. Rees (1973) questions the assumption that auditory processing skills are fundamental to language acquisition and academic learning. She does suggest that the area might be better approached on the basis of cognitive factors, especially in terms of syntactic skills.

FUTURE CONCERNS

Before discussing future directions, in terms of research and clinical interests, it is necessary to indicate that certain areas have not been covered in this chapter. Included would be areas such as speech reception tests for children, the effects of frequency transposition, and the effects of certain types of speech compression systems such as vocoders.

Research

The focus of research seems to be shifting from the "building block" approach to the study of speech perception to an approach that attempts to relate the perception of speech to the perception of various linguistic cues. The aim of such an approach is to provide a better understanding of the development of language and the factors that assist or detract from such development.

There is a need for more "solid" data in the area of auditory or central processing. Such research will involve the study of the role that memory and other cognitive factors play in such processing.

In addition, there will be continuing research in the perception of discrete elements of speech, but attention will be directed toward a study of the perception of distinctive features. Further research will be conducted on reactions to various forms of distorted speech.

Finally, there will be more attention paid to the development of models that can serve as starting poitns for a better understanding of speech perception.

Clinical and Educational

There will be a continuation of the present interest in auditory processing as it may relate to learning disabilities and language disorders. Also, efforts will be made to develop more sophisticated tests of speech perception, the results of which can provide relevant data in regard to the disorders discussed earlier.

It would seem that clinical audiologists will continue with their efforts to develop better tests of discrimination, especially ones that involve longer units of speech, such as sentence materials, or that are more representative samples of everyday speech. Also, much more clinical attention will be directed toward the use of the synthetic sentence tests.

Finally, greater efforts will be needed to evaluate the results of speech perception, in terms of particular tests and type of information required in prognostic approaches to rehabilitative approaches. In other words, if the real problem of rehabilitation is one of handling linguistic units and the behavioral accompaniments of speech perception, rather than a simple problem of increased amplification, then it will be necessary to relate prognostic evaluations to actual outcomes of therapy. It well may be that speech perception will assume more and more importance, especially if the purpose of diagnostic evaluations is to concentrate on the effects that hearing loss or difficulties in the perception of speech have on linguistic and academic performance.

REFERENCES

Antonelli, A., and C. Calearo. 1968. Further investigations on cortical deafness. Acta Otolaryngol. 66: 97–100.

Aten, J. 1972. Auditory memory and auditory sequencing. *In* D. L. Rampp (ed.), The Proceedings of the First Annual Memphis State University Symposium on Auditory Processing and Learning Disabilities, July 10–14, pp. 108–135. Memphis State University, Memphis.

Balas, R. F. 1971. Staggered spondaic word test: Support. Ann. Otol. Rhinol. Laryngol. 80: 132–134.

Beasley, D. S., B. S. Forman, and W. F. Rintelmann. 1972. Perception of time-compressed CNC monosyllables by normal listeners. J. Aud. Res. 12: 71–75.

Bennett, D. N., and V. W. Byers. 1967. Increased intelligibility in the hypacusic by slow-play frequency transposition. J. Aud. Res. 7: 107–118.

Black, J. W. 1952. Accompaniments of word intelligibility. J. Speech Hear. Disord. 17: 409–418.

Black, J. W. 1955. The prediction of the words of varied materials. Report 57. U.S. Naval School of Aviation Medicine, Naval Air Station, Pensacola, Fla.

Black, J. W. 1959. Equally contributing frequency bands in intelligibility testing. J. Speech Hear. Res. 2: 81–83.

Black, J. W. 1961. Aural reception of sentences of different lengths. Q. J. Speech. 47: 51–53.

Black, J. W. 1963. Language barriers and language training. In F. A. Geldard (ed.), Communication Processes. Proceedings of a Symposium Held in Washington, pp. 101–128, Pergamon Press, New York.

Black, J. W. 1968. Speech perception. In D. J. Sills (ed.), International Encyclopedia of the Social Sciences, pp. 556–560. Vol. 11. Macmillan and Free Press, New York.

Black, J. W., K. H. Lang, and S. Singh. 1967. Altering intelligibility through a self-administered procedure. Q. J. Speech. 53: 361–364.

Black, J. W., and H. M. Morrison. 1957. Prediction of missing words in sentences. J. Speech Hear. Disord. 22: 236–240.

Black, J. W., and S. Singh. 1968. The psychological basis of phonetics. In B. Malmberg (ed.), Manual of Phonetics, pp. 105–128. North-Holland, Amsterdam.

Black, J. W., and G. C. Tolhurst. 1955. The relative intelligibility of language groups. Q. J. Speech 41: 57–60.

Bocca, E. 1958. Clinical aspects of cortical deafness. Laryngoscope 68: 301–309.

Bocca, E., C. Calearo, and V. Cassinari. 1954. A new method for testing hearing in temporal lobe tumors, preliminary report. Acta Otolaryngol. 44: 219–221.

Bocca, E., C. Calearo, V. Cassinari, and F. Miglwacca. 1955. Testing 'cortical' hearing in temporal lobe tumors. Acta Otolaryngol. 45: 289–304.

Brandy, W. T. 1966. Reliability of voice tests of speech discrimination. J. Speech Hear. Res. 9: 461–465.

Broadbent, D. E. 1952. Listening to one of two synchronous messages. J. Exp. Psychol. 44: 51–55.

Broadbent, D. E. 1958. Perception and Communication, pp. 11–35. Pergamon Press, New York.

Broadbent, D. E. 1962. Attention and the perception of speech. Sci. Amer. 206: 143–151.

Broadbent, D. E. 1970. Psychological aspects of short-term and long-term memory. Proc. R. Soc. Lond. 175B: 333–350.

Bruce, D. J. 1955. The effects of context on the intelligibility of heard speech. Proceedings of the Third London Symposium on Information Theory. Butterworths, London.

Bryden, M. P. 1971. Attentional strategies and short term memory in dichotic listening. Cog. Psychol. 2: 99–116.

Carhart, R. 1967. Binaural reception of meaningful material. In A. B. Graham (ed.), Sensorineural Hearing Processes and Disorders, chap. 13. Little, Brown, Boston.

Carhart, R. 1970. Monaural vs. binaural speech perception. In C. Rojskjaer (ed.), Speech Audiometry. Second Danavox Symposium, pp. 218–225. Odense, Denmark.

Carhart, R., and T. Tillman. 1970. Interaction of competing speech signals with hearing losses. Arch. Otolaryngol. 91: 273–279.

Chaiklin, J. B. 1955. Native American listener's adaptation in understanding speakers with foreign dialect. J. Speech Hear. Disord. 20: 165–170.

Chalfant, J. S., and M. A. Scheffelin. 1969. Central processing dysfunctions in children: A review of research. NINDS Monograph 9. U.S. Department of Health, Education, and Welfare, Washington, D.C.

Chappell, R. G., J. F. Kavangh, and S. Zerlin. 1963. Monaural versus binaural discrimination of hearing aid evaluation. J. Speech Hear. Res. 6: 263–269.

Cherry, E. C. 1953. Some experiments on the recognition of speech, with one and with two ears. J. Acoust. Soc. Amer. 25: 975–979.

Crowder, R. G., and J. Morton. 1969. Precategorical acoustic storage (PAS). Percept. Psychophys. 5: 365–373.

Curtis, J. F. 1954. The rise of experimental phonetics. In K. W. Wallace (ed.), A History of Speech Education in America, pp. 348–369. Appleton-Century-Crofts, New York.

Denes, P. B. 1964. On the motor theory of speech perception. In Symposium on Models for the Perception of Speech and Visual Form, sponsored by Data Sciences Laboratory, Air Force Cambridge Research Laboratories, Office of Aerospace Research, U.S. Air Force, Bedford, Mass.; held in Boston, November 11–14.

DeQuiros, J. B. 1964. Accelerated speech audiometry. An examination of test results. Translations Beltone Inst. Hear. Res. No. 17. June. 48p.

Deutsch, J., and D. Deutsch. 1963. Attention: Some theoretical considerations. Psychol. Rev. 70: 80–90.

Dirks, D. D., and D. R. Bower. 1969. Masking effect of speech competing messages. J. Speech Hear. Res. 12: 229–245.

Doyne, M. P., and M. Steer. 1951. Studies in speech reception testing. J. Speech Hear. Disord. 16: 132–139.

Duffy, J. R., T. G. Giolas, and R. L. Sergeant. 1971. Studies in Navy communication: The effect of word predictability on sentence intelligibility. Report 672. U.S. Naval Submarine Medical Center, Groton, Conn.

Eakins, B. W. 1969. Research in slow-played speech: Listener training, consonant errors, and sex and age differences in speaker intelligibility. Cent. States Speech J. Winter: 302–307.

Egan, J. P. 1948. Articulation testing methods. Laryngoscope 58: 955–991.

Egan, J. P., and F. M. Weiner. 1946. On the intelligibility of bands of speech in noise. J. Acoust. Soc. Amer. 18: 435–441.

Epstein, A., T. G. Giolas, and E. Owens. 1968. Familiarity and intelligibility of monosyllabic word lists. J. Speech Hear. Res. 11: 435–438.

Fairbanks, G., W. L. Everitt, and R. P. Jaeger. 1954. Method for time or frequency compression-expansion of speech. Trans. Inst. Radio Engineers Prof. Group Audio. January-February: 7–12.

Fairbanks, G., N. Guttman, and M. S. Miron. 1957. Effects of time compression upon the comprehension of connected speech. J. Speech Hear. Disord. 22: 10–19.

Fairbanks, G., and F. Kodman, Jr. 1957. Word intelligibility as a function of time compression. J. Acoust. Soc. Amer. 29: 636–641.

Farrimond, T. 1962. Factors influencing auditory perception of pure tones and speech. J. Speech Hear. Res. 5: 194–204.

Feldmann, H. 1965. Experiments on binaural hearing in noise. Translations Beltone Inst. Hear. Res. No. 18. July. 42p.

Flanagan, J. L. 1965. Speech Analysis, Synthesis and Perception, pp. 212–213. Academic Press, New York.

Fletcher, H., and J. C. Steinberg. 1929. Articulation testing methods. Bell System Tech. J. 8: 806–854.

Foulke, E. 1964. The comprehension of rapid speech by the blind. Part 2. Cooperative Research Project 1370. Office of Education, U.S. Department of Health, Education, and Welfare, Washington, D.C.

Foulke, E., and T. G. Sticht. 1969. Review of research on the intelligibility and comprehension of accelerated speech. Psychol. Bull. 72: 50–62.

French, N. R., and J. C. Steinberg. 1947. Factors governing the intelligibility of speech sounds. J. Acoust. Soc. Amer. 19: 90–119.

Garvey, W. E. 1953. The intelligibility of abbreviated speech patterns. Q. J. Speech 39: 296–306.

Garvey, W. D., and R. H. Henneman. 1950. Practical limits of speeded speech. U.S. Air Force Technical Report 5917. Wright-Patterson Air Force Base, Dayton, Ohio.

Gerber, S. E. 1967. Phase and speech discrimination in noise: An expectation and first look. Int. Audiol. 6: 397–400.

Gillespie, M. E., and J. W. Black, 1967. A self administered technique in auditory training. Speech Monogr. 34. 98–101.

Giolas, T. G., H. S. Cooker, and J. R. Duffy. 1970. The predictability of words in sentences. J. Aud. Res. 10: 328–334.

Glucksberg, S., and G. N. Cowen, Jr. 1971. Memory for nonattended auditory material. Cog. Psychol. 2: 149–156.

Haagen, C. H. 1944. Intelligibility measurement: Techniques and Procedures Used by the Voice Communication Laboratory. Psychological Corporation. OSRD Report 3748.

Haagen, C. H. 1945. Intelligibility measurement: Twenty-four word multiple choice tests. Psychological Corporation. OSRD Report 5567.

Hauptmann, L. 1952. A study of the effects of listener adaptation on the change in the intelligibility of international students speaking English. Unpublished masters thesis. Ohio State University, Columbus.

Hawkins, J. E., Jr., and S. S. Stevens. 1950. The masking of pure tones and of speech by white noise. J. Acoust. Soc. Amer. 39: 1188–1189.

Hecker, M. H. L., K. N. Stevens, and C. E. Williams. 1966. Measurements of reaction time in intelligibility tests. J. Acoust. Soc. Amer. 39: 1188–1189.

Heffler, A. J., and M. C. Schultz. 1964. Some implications of binaural signal selections for hearing aid evaluation. J. Speech Hear. Res. 7: 279–289.

Hirsh, I. J., E. G. Reynolds, and M. Joseph. 1954. Intelligibility of difficult speech materials. J. Acoust. Soc. Amer. 26: 530–538.

Holloway, C. M. 1972. Some effects of noise on a speech communication task. Sound 6: 27–31.

Howes, D. 1957. On the relation between the intelligibility and frequency of occurrences of English words. J. Acoust. Soc. Amer. 29: 296–305.

Hudgins, C. V., J. W. Hawkins, J. E. Karlin, and S. S. Stevens. 1947. The development of recorded auditory tests for measuring hearing loss for speech. Laryngoscope 57: 57–89.

Hutton, C., and J. Weaver. 1959. PB intelligibility and word familiairty. Laryngoscope 69: 1443–1450.

Irwin, J. V. 1947. A Battery of Tests of Speech Hearing. Unpublished doctoral dissertation. University of Wisconsin, Madison.

248   John J. O'Neill

Jerger, J. 1960. Observations on auditory behavior in lesions of the central auditory pathways. Arch. Otolaryngol. 71: 797–806.

Jerger, J. 1964. Auditory tests for disorders of the central auditory mechanism. In W. Fields and B. Alford (eds.), Neurological Aspects of Auditory and Vestibular Disorders, pp. 77–93. Charles C Thomas, Springfield, Ill.

Jerger, J. 1970. Development of synthetic sentence identification (SSI) as a tool for speech audiometry. In C. Rojskjaer (ed.), Speech Audiometry. Second Danavox Symposium, 44–65. Odense, Denmark.

Jerger, J. F., R. Carhart, T. W. Tilman, and J. L. Peterson. 1959. Some relations between normal hearing for puretones and for speech. J. Speech Hear. Res. 2: 126–140.

Katz, J. 1968. The SSW test—An interim report. J. Speech Hear. Disord. 33: 132–146.

Katz, J. 1962. The use of staggered spondaic words for assessing the integrity of the central auditory nervous system. J. Aud. Res. 2: 327–337.

Katz, J., R. A. Basil, and J. M. Smith. 1963. A staggered spondaic word test for detecting auditory lesions. Ann. Otol. Rhinol. Laryngol. 72: 908–918.

Keith, R. W., and H. P. Talis. 1972. The effects of white noise on PB scores of normal and hearing impaired listeners. Aud. J. Aud. Commun. 11: 177–186.

Kryter, K. D. 1963. Hearing impairment for speech. Arch. Otolaryngol. 77: 598–602.

Kryter, K. D. 1970. Effects of Noise on Man, chap. 2. Academic Press, New York.

Kryter, K. D., C. Williams, and D. M. Green. 1962. Auditory acuity and the perception of speech. J. Acoust. Soc. Amer. 34: 1217–1223.

Kurtzrock, G. H. 1956. The effects of time and frequency distortion upon word intelligibility. Unpublished doctoral dissertation. University of Illinois, Urbana.

Lafon, Jean-Claude. 1969. Auditory basis of phonetics. In B. Malmberg (ed.), Manual of Phonetics, pp. 76–104. North-Holland, Amsterdam.

Licklider, J. C. R. 1946. Effects of amplitude distortion upon the intelligibility of speech. J. Acoust. Soc. Amer. 18: 429–434.

Licklider, J. C. R. 1948. The influence of interaural phase relations upon the masking of speech by white noise. J. Acoust. Soc. Amer. 20: 150–159.

Licklider, J. C. R., D. Bindra, and I. Pollack. 1948. The intelligibility of rectangular speech-waves. Amer. J. Psychol. 61: 1–20.

Licklider, J. C. R., and I. Pollack. 1948. Effects of differentiation, integration, and infinite peak clipping upon the intelligibility of speech. J. Acoust. Soc. Amer. 20: 42–51.

Luria, A. R. 1966. Higher Cortical Functions in Man, pp. 96–100. Basic Books, Consultants Bureau, New York.

MacKeith, N. W., and R. R. A. Coles. 1971. Binaural advantages in hearing of speech. J. Laryngol. Otol. 85: 213–232.

Malmberg, B. 1966. Structural Linguistics and Human Communication. 2nd Ed. Springer Verlag, Berlin.

Mason, H. M. 1946. Improvement of listener performance in noise. Speech Monogr. 13: 41–46.

Matzker, J. 1959. Two new methods for the assessment of central auditory functions in cases of brain disease. Ann. Otol. Rhinol. Laryngol. 68: 1185–1197.

Miller, G. A. 1947. The masking of speech. Psychol. Bull. 44: 105–129.

Miller, G. A. 1962. Some psychological studies of grammar. Amer. Psychol. 17: 748–762.

Miller, G. A., G. A. Heise, and W. Lichten. 1951. The intelligibility of speech as a function of the context of test materials. J. Exp. Psychol. 41: 329–335.

Miller, G. A., and S. Isard. 1963. Some perceptual consequences of linguistic rules. J. Verb. Learning Verb. Behav. 2: 217–228.

Miller, G. A., and J. C. R. Licklider. 1950. The intelligibility of interrupted speech. J. Acoust. Soc. Amer. 22: 167–173.

Moray, N. 1970. Attention. Selective Processes in Vision and Hearing. Academic Press, New York.

Moser, H. M., and J. J. Dreher. 1953. A comparison of the U.S., U.K. and ICAO phonetic alphabets. Report 38. Human Factors Operations Research Laboratory, Bolling Air Force Base, Washington, D.C.

Moser, H. M., and J. J. Dreher. 1955. Effects of training on listeners in intelligibility studies. J. Acoust. Soc. Amer. 27: 1213–1219.

Moser, H. M., J. J. Dreher, H. Oyer, and J. J. O'Neill. 1956. Effects of sequence upon the reception of related and nonrelated message elements. AFCRS TN 56–55. Technical Report 35. Air Force Cambridge Research Center, Bolling Air Force Base, Washington, D.C.

Moser, H. M., J. J. Dreher, H. J. Oyer, J. J. O'Neill, and L. J. Schwartzkopf. 1957. Expectation in message reception. Technical Report 44. Air Force Cambridge Research Center, Applications Laboratory, Bolling Air Force Base, Washington, D.C.

Nussbaum, D. 1927. An improved method for testing the hearing with the spoken voice. Laryngoscope 37: 176–183.

O'Neill, J. J. 1954. Listener judgments of speaker intelligibility. Joint Project NM001 064.01. Report 28. Ohio State University Research Foundation and U.S. Naval School of Aviation Medicine.

O'Neill, J. J. 1957. Recognition of intelligibiltiy test materials. J. Speech Hear. Disord. 22: 87–90.

Orr, D. B., H. L. Friedman, and J. C. C. Williams. 1965. Trainability of listening comprehension of speeded discourse. J. Educ. Psychol. 56: 148–156.

Owens, E. 1961. Intelligibility of words varying in familiarity. J. Speech Hear. Res. 4: 113–129.

Oyer, H. J., and M. Doudna. 1959. Structural analysis of word responses made by hard of hearing subjects on a discrimination test. Arch. Otolaryngol. 70: 357–364.

Oyer, H. J., and M. Doudna. 1960. Word familiarity as a factor in testing discrimination of hard-of-hearing subjects. Arch. Otolaryngol. 72: 350–355.

Peters, R. W. 1954a. Message reception as a function of the time of occurrence of extraneous messages. Joint Project Report 33. U.S. Naval School of Aviation Medicine, Naval Air Station, Pensacola Fla.

Peters, R. W. 1954b. Competing messages: The effect of interferring messages upon the reception of primary messages. Project NM 001 06 401. Report 27. U.S. Naval School of Aviation Medicine, Naval Air Station, Pensacola, Fla.

Peters, R. W. 1956. Listener responses to voice messages as a function of signal-to-noise ratio and experience with similar messages. Report 64. U.S. Naval School of Aviation Medicine, Naval Air Station, Pensacola, Fla.

Peters, R. W. 1967. Perceptual organization for speech and other auditory

250   John J. O'Neill

signals. AMRL-TR-68-31. Aerospace Medical Research Air Force Systems Command, Wright-Patterson Air Force Base, Dayton, Ohio.
Pickett, J. M., and K. D. Kryter. 1958. Prediction of speech intelligibility in noise. AFCRC TR 58–62. U.S. Department of Commerce, Office of Technical Services, Washington, D.C.
Pollack, I., and H. Rubenstein. 1963. Response times to known message-sets in noise. Lang. Speech 6: 57–62.
Pollack, I., H. Rubenstein, and L. Decker. 1959. Intelligibility of known and unknown message sets. J. Acoust. Soc. Amer. 31: 273–279.
Poulton, E. C. 1953. Two-channel listening. J. Exp. Psychol. 46: 91–96.
Poulton, E. C. 1954. Verbal extrapolation and interpolation. British J. Psychol. 45: 51–57.
Rampp, D. 1972. Auditory perceptual disturbances. In A. Weston (ed.), Communicative Disorders: An Appraisal. pp. 297–330. Charles C Thomas, Springfield, Ill.
Rees, N. S. 1973. Auditory processing factors in language disorders: The view from Procrustes' bed. J. Speech Hear. Disord. 38: 304–315.
Rhodes, R. C. 1966. Discrimination of filtered CNC lists by normals and hypacusics. J. Aud. Res. 6: 129–133.
Rosenzweig, M. R., and L. Postman. 1957. Intelligibility as a function of frequency of usage. J. Exp. Psychol. 54: 412–422.
Rubenstein, H., and I. Pollack. 1963. Word predictability and intelligibility. J. Verb. Learning Verb. Behav. 2: 147–158.
Schon, T. D. 1970. The effects on speech intelligibility of time-compression and expansion on normal-hearing, hard of hearing, and aged males. J. Aud. Res. 10: 263–268.
Schultz, M. C. 1964. Word familiarity influences in speech discrimination. J. Speech Hear. Res. 7: 395–400.
Sergeant, R. L. 1964. Interactions among bandwidth, center frequency, and type of distortion in speech intelligibility. U.S. Naval Medical Research Laboratory. Report 432.
Shannon, C. E. 1951. Prediction and entropy of printed English. Bell Syst. Tech. J. 30: 50–64.
Shaw, W. A., E. B. Newman, and I. J. Hirsh. 1947. The difference between monaural and binaural thresholds. J. Exp. Psychol. 37: 229–242.
Siegenthaler, B. 1949. A study of the relationship between measured hearing loss and intelligibility of selected words. J. Speech Hear. Disord. 14: 111–118.
Siegenthaler, B. 1951. Formulation of a diagnostic word test of hearing. Unpublished doctoral dissertation. University of Michigan, Ann Arbor.
Silverstein, B., R. C. Bilger, T. D. Hanley, and M. D. Steer. 1953. The relative intelligibility of male and female talkers. J. Educ. Psychol. 44: 418–428.
Smith, B. B., and D. M. Resnick. 1972. An auditory test for assessing brain stem integrity: Preliminary report. Laryngoscope 82: 414–424.
Speaks, C. 1967. Performance-intensity characteristics of selected verbal materials. J. Speech Hear. Res. 10: 344–347.
Speaks, C., and J. Jerger. 1965. Method for measurement of speech identification. J. Speech Hear. Res. 8: 185–194.
Speaks, C., J. Jerger, and S. Jerger. 1966. Performance-intensity characteristics of synthetic sentences. J. Speech Hear. Res. 9: 305–312.
Speaks, C., J. L. Karmen, and L. Benitez. 1967. Effect of a competing

message on synthetic sentence identification. J. Speech Hear. Res. 10: 390–397.

Stevens, K. N., and A. S. House. 1972. Speech perception. *In* J. V. Tobias (ed.), Foundations of Modern Auditory Theory, pp. 3–62. Vol. 2. Academic Press, New York.

Sticht, T. G., and B. B. Gray. 1969. The intelligibility of time compressed words as a function of age and hearing loss. J. Speech Hear. Res. 12: 443–448.

Stuckey, C. W. 1963. Investigation of the precision of an articulation-testing program. J. Acoust. Soc. Amer. 35: 1782–1787.

Stuntz, S. E. 1963. Speech-intelligibility and talker recognition tests of Air Force voice communication systems. Technical Documentary Report ESD-TDR-63-224. Operational Applications Laboratory, ESD, AFSC, L. G. Hanscom Field, Bedford, Mass.

Teatini, G. P. 1970. Sensitized speech tests: Results in school children. *In* C. Rojskjaer (ed.), Speech Audiometry. Second Danavox Symposium, pp. 102–111. Odense, Denmark.

Thomas, I. B. 1966. Dynamic analysis of speech signals. Unpublished doctoral dissertation. University of Illinois, Urbana.

Tiffany, W., and D. Bennett. 1961. The intelligibility of slow-played speech. J. Speech Hear. Res. 4: 248–258.

Tillman, T. W., and R. Carhart. 1965. Monaural versus binaural discrimination for filtered CNC materials: The normal auditory mechanism. SAM-TR-65-79. U.S. Air Force School of Aerospace Medicine, Brooks Air Force Base, Texas.

Tillman, T. W., and W. O. Olsen. 1973. Speech audiometry. *In* J. Jerger (ed.), Modern Developments in Audiology, pp. 37–70. 2nd Ed. Academic Press, New York.

Tolhurst, G. C. 1954. The effect on intelligibility scores of specific instructions regarding talking. Joint Project NM 001 064.01. Report 35. Ohio State University Research Foundation and U.S. Naval School of Aviation Medicine.

Tolhurst, G. C., and R. W. Peters. 1956. The effect of attenuating one channel of a dichotic circuit upon the reception of dual messages. J. Acoust. Soc. Amer. 28: 602–605.

Traul, G. N., and J. W. Black. 1965. The effect of context on aural perception of words. J. Speech Hear. Res. 8: 363–369.

Treisman, A. M. 964. Selective attention in man. Brit. Med. Bull. 20: 12–16.

Voor, J. M., and J. M. Miller. 1965. The effect of practice on the comprehension of speeded speech. Speech Monogr. 32: 452–455.

Webster, J. C. 1969. Effects of noise on speech intelligibility. *In* Noise as a Public Health Hazard, pp. 49–73. ASHA report 4.

Webster, J. C., and P. O. Thompson. 1953. Some audio considerations in a control tower. J. Aud. Engineer. Soc. 1: 171–175.

Weener, P. D. 1972. Toward a developmental model of auditory processes. *In* D. L. Rampp (ed.), The Proceedings of the First Annual Memphis State University Symposium on Auditory Processing and Learning Disabilities, July 10–14.

Weston, P. B., J. D. Miller, and I. J. Hirsh. 1965. Release from masking for speech. J. Acoust. Soc. Amer. 38: 1053–1054.

Wickelgren, W. A. 1973. The long and short of memory. Psychol. Bull. 80: 425–438.
Wolf, O. 1874. New investigations on the methods of examination and the derangements of hearing. Arch. Opthalmol. Otol. 4: 67–86.
Zelnick, E. 1970. Comparison of speech perception utilizing monotic and dichotic modes of listening. J. Aud. Res. 10: 87–97.

Measurements of the Response of the Ear to Excess Acoustic Energy

Charles W. Nixon, Ph.D.
Chief, Biological Acoustics
Aerospace Medical Research Laboratory
Wright-Patterson Air Force Base

CONTENTS

INTRODUCTION

Virtually all environments contain acoustic energy at sufficient intensity levels to be processed by the auditory mechanism and perceived by man. Man is critically dependent on environmental information processing by the auditory system for the maintenance of normal activities in everyday living situations. It is curious that this pressure-sensitive system, designed to respond optimally to acoustic energy, is so susceptible to sound exposure that aural damage and corresponding loss of function are commonplace. Noise-induced hearing loss and associated problems are clearly the most critical and widespread of the various consequences of noise exposure. The impressive amount of research on this problem over the years has attempted to relate quantities that describe acoustic environments to other quantities that describe changes in the ears of persons who experience the environments. Quantities describing the character, magnitude, and duration of the exposure are utilized to specify the physical environment. Auditory function is measured and described in such a way that schemes may be formulated for predicting the response of the ear to any noise environment. Noise exposures which constitute a threat to hearing must be unambiguously defined and identified for preventive measures in hearing conservation programs.

This chapter presents an overview of measurements of adverse effects on the ear from excessive noise exposure to a wide variety of acoustic energy. Some attributes of normal auditory function are related to noise exposure effects. Characteristics of the physical stimuli and of auditory response factors determine the nature and magnitude of the influences on the ear. Recently collected data are presented on auditory effects of infrasound, impulsive sound, ultrasound, and long duration exposures. Major emphasis is on the state-of-the-art of exposure criteria for various categories of acoustic energy.

AUDITORY SENSITIVITY

The human ear is sensitive to a wider frequency range than the generally accepted one of 20 Hz–20 kHz. However, the frequency range of 500–5,000 Hz contains the sounds most important to man. Hearing function for the audiofrequency region (20 Hz–10 kHz) is well defined for discrete tones, bands of noise, a wide variety of speech materials, loudness, comfort, pitch, and even acceptability of sounds. For most of these attributes, individual responses may be evaluated against group data that have been collected using well defined and widely accepted procedures. Auditory responses to acoustic energy in the infrasonic region, below about 20 Hz, and in the ultrasonic region, energy above about 10 kHz, have not been extensively examined.

Infrasound, acoustic energy below the audiofrequency range, is not detected by the ear except at very high sound pressure levels. A number of investigators, using a wide variety of instrumentation, have independently measured hearing thresholds for infrasound (von Békésy, 1960; Whittle, Collins, and Robinson, 1972; Yeowart, Bryan, and Tempest, 1969). These are summarized in Figure 1. The agreement among the values shown is very good, and it provides some confidence that the general sensitivity curve for the human ear may have been described for this frequency region.

The sensitivity of the human ear decreases sharply at frequencies above 10 kHz. Data from Northern et al. (1972) for frequencies from 8,000 Hz to 18 kHz are included in Figure 1. The data from 10 kHz to about 95 kHz were adapted from the bone conduction data of Corso (1963). The bone conduction threshold at 10 kHz is 40 dB above the corresponding air conduction value. Consequently, 40 dB was subtracted from all bone conduction values (see Figure 1). The data from Corso are consistent with those of Northern et al. for the 10–20 kHz region. Thus the hearing function pattern represented by the curve in Figure 1 for frequencies above 10 kHz also seems reasonable.

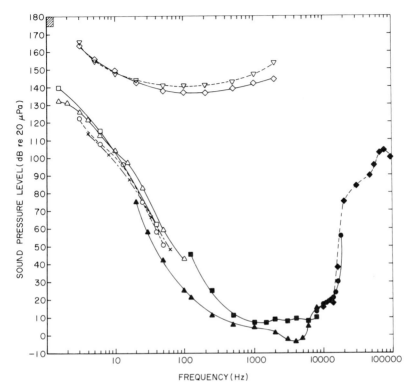

Figure 1. Human auditory sensitivity and pain threshold levels. □, von Békésy (1960) data—minimum audible pressure (MAP); ○, Yeowart, Bryan, and Tempest (1969) data—MAP; △, Whittle, Collins, and Robinson (1972) data—MAP; ×, Yeowart, Bryan, and Tempest (1969) data—MAP for bands of noise; ■, Standard reference threshold values—MAP (American National Standard on Specifications for Audiometers, 1969); ▲, ISO R226—minimum audible field (1961); ●, Northern et al. (1972) data; ♦, Corso (1963) data—bone conduction minus 40 dB; ◇, von Békésy (1960) data—tickle, pain; ▼, Benox Report—pain; ▨, static pressure-pain.

Presbyacusis is the gradually increasing loss of hearing sensitivity for high frequency sounds ascribed solely to advancing age. Central as well as peripheral components of the auditory system are affected. The highest frequencies customarily measured by conventional audiometry are affected first, and both ears show about the same threshold values. The amount of the loss gradually accelerates with increasing age as it moves down to affect frequencies as low as 500 Hz. Although individual patterns of presbyacusis growth vary widely, normative data describing hearing and aging have been compiled for our society.

Sociacusis is hearing loss attributed to the acoustic exposures man typically encounters in his everyday living experiences. It does not include presbyacusis or hearing loss resulting from occupational noise exposure.

Sociacusis effects may vary significantly from person to person. Standardized curves relating hearing loss to the noises of everyday living have not been formulated in the same manner as for hearing loss attributable to aging. The numerous medical factors that also may contribute to hearing loss—such as drugs, infections, circulatory disorders, heredity, head injury, and the large category of unknown causes—are not included in these definitions.

HEARING FOR SPEECH

Perhaps the most important function of the human auditory system is the role it plays in understanding everyday speech. Hearing for speech may be assessed with audiometry, which utilizes speech or speech-like materials as the test stimuli. Speech audiometry is generally more complicated and time consuming than discrete frequency testing. Although differential diagnosis and hearing aid evaluations still require good speech audiometry, pure tone assessment of speech function has become widely accepted, particularly for applications such as industrial audiometry, where the hearing of many employees is measured periodically as part of hearing conservation programs. Although hearing loss for discrete tones does not provide a valid description of a person's actual impairment, procedures have been formulated which reliably relate impairment to hearing for pure tones.

In 1959, the American Academy of Ophthalmology and Otolaryngology (AAOO) published a *Guide for Evaluation of Hearing Impairment.* Impairment is functionally defined as the inability to hear everyday speech under everyday conditions. Impairment is determined on the basis of the average hearing level (AHL) at 500, 1,000, and 2,000 Hz and is defined as beginning at an AHL of 25 dB relative to the normative hearing reference data in the American National Standard on Specifications for Audiometers (1969). Total percentage of hearing impairment is derived by multiplying the number of decibels above 25 dB AHL by 1.5%, with binaural impairment based on a 5 to 1 weighting of the better ear over the poorer ear. Total hearing impairment is defined as 92 dB AHL.

This AAOO formula for calculating hearing impairment based on discrete frequency hearing levels has become widely adopted and extensively used, especially in hearing compensation cases. In recent years, however, this formula has been questioned on at least two merits. First, many persons who have no hearing impairment according to the AAOO definition but who have losses above 2,000 Hz, subjectively report difficulty with speech communication in the noises of everyday situations. The incidence of this type of report has prompted proposals that the AAOO formula be changed to include a frequency above 2,000 Hz in order to better predict speech discrimination in noise. Some proposed changes are to use the average of 1,000, 2,000, and 3,000 Hz or 1,000, 2,000, and 4,000 Hz, or just to add 3,000 Hz to the present method to yield an average hearing level at 500, 1,000, 2,000, and

3,000 Hz to define impairment. Although there is merit to the question, data are not sufficient for selecting a significantly better formula for compensation purposes than the current one.

The second question arises from the use of the AAOO formula as a criterion to be applied in the prevention of noise-induced hearing loss. Application of this criterion as a preventive standard allows noise-induced hearing loss to develop until it reaches an AHL of 25 dB (using the American National Standard on Specifications for Audiometers (1969)), where it is then defined as impairment. This application of the AAOO low fence is inappropriate. Ideally, any noise-induced hearing loss should be prevented, and any observed changes in hearing level should be interpreted as warnings that the individual needs special attention. In the final analysis, however, the individual may choose to accept some noise-induced hearing loss in preference to changing jobs or giving up noisy recreational activities. Although the AAOO formula is considered appropriate as a means of determining degree of impairment for compensation purposes, it is at the same time considered inappropriate and too lenient as a standard for the prevention of noise-induced hearing loss.

CHARACTERISTICS OF NOISE EXPOSURE

Excessive exposure of the ear to acoustic energy is a common cause of both temporary and permanent losses of hearing sensitivity. Noise-induced temporary threshold shift (NITTS) returns to preexposure hearing levels following the experience. Noise-induced permanent threshold shift (NIPTS) does not recover to preexposure levels regardless of recovery time. Hearing loss induced by intense or long duration noise exposure may involve both a temporary and a permanent component. Presumably, noise exposure produces a change in auditory sensory hair cell function which recovers with rest in the case of NITTS and which does not recover in the case of NIPTS. No medical treatment is known that can improve or cure noise-induced sensorineural hearing loss. Some relationships have been established between noise exposure and NITTS and between noise exposure and NIPTS experienced daily over many years. It is assumed that NITTS is an integral part of and an essential precursor to NIPTS. It is further assumed that without NITTS no NIPTS will occur; that NIPTS develops similarly to NITTS but on a different time scale; and that all noise exposures with equal amounts of NITTS are considered to be equally noxious with respect to NIPTS. On the bases of these assumptions, of NITTS data from the laboratory and NITTS/NIPTS data from actual everyday noise exposures, hearing risk criteria were formulated which relate noise exposure to hearing loss (Kryter, 1965).

Experimentally noise-induced temporary threshold shift is a widely used research tool for the study of responses of the ear to acoustic energy. Both the incidence and magnitude of NITTS may be predicted statistically for exposures to specific noises at known levels and durations. The growth and recovery of NITTS follows predictable patterns for TTS values of about 40 dB or less whereas threshold changes greater than 40 dB are more erratic and more likely to involve permanent changes. On this basis alone it is not unreasonable to consider limiting the TTS incurred by laboratory study volunteers to a maximum of 30 dB, as an added safety factor.

Growth of NITTS

Some of the characteristics of the growth of NITTS during continuous exposure may be observed in the hypothetical curves of Figure 2 (Guignard,

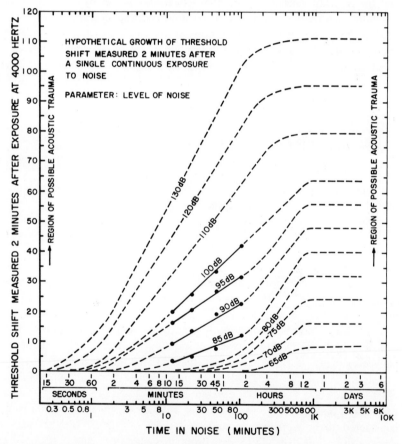

Figure 2. Hypothetical predictions of threshold shift for an average, normally hearing young adult exposed to a band of noise or pure tone centered near 4,000 Hz, where the ear is most susceptible. Curves were drawn to be consistent with current facts and theory, and in many cases extrapolations had to be made from appropriately corrected data from animals (cats and chinchillas). Adapted from Guignard (1973). Data points are from Ward, Glorig, and Sklar (1959).

1973). Magnitude of TTS grows as the level of the noise is increased and as the duration of the exposure is lengthened. Noise levels as low as 65 dB may produce TTS in the sensitive 4,000-Hz region of hearing when the duration of the continuous exposure exceeds a couple of hours. Noise levels must exceed 60 dB for most people to experience any TTS even for long exposures.

The growth of TTS from continuous noise reaches an asymptote or plateau during long duration exposures. Once this asymptotic level is reached, additional TTS is not observed for total exposure durations of up to 24 hr. The growth curves in Figure 2 reveal that asymptotic TTS occurs between 8 and 16 hr for noise exposures of around 100 dB and below, and at much earlier times during exposure to levels above 100 dB. Threshold shifts in excess of 40 dB measured 2 min after exposure are considered to be in a region of possible acoustic trauma.

Noises with energy concentrated in the 2,000–6,000 Hz frequency range produce the greatest effect on the ear at around 4,000 Hz. The maximal effect for other bands of noise and for tonal signals is usually found at about 0.5–1.0 octave above the exposure frequency. Intermittent noise exposures produce less TTS than continuous energy over the same time period. The greater the number of interruptions and corresponding rest periods, the smaller is the amount of the TTS.

Individual susceptibility to noise exposure varies greatly. A specific exposure which produces a marked NITTS in one person may produce no NITTS in another. Measurements of the noise susceptibility of an individual would be most valuable. However, in spite of considerable research on the subject, a satisfactory method for arriving at such a decision is not available. Exposure criteria have not incorporated a susceptibility factor because of the variability from person to person and the inability to reliably predict TTS for a specific ear.

In general, the hearing of women is better than that of men. However, women show significantly more NITTS for stimuli higher than 2,800 Hz and less NITTS for frequencies below 1,000 Hz than men when exposed to high intensity tones and noises (Ward, 1966). No sex differences were observed in rate of recovery or in TTS produced by impulse noises. No differences in susceptibility to TTS were measured as a function of time of day or night (Nixon, unpublished data). No data are available on differences in NITTS because of age, nationality, or race.

Protective Mechanisms of the Ear The human auditory mechanism reacts in the presence of intense sound with a number of protective actions that reduce acoustic transmission to the inner ear (von Békésy, 1960). The mode of vibration of the middle ear system is altered during intense exposure, and the ossicular action of the stapes in the oval window changes from a piston-like movement to a rocking motion. In addition, the stapedius and tensor tympanic muscles contract, producing an increase in stiffness and possibly in damping of the ossicular chain (Nixon, Sommer, and Cashin,

1963). This aural reflex action fails to provide protection from sudden and impulsive sounds of less than 15–25 msec because of its response latency, nominally ranging from about 25 to as many as 200 msec depending on the person. The protective value of the aural reflex gradually decreases during exposure to sustained and repetitious stimuli simply because the muscles become fatigued. Any effort to utilize the aural reflex as a protective mechanism against noise should consider the use of an acoustic signal to induce the reflex prior to the noise exposure.

Tinnitus Tinnitus is a sound or sounds perceived by the individual as hissing, ringing, roaring, etc., for which there is no external stimulus reaching the ear. Although it is speculated that tinnitus may be caused by spontaneous neural discharge somewhere along the auditory pathways or to some unknown hair cell activity in the cochlea, no specific cause has been proved. Tinnitus may occur spontaneously or in response to noise exposure. It may occur during and/or after noise exposure and is commonly reported by persons who work in noisy industries or participate in noisy nonoccupational activities. Tinnitus may appear as the only indication or warning of an intense acoustic exposure. However, it is not experienced by all persons. Although several different factors may produce tinnitus, when it does occur during and after a noise exposure, that exposure should be recognized as excessive; it should be terminated and avoided in the future.

Recovery of NITTS

Recovery of NITTS to preexposure hearing threshold levels is generally linear with the logarithm of the postexposure time. This pattern of recovery applies to moderate and to high level exposures of short duration. When an exposure is severe in terms of either level or duration, rate of recovery is slower and the TTS persists for longer periods of time. Recovery of TTS induced by long duration exposures of 12–24 hr, and more, as well as TTS values in excess of 40 dB, tends to be quite slow. Neither acquisition nor recovery of NITTS following exposure to impulse sounds necessarily follows the general patterns found for continuous noise exposure.

Response of the Auditory Mechanism

Noise exposure can produce injury and damage to the ear, resulting in hearing loss associated with two general syndromes that involve the eardrum membrane-middle ear system or the cochlear section of the inner ear. Combined losses occur in which both the mechanical and sensorineural elements are affected.

Middle Ear System Very intense noises of either a continuous or impulsive character may drive the middle ear system beyond the mechanical limits of its normal modes of operation. Damage may occur as drum membrane rupture, as dislocation, or even as fracture of the ossicles. Hearing loss caused by this type of damage is characteristically about the same amount for all frequencies, assuming no sensorineural involvement. Drum membrane ruptures that are not too severe and have no ossicular chain involvement will likely heal with little or no persistent hearing loss. Ossicular chain damage may be amenable to surgery or prosthetic device reconstruction. Sensorineural involvement, if it is also present, may not be determined for many months. The threshold of damage for eardrum membrane rupture involves average pressure changes of around 6–8 pounds/sq. inch.

Aural pain is localized in the middle ear. It is not related to sensitivity, as evidenced by the fact that normal hearing and hard-of-hearing persons have the same average aural pain thresholds for sound. It occurs in response to sound almost independent of frequency at levels between about 135 and 144 dB, except for infrasound, which is more tolerable. Aural pain seems to be associated with excessive distortion or mechanical displacement of the middle ear system and is believed to occur near the threshold for damage. It therefore acts as a warning mechanism to the individual of an overexposure. The inner ear has no such warning system, so that sensorineural hearing loss can become severe without any experience of aural pain. Representative thresholds for aural pain caused by intense sound are summarized in Figure 1. The threshold values are elevated above about 140 dB re 20 μPa for frequencies below 20 Hz. The threshold of aural pain for static pressures is in the region of 180 dB re 20 μPa (von Békésy, 1960; von Gierke et al., 1953).

Inner Ear System Overexposure of the inner ear system is associated with damage to sensory hair cells in the cochlea. Vivid confirmation of the destructive force of excessive acoustic energy on hair cell integrity is revealed through electron microscope techniques. Normal hair cell structure is shown in Figure 3A, along with single hair cell destruction in 3B, and extensive hair cell destruction in 3C, produced by noise exposure (Lim and Melnick, 1971). Hair cell pathology is nonreversible, and hearing loss associated with this condition does not recover. These effects are confined to the inner ear and extracochlear mechanisms are not involved.

Sensorineural hearing loss resulting from acoustic exposure is typically a high frequency loss and usually is observed first between 2,000 and 6,000 Hz with the greatest decrease in sensitivity at 4,000 Hz. It is frequently accompanied by recruitment, which is an abnormally large growth of loudness for a typical increase in intensity. With continued exposure the loss of sensitivity spreads to adjacent frequencies and increases in magnitude at least to its asymptotic level. Studies of long-term industrial exposures show that for a constant exposure to hazardous levels of noise, hearing loss increases with number of years on the job. The vast majority of hearing damage risk criteria and standards are directed to the prevention of noise-induced sensorineural hearing loss in the occupational situation.

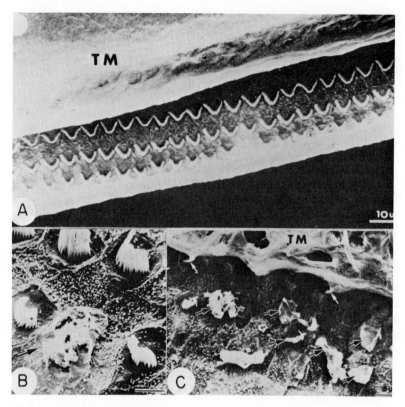

Figure 3. Noise-induced hair cell pathology. A, normal appearance of three rows of outer hair cells and tectorial membrane (TM); B, a single degenerated outer hair cell, indicated by arrow; C, degenerated outer hair cells with apparent loss of orderly arrangement in the third turn of cochlea. Reprinted with permission: Lim and Melnick; 1971; Arch. Otolaryngol. 94: 294–305.

DAMAGE RISK CRITERIA

Environmental noise sources generate acoustic energy over a very wide spectrum ranging from below 1 Hz to 100 kHz. Exposure to various segments of this acoustic continuum produce differential effects on man. To ensure that the overall exposures are safe, definitions of limiting levels and durations of exposure must be provided for a number of specific purposes of the spectrum. Generally, limiting values based on relationships of noise exposure to effects on the auditory system may be defined specifically for infrasound (1–20 Hz), audiofrequencies (20 to about 8,000 Hz), ultrasound (8,000 Hz to about 40 kHz), and impulsive sound. Some of the exposure limits discussed are well substantiated by experimental evidence and experience, but others must be considered tentative until there is more evidence.

Infrasound (Range 1–20 Hz)

Quantitative relationships between human exposure to infrasound and hearing loss are not well established. Investigations are few because of technical problems involved in the measurement of hearing thresholds for infrasound and the inability to generate infrasound stimuli without audible overtones produced by distortion. Nevertheless, the consistency of the findings and the relatively innocuous effect of infrasound on the ear at the levels and durations examined suggest that tentative limiting levels based on the short duration exposures investigated are appropriate. Maximal permissible levels of infrasound are formulated from available experience in noise fields with intense infrasound components and from laboratory investigations. Factors such as temporary auditory threshold shift, aural pain, middle ear response, and whole body effects influence such criteria. Tentative limiting sound pressure levels are indicated in Figure 4, based in part on the data contained in Figure 5. Various exposure parameters and corresponding effects on hearing are summarized for a series of laboratory studies in Figure 5 (Johnson, 1973a; Nixon, 1973; Nixon and Johnson, 1973). About 100 ear exposures are represented by these data. It is clear that exposure durations of 8 min or less at levels up to 150 dB caused essentially no TTS. These tentative limiting levels apply to discrete frequencies or octave bands centered about the stated frequencies. The use of good insert earplugs may increase the permissible levels by 5 dB for the same exposure times and are strongly recommended for all intense infrasound exposures to minimize subjective

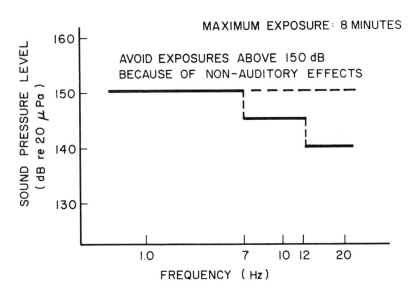

Figure 4. Tentative limiting exposures for infrasound.

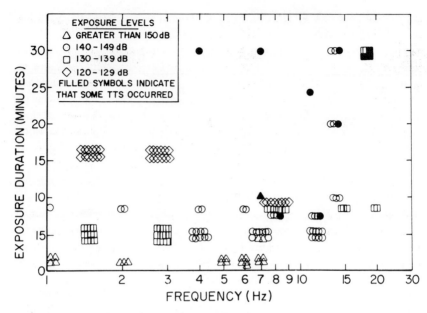

Figure 5. Infrasound exposure effects on hearing.

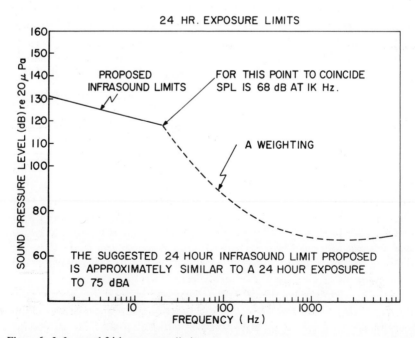

Figure 6. Infrasound 24-hr exposure limits.

sensations. Levels above 150 dB should be avoided even with maximal hearing protection until additional technical data are accumulated.

To specify criteria for long duration exposures to infrasound requires some extrapolation in the absence of complete data. The data contained in Figure 5 show essentially no effects at 20 Hz for exposures of 8 min at levels up to 141 dB. Using the equal energy rule of 3 dB per doubling or halving of time and some extrapolation from 8 min to 24 hr, the limiting level is reduced to about 118 dB at 20 Hz (Figure 6). (Details of calculations used to derive limiting levels for infrasound are described in Nixon and Johnson, 1973.)

Audiofrequencies

A substantial body of knowledge exists from laboratory and field investigations and audiometric surveys which describes effects of various types of noise exposure on hearing for audiofrequencies. The vast majority of these data concern continuous noise exposures of 8 hr and less as experienced in occupational situations. Recent emphasis on environmental quality has stimulated interest in nonoccupational noises as well as long duration exposures of 8–24 hr. As a consequence, the question of impairment or significant loss of hearing because of occupational noise is being considered as part of the total environmental noise exposure.

Perhaps the most widely used criteria for audiofrequencies which specify tolerable exposures are those which were published in 1965 by the National Academy of Sciences-National Research Council, Committee on Hearing, Bioacoustics, and Biomechanics (CHABA) (Kryter, 1965). This method described noise exposure in terms of pure tones or one third and full octave bands, and it applied to the frequency range of 100–7,000 Hz. The basic criteria considered an environmental noise to be acceptable if it produced, on average, a NIPTS in people after 10 years or more of near daily exposure of no more than 10 dB at 1,000 Hz and below, 15 dB at 2,000 Hz, and no more than 20 dB at 3,000 Hz and above. This standard was based on a number of assumptions concerning NITTS and probable relationships between NITTS and NIPTS. Growing acceptability of the A-weighted sound level as a descriptor of noise effects on man and the desire for hearing risk criteria which were simple to use, resulted in the formulation from the CHABA contours of permissible exposure criteria in terms of A-weighted sound level. Although the relationships described in the CHABA method are no less accurate than at the time of its publication, most hearing risk criteria have been converted to A-weighted sound level for simplicity and ease of application.

The Noise Control Act of 1972 required the Environmental Protection Agency (EPA) to provide to Congress the best scientific knowledge on all identifiable noise effects on public health and welfare and also to provide information on levels of environmental noise requisite to protect public health and welfare with an adequate margin of safety. These requirements were satisfied with the publication of two key documents by the EPA, the Noise Criteria document in 1973 and the Environmental Noise Levels document in 1974. Preparation of these documents and the scientific concepts presented therein are milestones in the long history of noise research. Consideration was given to all available data, from which a unified position was established, including authoritative studies; inputs from scientific, technical, and professional groups; individual experts; and public hearings. This position involved selection of a universal method for describing noise exposure which would reflect the total noise exposure of the public, specifically, levels below which no permanent health effects would occur. Health effects to be protected were hearing, speech communication, and general well-being (relaxation, sleep, etc.). Long-term effects were of primary concern; however, short-term effects may be determined from the total noise exposures. The levels identified in these documents are not to be interpreted as standards or regulatory values, but as guidelines or long range goals toward which noise research and activities should be directed.

Equivalent continuous sound level (Leq) was selected as the most reliable descriptor of noise exposure. Leq is the constant sound level in a specified time period equivalent to the total A-weighted sound energy received from the actual time-varying noise exposure. This means that any noise exposure can be converted to the quantity, Leq. Leq for 8 hr is numerically equal to A-weighted sound level in decibels. (The calculation of Leq is described in detail in appendix 8 of the Noise Criteria document.) This quantity is simple and predictable. It measures all conditions over long time periods and correlates well with effects on man and with other physical descriptors, and measurement equipment is currently available. It does not incorporate a pure tone correction nor does it completely handle all short duration, high intensity noises. Overall, it is considered, with few exceptions, as a best choice for describing all types of environmental noise exposure.

Numerous researchers, on the basis of hearing survey studies, have attempted to develop predictive schemes relating hearing loss to the 8-hr working day noise exposure. Three authoritative studies were selected and integrated into a unified method for describing NIPTS as a function of noise exposure. All three methods, Baughn (1973), Passchier-Vermeer (1971), and Robinson (1971), have shortcomings as well as strong points. However, when the predicted NIPTS data were tabulated for each method and compared, differences no larger than ± 5 dB were observed. Consequently, the final predictive scheme is the average of the NIPTS of the three methods (Johnson, 1973b).

Noise exposure criteria selected to protect hearing will vary with the administrative positions taken with regard to such questions as what is hearing impairment, how much hearing should be protected, and what percentage of the population is to be protected. The AAOO formula discussed earlier considers impairment as inability to hear everyday speech under everyday conditions. The amount of loss allowed is an AHL of 25 dB for the 500-, 1,000-, and 2,000-Hz test signals. However, if impairment is defined as no noise-induced loss at any test frequency, the most sensitive region of the ear must be protected, namely, 4,000 Hz, and the amount of allowable loss would be 5 dB, which is the error typically associated with hearing threshold measurement. Any change greater than 5 dB at 4,000 Hz would constitute impairment by the latter definition. This differs significantly from the AAOO formula. The percentage of the population to be protected is decided, and the corresponding permissible exposures are selected from data relating noise exposure to hearing loss. Obviously, a standard that protects the most sensitive portion of the hearing function will allow less noise exposure than more liberal standards. It has been customary to establish a basic criterion for the permissible level of exposure for an 8-hr period, which corresponds to a typical work day.

Once the standard is determined for 8-hr exposures, other permissible exposures are calculated, using an appropriate rule for allowing a higher level of exposure for shorter and a lower level for longer durations. The "equal energy" rule of 3 dB/doubling or halving of time is the most conservative rule, and incidentally, is widely used throughout Europe for hearing conservation. This rule essentially protects hearing at 4,000 Hz. The 5-dB rule, currently used by the Department of Labor, Office of Occupational Safety and Health (OSHA)(1969), essentially protects hearing for the conventional speech frequencies of 500, 1,000, and 2,000 Hz. It is of interest that the United States Air Force (1973), in its expanded regulation of noise control, adopted a 4-dB rule for calculating exposures less than 8 hr.

The EPA Noise Criteria document presents limiting levels of noise exposure for the conversational speech frequencies and also for the most sensitive frequency for humans, which is 4,000 Hz. It is demonstrated that to protect hearing for these speech frequencies in 90% of the population, daily exposures to continuous noise should not exceed 85 dB(A) for 8 hr. Continuous daily exposures should not exceed 75 dB(A) for 8 hr (70 dB(A) for 24 hr) to protect hearing at the 4,000-Hz test frequency. The present OSHA requirement specifies 90 dB(A) for 8 hr. Table 1 contains the permissible levels of noise as a function of duration as regulated by the OSHA, the Air Force, and the Army (1972). All three of these standards are based on essentially the same data. The differences are attributable to various interpretations of data and assumptions by the formulating agency relative to the questions posed earlier as to how their respective populations are to be protected.

The criteria in Table 1 display different limiting levels for 8-hr exposures as well as different trade-off rules. OSHA and the Army employ 5-dB rules whereas the Air Force utilizes a 4-dB rule. Column 2 describes permissible noise levels when the equal energy rule of 3 dB is applied to the basic OSHA 8-hr exposure level of 90 dB(A). Each of these criteria allows some noise-

Table 1. Permissible noise exposures in A-weighted sound pressure level (dB) for cited agencies

Duration of exposure (hr)	Equal energy[a]	OSHA	U.S. Army	U.S. Air Force	EPA
16				80	
8	90	90	85	84	75[b]
4	93	95	90	88	
2	96	100	95	92	
1	99	105	100	96	
0.5	102	110	105	100	
0.25	105	115[c]	110[c]	104	

[a]Equal energy rule of 3 dB applies to a basic 8-hr criterion of 90 dB(A).
[b]Threshold for detectable NIPTS at 4,000 Hz; exposures exceeding 75 dB(A) may cause NIPTS exceeding 5 dB in 10% of the population after cumulative noise exposure of 10 years.
[c]Ceiling on exposure.

induced hearing loss in a portion of the exposed population. There is some agreement that an exposure of 115 dB(A) for 15 min is excessive. The single limiting value of the EPA standard for 8 hr is described as the threshold for detectable NIPTS at 4,000 Hz. Noise exposures exceeding 75 dB(A) may cause NIPTS exceeding 5 dB in 10% of the population after cumulative noise exposure of 10 years.

Noise exposures that are interrupted or intermittent affect hearing less than continuous exposures do over comparable time periods. Noise exposure standards, such as those summarized in Table 1, provide procedures for assessing interrupted exposures whereby the individual on-times are compared to the corresponding values in the table and are combined to provide a total daily exposure description. Specifically, the ratio of actual exposure duration to permissible exposure duration is calculated at each level for each exposure and the ratios are summated. The total daily exposure should not exceed a value of 1 to be permissible.

Long Duration

Noise exposure durations greater than 8 hr are typical of some work assignments as well as of situations in which occupational noise is supplemented by large amounts of environmental noise after working hours, such as household noises, recreational noises, noises from second jobs, from transportation, and from proximity to industry. Most hearing risk criteria in use today do not include exposures longer than 8 hr. The development of allowable occupational noise doses of up to 8 hr assumes that recovery of any NITTS occurs during the interval prior to the next exposure. This opportunity for recovery does not exist for exposures in excess of 8 hr. The validity of extrapolating from present noise exposure criteria for 8 hr to longer duration exposures is

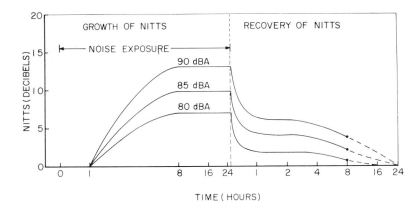

Figure 7. Growth and recovery of NITTS. Noise band (one third octave) centered on 1,000 Hz. Data: average hearing levels at 1,000, 1,500, and 2,000 Hz. Test frequencies measured at times marked on abscissa.

not known. However, some agencies have adopted the practice of reducing the permissible level by 3 dB to 5 dB for each doubling of exposure time for up to 16 hr. Clearly, additional data are required to establish long duration limiting levels.

The number of studies is small in which long duration exposure to sound and NITTS have been observed in man (Melnick, 1972; Mills et al., 1970; Smith et al., 1970). Agreement among the results of the various studies is quite good in terms of NITTS magnitudes. Exposures to narrow- and to broad-band acoustic energy for 24-hr durations at levels of 75 dB to over 95 dB show maximal average NITTS values ranging from 10 dB to 25 dB with reasonably short recovery times. The acquisition of NITTS during exposure seems to asymptote between 8 and 16 hr for levels up to about 90 dB(A) as shown in Figure 7 (Nixon, unpublished data). No increase in NITTS is observed during the last 16 hr of the exposure. It is not known if the NITTS remains stable for exposure durations longer than 24 hr. The postexposure data clearly show that recovery is not a function of log time, as in the case of moderate exposures of 8 hr and less. An initial rapid increase in sensitivity seems to stabilize for a period of time prior to complete return to threshold. The magnitude of the shifts in the studies represented in Figure 7 were small, and recovery was complete by 24 hr postexposure.

Ultrasound

The incidence of ultrasonic sound sources in our society has increased at an accelerating pace in the past decade, in the form of ultrasonic cleaning and measuring devices, drilling and welding processes, repellents for birds and other creatures, alarm systems, power and communication control applications, and a wide range of medical applications. Although the number of personnel exposed to airborne ultrasound is quite large, documented evidence of detrimental effects on man are scarce. In the late 1940's, alarm over "ultrasonic sickness" prompted investigations that identified the causes as being psychosomatic or subjective (Parrack, 1969), but no efforts were made to establish ultrasound exposure criteria.

Recent evidence (Acton, 1973; Grigor'eva, 1966; Michael et al., 1974) provides some correlation of subjective symptoms with exposure to specific ultrasound conditions. Energy at frequencies above about 17 kHz and at levels in excess of 70 dB may produce adverse subjective effects experienced as fatigue, headache, and malaise. These effects are related to hearing ability because persons who do not hear in this frequency range do not experience the subjective symptoms. Women experience the symptoms more often than men, and younger men report them more often than older men do. This is consistent with the relative hearing abilities of the three groups. Although most ultrasound is very narrow band or pure tone in nature, substantial lower frequency energy is also frequently present in the exposure. Acton (1973), Grigor'eva (1966), and Parrack (1969) independently report that effects attributed to ultrasound, especially for hearing sensitivity, are actually attributable to this high audiofrequency energy. Reducing the level of the audio portion of such exposures usually results in the disappearance of the auditory and subjective symptoms.

Limiting levels of ultrasound to control auditory and subjective effects are summarized in Figure 8. Agreement among the three sets of criteria is

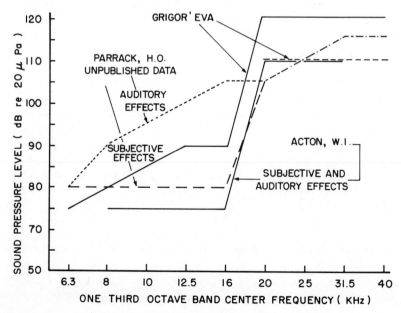

Figure 8. Proposed criteria for subjective and auditory effects of ultrasound.

good. Limiting effects above 20 kHz are confined to the subjective symptoms described earlier. Compliance with these proposed values should greatly minimize or eliminate adverse effects of ultrasound. The criteria refer to levels at the head of the exposed person, because ultrasound is not propogated well in air and it diminishes rapidly as distance from the source is increased. In addition, personal hearing protective devices are very efficient against airborne energy above about 8,000 Hz. The use of hearing protection by personnel in ultrasound noise fields usually eliminates overexposure problems relating to hearing as well as to subjective symptoms of ill feeling.

A comprehensive evaluation of ultrasound sources, effects on personnel, and proposed criteria was recently conducted by Michael et al. (1974). Among the conclusions, it was noted that relatively few people are exposed to a constant level of ultrasound above 10 kHz, that individual differences in sensitivity to ultrasound are quite large, and that subjective symptoms (psychological may lead to physiological effects) were real. The authors supported the limiting levels of ultrasound proposed by Acton (1973) and Parrack (1969), and pointed out that better methods are needed for predicting ultrasound exposures and for gaining knowledge of the response of the ear to ultrasound.

Impulse

An impulsive or impact noise is described as a sudden, brief sound or short burst of acoustic energy and is defined as a pressure rise at a rate of 40 dB/0.5 sec or faster. Impulse noises may occur singly or as a series of events. When the repetition rate of a series of impulsive noises exceeds 10/sec and the decay from the individual peaks to the minima does not exceed 6 dB, the noise may be treated as steady state and measured with a sound level meter. Otherwise, the rapid rise times of very short duration impulse noises cannot be adequately measured by conventional sound level meters and octave band analyzers. Performance limitations of the microphones and the meter ballistics as well as other characteristics of the instruments may result in underestimations of the actual levels of impulse noises. Impulse noises are usually measured using impulse meters or with oscillographic techniques which provide pressure-time histories of the signal.

A number of factors describing the impulsive stimulus have been identified as possibly relating to effects on the ear, including frequency spectrum, duration, peak pressure level, total energy, background noise, type of impulse, and rise time. Among these factors, only peak pressure level, duration, and type of impulse have been incorporated into standards describing safe levels of exposure.

Relationships between impulse noise exposures and hearing have been measured for a variety of impulse noises. The largest body of data has been collected for the very short duration impulses generated by weapons fire. Two extensive programs independently carried out in the United Kingdom

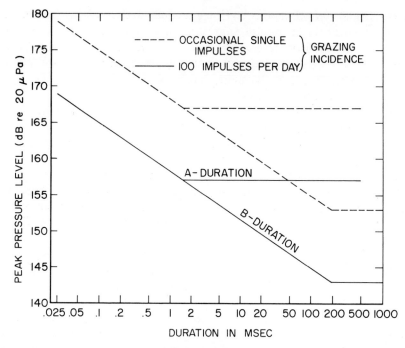

Figure 9. Proposed damage risk criteria for impulse noise.

and in the United States have examined a large range of exposure to gunfire conditions which were integrated into a proposed standard (Coles et al., 1968). The CHABA reviewed and essentially adopted this work in its proposed damage risk criterion for impulse noise (Ward, 1968).

Limiting noise exposure values for impulsive stimuli are shown in Figure 9. Exposures which comply with these criteria should produce, on the average, no more NITTS than 10 dB at 1,000 Hz, 15 dB at 2,000 Hz, and 20 dB at 3,000 Hz and above, in 95% of the exposed ears. These curves represent criteria for daily exposure of 100 impulses during any time period ranging from about 4 min to several hours. The criterion values are increased for fewer and decreased for more than 100 impulses/day by a factor of 1.5 dB for each doubling or halving of the number of impulses. The allowable level must be decreased by 5 dB for impulses that strike the ear at perpendicular incidence. The A duration curve is used to evaluate simple, nonreverberating impulses which occur in open spaces. The B duration curve is applied to oscillatory-type impulses that occur under reverberant conditions. The 138-dB floor at 200 msec reflects the action of the aural reflex, whereby energy entering the ear after 200 msec will be greatly reduced.

The comprehensive damage risk criteria displayed in Figure 9 require information on peak pressure level, duration, and type of impulse. Data on duration and type of impulse are not provided by impulse meters but require complex oscillographic instrumentation not usually available to field personnel responsible for noise measurement and hearing conservation. Consequently, most agencies have adopted an impulse criterion of 140-dB peak pressure level that can be measured in the field by impulse meter and used to identify hazardous impulse noise.

Sonic booms, generated by aircraft in supersonic flight, are impulsive sounds with the maximal energy in the infrasound region. Field investigations and laboratory studies with human exposures reveal no adverse effects on hearing from the levels of sonic booms experienced in the community (Nixon, 1965). Similarly, extremely intense sonic booms ranging in level from about 50 pounds/sq. foot to 144 pounds/sq. foot were experienced by persons in a field study with no adverse effects on hearing (Nixon et al., 1968). Sonic booms do not constitute a problem for the human auditory system.

Air bag systems, a new concept in automobile safety devices, utilize hollow cushions that inflate in front of occupants to cushion their forward motion when the car encounters a forward impact. The extremely rapid deployment of prototype air cushion systems was accompanied by intense impulsive noise inside the car. In one study, 91 volunteers experienced this air bag inflation noise inside a test automobile at a median peak pressure level of 168 dB (Nixon, 1969). About 50% of the subjects experienced some TTS with about 95% of the these recovering preexposure threshold on the same day. About 5% required a little longer for recovery, with one subject showing a gradually returning shift at one frequency that persisted for several months. The impulsive noise which accompanies present generation automobile air bag system inflations is loud. However, the levels are significantly lower than those generated by the early prototype system.

HEARING PROTECTION

Personal hearing protection must be provided when the preferred methods of noise control, which are reduction at the source and at the propagation media, do not reduce the exposure of the person to within safe limits. Personal hearing protective devices consist of items that are inserted into the external ear canal, items that cover the external ear, and even antinoise suits or whole body enclosures. The nominal range of hearing protection provided by good devices is summarized in Figure 10. Data are mean hearing protection values. Some methods of evaluating protector effectiveness in noise have subtracted one or two standard deviations from mean values in order to protect larger proportions of the population. Hearing protectors permit subjects to experience more intense and longer duration exposures than with unprotected ears and still remain within established health standards. The

HEARING PROTECTION	FREQUENCY RANGE IN HERTZ				
	1-20	20-100	100-800	800-8000	> 8000
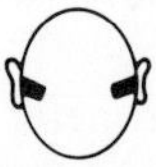 EARPLUGS	5-10	5-20	20-35	30-40	30-40
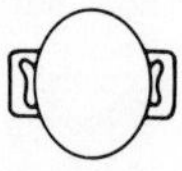 EARMUFFS	0-2	2-15	15-35	30-45	35-45
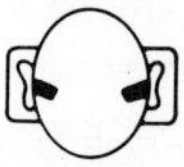 EARPLUGS AND EARMUFFS	10-15	15-25	25-45	30-60	40-60
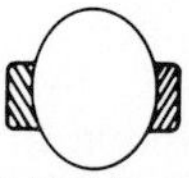 COMMUNICATION HEADSETS	0-2	2-10	10-30	25-40	30-40
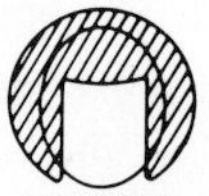 HELMETS	0-2	2-7	7-20	20-50	30-50
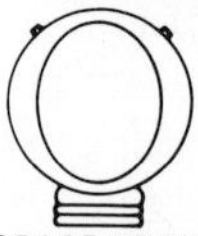 SPACE HELMET (TOTAL HEAD ENCLOSURE)	3-8	5-10	10-25	30-60	30-60

Figure 10. Expected range of hearing protection (on average) of good protective devices. Entries show approximate minimal and maximal protection available.

maximal amount of protection obtainable with ideal devices is limited by the tissue and bone properties of the head; that is, sound bypasses the protector and reaches the inner ear through tissue and bone pathways of the head (Nixon and von Gierke, 1960). Other features that reduce protective properties are air leaks, poor transmission loss of the material, and noise-induced motion of the device, which itself produces sound under the protector. Total head enclosures increase the available protection at the high frequencies by about 10 dB. Antinoise suits and whole body enclosures provide protection for hearing as well as against nonauditory effects on the abdomen, the chest, respiration, and vibrotactile sensitivity.

Personal hearing protection is critical to the maintenance of an effective hearing conservation program. Selection of an appropriate hearing protector should be made in accordance with the needs of the particular noise exposure situation because each type of protective device has advantages and disadvantages. Earplugs are small, more easily lost, more difficult to insert, and require a specific size and a healthy ear canal. However, they are less expensive, provide better low frequency protection than muffs, and are compatible with other personal items including eyeglasses, hats, some safety equipment, and long hair, without losing their effectiveness. Earmuffs are more costly, more cumbersome to carry around, may be too bulky in tight work places, may be too hot, do not fit well over eyeglasses and other obstacles such as hats and long hair. However, they are easier to put on, one size fits all, and they provide better high frequency sound protection. Earmuffs provide essentially no protection against infrasound (Nixon, Hille, and Kettler, 1967). An excellent discussion of personal protective devices and their relationship to hearing conservation is contained in Sataloff and Michael (1974).

SUMMARY

Although an impressive quantity of work has been accomplished on the effects of noise on man, particularly since World War II, and problems still persist, substantial gains have been made in virtually all aspects of noise control. Programs underway range from land use planning for compatibility with existing noises, and aircraft certification for noise, to extensive hearing conservation programs in the government and in industry. The immediate goal of all noise control activities is to reduce exposures to safe levels. The emphasis in this chapter has been on exposure criteria for the prevention of noise-induced hearing loss.

Hearing damage risk criteria have been described for a wide range of acoustic exposures including infrasound, audiofrequencies, ultrasound, impulsive sounds, and long duration exposures. The criteria represent interpretations by experts of available data relating noise exposures to hearing loss of both a temporary and a permanent nature. These data are much more tentative for some types of noise exposures than for others. Nevertheless, the guidance provided by these descriptions of permissible noise exposures is the basis for the prevention of noise-induced hearing loss. A major problem that has persisted for some time is lack of implementation of what is already known about noise-induced hearing loss and its prevention. The blame must be shared by all, even the individual employee who elects not to wear the hearing protection provided to him. Perhaps one of the contributions to be made by the Noise Control Act of 1972, will be that of requiring the systematic organization, integration, and implementation of the state of the noise control art as it is known today. Ongoing research will refine the technology base from time to time. However, the final guidelines and standards that define permissible noise exposures to assure the health and well-being of the individual will continue to be based upon administrative decisions.

REFERENCES

Acton, W. I. 1973. The effects of airborne ultrasound and near ultrasound. *In* Proceedings of the International Congress on Noise as a Public Health Problem. 550/9-73-008. Environmental Protection Agency, Washington, D.C. p. 349.

American National Standard on Specification for Audiometers. 1969. 53.6., American National Standards Institute, New York.

Baughn, W. L. 1973. Relation between daily noise exposure and hearing loss based on the evaluation of 6,835 industrial noise exposure cases. TR 73–53. Aerospace Medical Research Laboratory, Wright-Patterson Air Force Base, Dayton, Ohio.

von Békésy, G. 1960. Experiments in Hearing. McGraw-Hill, New York. 745p.

Coles, R. R. A., G. R. Garinther, D. C. Hodge, and C. G. Rice. 1968. Hazardous exposure to impulse noise. J. Acoust. Soc. Amer. 43: 336–343.

Corso, J. F. 1963. Bone-conduction thresholds for sonic and ultrasonic frequencies. J. Acoust. Soc. Amer. 35: 1738–1743.

von Gierke, H. E., H. Davis, D. H. Eldredge, and J. D. Hardy. 1953. *In* Benox Report: An Exploratory Study of the Biological Effects of Noise. University of Chicago Press, Chicago.

Grigor'eva, V. M. 1966. Effect of ultrasonic vibration on personnel working with ultrasonic equipment. Sov. Phys. Acoust. 11: 426–427.

Guide for Evaluation of Hearing Impairment. 1959. American Academy of Opthalmology and Otolaryngology, Rochester, Minn.

Guignard, J. C. 1973. A basis for limiting noise exposure for hearing conservation. 550/9-73-001-A. Environmental Protection Agency, Washington, D.C.

ISO Recommendation R226, Normal Equal-Loudness Contours for Pure Tones and Normal Threshold of Hearing Under Free Field Listening Conditions, 1961, 150 Central Secretariat, Geneva, Switzerland.

Johnson, D. L. 1973a. Various aspects of infrasound. *In* International Colloquium on Infrasound, pp. 339–351. Le Centre National de la Recherche Scientifique, Paris.

Johnson, D. L. 1973b. Prediction of NIPTS due to continuous noise exposure. TR 73-91. Aerospace Medical Research Laboratory, Wright-Patterson Air Force Base, Dayton, Ohio.

Kryter, K. D. 1965. Hazardous exposure to intermittent and steady-state noise. National Academy of Sciences-National Research Council, Committee on Hearing, Bioacoustics and Biomechanics, Washington, D.C.

Lim, D. J., and W. Melnick. 1971. Acoustic damage of the cochlea. Arch. Otolaryngol. 94: 294–305.

Melnick, W. 1972. Investigation of human temporary threshold shift (TTS) from noise exposure of 16 hours duration. Presented at the Annual Convention of the American Speech and Hearing Association, November 18–21, San Francisco.

Michael, P., R. L. Kerlin, G. R. Bienvenue, and J. Prout. 1974. An evaluation of industrial acoustic radiation above 10 kHz. Environmental Acoustics Laboratory, Pennsylvania State University, State College, University Park, Pa.

Mills, J. H., R. W. Gengel, C. S. Watson, and J. D. Miller. 1970. Temporary changes of the auditory system due to exposure to noise for one or two days. J. Acoust. Soc. Amer. 48: 524–530.

Nixon, C. W. 1965. Human response to sonic boom. Aerosp. Med. 36: 399—405.

Nixon, C. W. 1969. Human auditory response to an air bag inflation noise. Clearinghouse for Federal Scientific and Technical Information. PB-184-837. Arlington, Va.

Nixon, C. W. 1973. Human auditory response to intense infrasound, pp. 315—336. Le Centre National de la Recherche Scientifique, Paris.

Nixon, C. W., and H. E. von Gierke. 1960. Experiments on the bone conduction threshold in a free sound field. J. Acoust. Soc. Amer. 31: 1121—1125.

Nixon, C. W., H. Hille, and K. Kettler. 1967. Ear protector performance at low audio and infrasonic frequencies. TR 67-27. Aerospace Medical Research Laboratory, Wright-Patterson Air Force Base, Dayton, Ohio.

Nixon, C. W., H. K. Hille, H. C. Sommer, and E. Guild. 1968. Sonic booms resulting from extremely low altitude supersonic flight: Measurements and observations on houses, livestock and people. TR 68-52. Aerospace Medical Research Laboratory, Wright-Patterson Air Force Base, Dayton, Ohio.

Nixon, C. W., and D. L. Johnson. 1973. Infrasound and hearing. In Proceedings of the International Congress on Noise as a Public Health Problem. Dubrovnik. p. 329. U.S. Government Printing Office, Washington, D.C.

Nixon, C. W., H. C. Sommer, and J. L. Cashin. 1963. Use of the aural reflex to measure ear protector attenuation in high level sound. J. Acoust. Soc. Amer. 35: 1535—1543.

Northern, J. L., M. P. Downs, W. Rudmose, A. Glorig, and J. L. Fletcher. 1972. Recommended high-frequency audiometric threshold levels (8000 Hz—18,000 Hz). J. Acoust. Soc. Amer. 52: 585—595.

Parrack, H. O. 1969. Proposed standard acceptable levels of high frequency airborne sound fields around ultrasonic equipment. Technical Memorandum to Sub-Group of Working Group S3-40. American National Standards Committee on Bioacoustics, New York.

Passchier-Vermeer, W. 1971. Steady-state and fluctuating noise: Its effects on the hearing of people. In D. W. Robinson (ed.), Occupational Hearing Loss, pp. 43—62. Academic Press, London.

Robinson, D. W. 1971. Estimating the risk of hearing loss due to exposure to continuous noise. In D. W. Robinson (ed.), Occupational Hearing Loss, pp. 43—62. Academic Press, London.

Safety and Health Standards. 1969. Fed. Register 34 (no.96, part 2):7448-7449.

Sataloff, J., and P. L. Michael. 1974. Hearing Conservation. Charles C Thomas, Springfield, Ill. 365 p.

Smith, P. F., M. S. Harris, J. S. Russotti, and C. K. Myers. 1970. Effects of exposure to intense low frequency tones on hearing and performance. Submarine Medical Research Laboratory Report 610. U.S. Naval Submarine Medical Center, Groton, Conn.

U.S. Air Force. 1973. Hazardous Noise Exposure. Air Force Regulation 161—35.

U.S. Army. 1972. Noise and Hearing Conservation. Technical Bulletin 251. Department of the Army, Washington, D.C.

Ward, W. D. 1966. Temporary threshold shift in males and females. J. Acoust. Soc. Amer. 40: 478—485.

Ward, W. D. 1968. Proposed damage-risk criterion for impulse noise (gunfire). National Academy of Sciences-National Research Council, Committee on Hearing, Bioacoustics and Biomechanics. Washington, D.C.

Ward, W. D., Glorig, A., and Sklar, D. L. 1959. Temporary threshold shifts from octave-band noise: Application to damage risk criteria. J. Acoust. Soc. Amer. 31: 522–528.

Whittle, L. S., S. J. Collins, and D. W. Robinson. 1972. The audibility of low-frequency sounds. J. Sound Vib. 21: 431–448.

Yeowart, N. S., M. E. Bryan, and W. Tempest. 1969. Low-frequency noise thresholds. J. Sound Vib. 9: 447–453.

The Measurement
of Middle Ear Function

Jon K. Shallop, Ph.D.
Professor of Hearing and Speech Sciences
Ohio University

CONTENTS

INTRODUCTION

The function of the middle ear is well understood, but the techniques for measuring this function probably will continue to be a most interesting topic. The task of the middle ear is conceptually simple: conduct energy from a low impedance (acoustic) medium to a high impedance (fluid) medium containing the sensory receptors of hearing. The density of air compared to the density of the cochlear fluids represents an impedance "mismatch" of about 30 dB (Kobrak, 1959, p. 64). Although the transformer action of the middle ear may be apparent to the modern reader, the changing history of the concept of middle ear function is well worth recounting.

279

HISTORICAL ASPECTS

Until about the middle of the 18th century, anatomists believed that "implanted air" played an essential role in the reception of sound. This theory hypothesized that the receptor must resemble, in some form, the original medium. For hearing, this simply meant that somewhere beyond the tympanic membrane there must be some air specifically implanted for the purpose of receiving the sound energy. Plato suggested that the air was implanted permanently during fetal development (Wever, 1949, p. 6). Galen, in the 2nd century, apparently identified the auditory and facial nerves but did not discount implanted air (Wever, 1949, p. 6). The implanted air concept carried on for centuries until anatomic and physical discoveries of the last 5 centuries disproved its merit.

As anatomists of the 16th century began to define more precisely the structures of the middle ear, the theory of implanted air persisted. During that period, cadavers were routinely placed in a fluid preservative. Any fluid subsequently observed in the cochlea was presumed to be a preservative rather than cochlear fluids. Hence, the anatomists assumed the cochlear space to be air filled rather than fluid filled during life. Incidentally, their rationale for the implanted air theory is strikingly simple: air in the cochlea would result in the middle ear being an optimal impedance matching device, i.e., air to air rather than air to fluid.

Wever (1949) reports that during the 16th century the essential structures of the middle ear were identified. The malleus and incus were described by Berengario da Carpi (c. 1514) and Vesalius (c. 1543). The stapes, the oval window, and the round window were identified by Ingrassia (c. 1546). The detailed articulations of the ossicles and the two divisions of the inner ear were described by Fallopius (c. 1561). The connecting (Eustachian) tube from the pharynx to the middle ear and the tensor tympani muscle were accurately described by Eustachio (c. 1564). The stapedius muscle was identified by Varolius (c. 1591). With the discovery of a passage for air in and out of the middle ear began the demise of the theory of implanted air within the middle ear. For reference, an illustration of the middle ear is presented in Figure 1.

Duverney (c. 1683), perhaps more than any other author of the 17th century, convinced his contemporaries that implanted air was within the "two separate" parts of the cochlea. We are fortunate to have his classical book, *Traite de l'organe de l'ouie,* available in reprinted form (see under Duverney, 1683). For additional understanding of the development of the theories of hearing, John W. Black's preface to this reprinted version and the text itself provide the reader with valuable information.

The concept of implanted air within the cochlea was also promulgated during the 17th century by Perrault (c. 1680). Although Schelhammer (c. 1684) convincingly opposed Perrault's theory, the implanted air hypothesis persisted in spite of his explanations (Wever, 1949, p. 8).

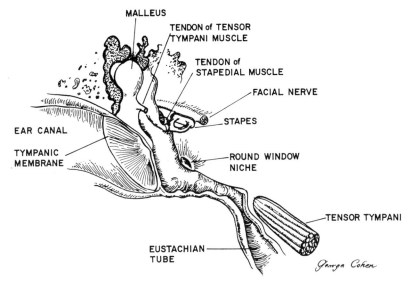

MALLEUS

TENDON of TENSOR
TYMPANI MUSCLE

TENDON of
STAPEDIAL MUSCLE

FACIAL NERVE

STAPES

EAR CANAL

TYMPANIC
MEMBRANE

ROUND WINDOW
NICHE

TENSOR TYMPANI

EUSTACHIAN
TUBE

Figure 1. The major structures of the middle ear.

The theory of implanted air within the cochlea was banished to the auditory museum during the 18th century by Valsalva (c. 1700), but he still contended that some air was present to account for the reception of sound (von Békésy and Rosenblith, 1948). It was finally Cotugno (1774) who confirmed that the inner ear contained only fluid (Wever, 1949, p. 9). This fact more clearly defined a new problem for investigation. How does the middle ear transform vibratory energy from air to a fluid in an efficient manner? Without the middle ear acting as an impedance match between these two mediums, 99.9% of the vibratory energy could not be transferred to the cochlear fluids (Gulick, 1971). This would amount to a 30-dB difference, which is compensated for by the mechanical advantages provided by the middle ear. This function was reported by Müller (1840) and one of his students, Helmholtz (1885).

Helmholtz (1885) emphasized the importance of the middle ear as a conductor of vibrations to the inner ear while recognizing some of the mechanical problems that were inherent in the transfer of energy from a low to a high density medium. He felt that the successful transduction of sound energy to the cochlear fluids was attributable to complex movements of the tympanic membrane, lever actions of the ossicles, and the areal ratio of the tympanic membrane to the stapes footplate. Later investigators reported the mechanical advantage of the combined lever action and the actual areal ratio to be $1.31 \times 14 = 18.3$ (Gulick, 1971). This represented a mechanical gain of 25 dB, assuming the average lever ratio of the ossicles to be about $1:1.3$ and the average areal ratio of the tympanic membrane to the stapes to be about 84:6 or 14:1.

Thus, during the 19th century the structure and function of the middle ear were fairly well understood. However, a typical description of the middle ear, such as the following one by the British aural surgeon Yearsley (1863), might be altered somewhat with today's knowledge.

The tympanum, then, may be said to be bounded externally by the membrana tympani, and internally by the labyrinth. Posteriorly by a short canal, which leads to the mastoid cells; and anteriorly by the opening of the Eustachian tube, which connects the ear with the throat.

Within the tympanum is seen a chain of four small bones, the *malleus, incus, os orbiculare,* and the *stapes.* They are thus named from their shape. The *malleus,* for instance, from its supposed resemblance to a hammer or mallet; the *incus,* from its resemblance to a blacksmith's anvil; and the *stapes,* from being shaped like a stirrup. It must be allowed that no bones of the skeleton are more appropriately or descriptively named. Ligamentous attachments connect them together so as to form an un-interrupted chain between the membrana tympani and the membrane of the fenestra ovalis, by means of which the impressions of sound are strengthened and conveyed from the former to the internal ear.

The Eustachian tube, so called after its discoverer, Eustachio, com-mences at the anterior and lower part of the tympanum, and proceeds forwards, downwards, and inwards, till it terminates at the upper and lateral part of the throat in an oblique and elliptic orifice, sufficiently large to admit the insertion of a quill. (Yearsley, 1863, p. 14)

Yearsley's reference to inserting a quill into the orifice of the Eustachian tube does not seem to be a pleasant experience.

Detailed information concerning the functions of the middle ear has been advanced considerably during the present century by the research of Nobel laureate Georg von Békésy. He demonstrated that the middle ear has an amplifying pressure transformation value of 22 (times greater than the input), which was determined by dividing the effective area of the eardrum by the area of the stapes and multiplying this quotient by the lever ratio of the ossicles. In addition, he has shown that the fluid behind the stapes is set into motion and thereby transmits the usually complex vibrations of sound along the cochlear partition as traveling waves. These complex waves then stimulate the receptor hair cells along the basilar membrane in a manner not yet completely understood.

Von Békésy (1960) used temporal bones of cadavers and determined that the absence of the middle ear structures, i.e., the ossicles, resulted in a decrease of the effective mechanical pressure transfer to the inner ear. This decrement was equivalent to an average hearing loss of approximately 55 dB from 250 to 3,000 Hz. Wever (1962) obtained similar results, reporting an average intensity loss of 42 dB in cats, using the cochlear microphonic procedure as a criterion measure. In another study, Wever and Lawrence (1950) demonstrated a less severe loss of 28 dB in the hearing sensitivity of cats when sound stimuli were directed through a flexible tube to the stapes footplate in the oval window rather than being directed into the entire open

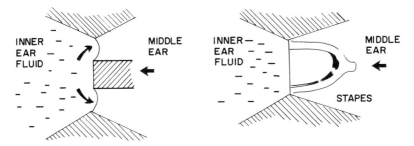

Figure 2. A schematic cross section drawing showing the close approximation of the stapes footplate within the oval window on the right. On the left is an illustration of the resultant backset of fluid pressure when a stapes replacement is too small. Adapted from von Békésy (1960).

middle ear. This latter procedure (flexible tube) reduces the effect of phase cancellation of the pressure waves.

According to von Békésy (1960), the footplate of the stapes must provide adequate closure of the oval window to prevent a loss of pressure, as illustrated in Figure 2. He indicated that the maximal width of the annular ligament circumscribing the footplate of the stapes is 0.1 mm, and that if the clearance between the footplate and the perimeter of the oval window is excessive, the transfer of sound to the inner ear is reduced by a backset of fluid pressure. In a similar vein, Wever (1962) compared the motion of the stapes with the piston of an engine. This analogy for the motion of the stapes is not entirely correct, since the stapes pivots about the posterior margin of its footplate. Onchi (1961) had attributed this movement to the stiffness of the posterior margin of the supporting ligament. Von Békésy (1960) has pointed out two rotational axes of the stapes, one at low and one at high intensities, attributable to the influence of the stapedius muscle.

METHODS OF EVALUATING MIDDLE EAR FUNCTION

There are several methods of evaluating middle ear function. Whatever method is selected must meet the following criteria to be continually useful: 1) easy to administer, thus having wider application; 2) able to produce valid and reliable measurements; 3) able to provide information that is readily conceptualized by the observer (primarily a clinical concern); and 4) not causing major physical discomfort to the subject.

Direct Observation

With the aid of a good light source, suitable speculum, magnification, and a skilled observer, essential information about the status of a middle ear can be assessed. The otoscope is commonly used for this purpose, and when it is accompanied by pneumatic pressure variations in the external auditory meatus, an observer may be able to detect abnormal middle ear functioning. It is doubtful that any measurement will ever totally replace this method; however, other methods have and will continue to make such direct observations more accurate.

Tuning Fork Tests

The use and significance of various tuning fork tests should not be overlooked. These tests are less quantitative than might be desired at times, but they are of definite value in the evaluation of the middle ear. The reader should be familiar with such tests as Weber, Rinne, and Schwabach and perhaps less familiar with the Pomeroy (Beatty, 1932) and Bing tests. Suitable masking for tuning fork tests can be obtained with a mechanical source such as the Barany Noise Box or with acoustic masking from an audiometer. Essentially, tuning fork tests try to differentiate qualitatively among normal hearing, conductive hearing loss, and sensorineural hearing loss. An interesting description of the use of a pocket watch in this regard is presented by Yearsley (1863).

> If we scrutinise the meaning of the term *nervous deafness,* it can only mean deafness in which paralysis of the auditory nerve is produced by some change in the nerve on the brain; but this is really the case in but a small minority of deaf patients. A simple test will show the fallacy of the usual diagnosis in diseases of the ear. If the ticking of a watch can be heard when applied closely to the auricle, or held between the teeth, it cannot be the auditory nerve that is in fault, but must be some part of the acoustic apparatus serving to transmit sound from the external air to the nerve of hearing. This test is unequivocal; because, the nerve being in contact with them, it is much the same as though the sonorous impulse was imparted directly to the nerve. If any deaf readers will try this experiment, very few will find themselves deaf to a watch held between the teeth. (Yearsley, 1863, p. 132)

Such methods demonstrate the insight and curiosity of Yearsley and others in the study and treatment of middle ear disease.

Tuning fork tests, when done properly, will provide good qualitative but limited quantitative information. More specific methodologies can be found elsewhere (DeWeese and Saunders, 1960; Kobrak, 1959).

Audiometry

Properly masked air and bone conduction thresholds to acoustic and vibratory signals provide a more quantitative assessment of middle ear function than do tuning forks. Audiometry is, in principle, the most accurate method of obtaining behavioral thresholds from a cooperative listener. The bulk of the basis of our present understanding about audition is obtained behaviorally with good psychoacoustic methodologies and is applied clinically through audiometry. Behavioral audiometry will continue to be a basic method of measuring hearing and assessing middle ear function through comparison of air and bone conduction thresholds. An adequate discussion of bone conduction theory is presented by Fournier (1959).

Audiometry plays an important role in the assessment of middle ear function. However, one must be aware of the possible changes in bone conduction thresholds (Carhart, 1962) resulting from middle ear pathology, such as stapes fixation. The explanation of these changes is a reflection of the complexity of middle ear mechanics. In the case of stapes fixation, Tonndorf (1966) describes the decreased bone conduction sensitivity maximized at 1,000–2,000 Hz as being the result of altering the resonance characteristic of the middle ear. The "Carhart notch" is the result of decreased resonance of the middle ear, which normally has a prominent resonance in the area of 1,200–1,500 Hz. A good discussion of middle ear mechanics is presented by Lawrence (1962).

Other Observations

Von Békésy (1960) performed numerous mechanical observations of middle ear function. He carefully studied the transformer effect of the middle ear with complex electromechanical measurement systems. Among his important findings are the equal amplitude contours of the tympanic membrane and the two forms of vibration of the ossicles. In the latter instance von Békésy noted that the stapes footplate vibrates with a posterior-to-anterior rocking motion at low to moderate intensities. At high intensities he noted that the motion of the footplate changes to an inferior-to-superior rocking motion. The net effect is a reduction of transmitted energy to the cochlea. He concluded that the articulation of the ossicles and the action of the middle ear muscles serve to protect the inner ear from intense stimulation.

Wilska (1959) observed the action of the tympanic membrane by coupling a small wood rod to the tympanic membrane. The other end of the rod was connected to a sensitive electromechanical system that measured the vibratory amplitudes by microscope. It was possible to present the signal in a vibratory or acoustic mode. He reported the familiar auditory threshold curve (Sivian and White, 1933) with increasing sensitivity as a function of frequency. Interestingly, he noted: "These experiments showed that the threshold values with air conduction were approximately ten times higher than those when the oscillations were conducted directly to the eardrum by means of a wooden rod." (Wilska, 1959, p. 78). This is a unique measurement of middle ear function, demonstrating the protective function of the tympanic membrane itself as well as the elastic control of the middle ear below about 1,000 Hz.

Some techniques other than the capacitive probe technique (von Békésy, 1941, 1960; Fischler et al., 1967) and the Wilska (1959) procedure have been used recently for measurement of vibratory patterns of the middle ear structures. Khanna and Tonndorf (1971, 1972) have shown the vibratory patterns of the tympanic membrane and the round window of cats by time-averaged holography. Their findings refute the "stiff-plate" hypothesis of von Békésy as the vibratory mode of the tympanic membrane. Rather Khanna and Tonndorf suggest that the tympanic membrane vibrates in complex isoamplitude contours parallel to the malleus. Their experiments were conducted with cats, and in this instance they proposed that the tympanic membrane vibrates as a curved membrane, as proposed by Helmholtz. Their holographic studies of the round window at high intensities raises the question of an inner ear mechanism for protection at high sound levels (Khanna and Tonndorf, 1971). Their studies with holography have also led to a reconsideration of the middle ear transformer ratio.

The Mössbauer technique has been applied to the study of auditory mechanical functioning (Gilad et al., 1967; Johnstone and Boyle, 1967; Johnstone, Taylor, and Boyle, 1970; Rhode, 1971). With this procedure, minute displacement and velocity values have been obtained for the middle and inner ear structures. Guinan and Peake (1967) utilized stroboscopic illumination for their study of the middle ear characteristics of cats. Laser inferometry has also been used in the study of these structures (Dragsten et al. 1974; Tonndorf and Khanna, 1968). Dragsten et al. report measurements of the cricket tympanic membrane covering amplitudes of 0.1 to 500 Å over the frequency range of 2–20 kHz. Techniques such as those just described provide precise measurements of middle ear function. It is interesting to note the continued acknowledgments to von Békésy among these contemporary authors, an honorable tribute to his exceptional scientific abilities.

ACOUSTIC IMPEDANCE, ADMITTANCE, AND TYMPANOMETRY

Acoustic impedance and admittance measures provide an essentially objective method of determining middle ear function. These measurements can be obtained at ambient atmospheric pressure (static measurements) or under induced changes of middle ear state (dynamic measurements). During the last 20 years, these measurements have provided a new methodology that has permitted more precise measurement of middle ear function. In fact, however, the principles of middle ear mechanics have been understood at least since the time of Müller (1840), who developed a hydromechanical model of the middle ear. He demonstrated the importance of the middle ear by removing the analagous middle ear structures. Such manipulations reduced the pressure delivered to the "inner ear" of the model. Lawrence (1962) has presented a reproduction and a more detailed description of Müller's middle ear model. Helmholtz (1863), one of Müller's students, continued the study of the middle ear, demonstrating his understanding of the principles of impedance.

Webster (1919) and Schuster (1934) described the principles of acoustic impedance. The first apparent studies of middle ear impedance were published by Sivian and White (1933) and von Békésy (1936). Von Békésy's original manuscript on middle ear impedance was translated from German into English in 1969. The first auditory clinical applications of acoustic impedance were described by Metz (1946). His instrument was a mechanical bridge designed in principle after Schuster's bridge. The Metz acoustic impedance bridge was not further utilized primarily because of its awkwardness and limited development. (Only two instruments were produced and they remain in Copenhagen.) The design and craftsmanship of these instruments is impressive. Zwislocki (1963) described a smaller, refined version of the Metz bridge. The Zwislocki acoustic bridge became commercially available in the 1960's but has been used less frequently in recent years because of advances in electroacoustic impedance and admittance instrumentation. Practical electroacoustic instruments were introduced in Europe by Thomsen (1955) and Terkildsen and Thomsen (1959).

Definition of Acoustic Impedance

The concept of acoustic impedance requires diligent study, and investigators should be aware of the entire concept, as a complex mathematical solution is required.

First, assume a simple mechanical system, as illustrated in Figure 3, which consists of a spring (S), mass (M), and frictional resistance (R_m) primarily between the surface of the mass and its support surface. The mechanical impedance (Z_m) of this system in response to a sinusoidal (back and forth) force (F) can be described as the ratio of the force (F) divided by the velocity (V) of the mass. The opposition to the applied force is the impedance of the system. The total impedance in this situation results from three interacting factors, the so-called "real" component, the frictional resistance, and the two "imaginary" components, the elastic reactance of the spring and the mass reactance of the mass.

The imaginary (reactive) components of impedance are so named because they do not coincide with the phase of the applied sinusoidal force. The resistive component, however, is in phase with the force. The physical

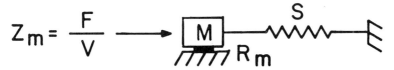

Figure 3. The mass M is being driven for an applied sinusoidal force F. The mass is attached to a stationary surface through spring S. The mass rests on a surface, with an intermediate mechanical resistance (friction) R_m. The impedance Z_m of the system is the ratio of the applied force divided by the velocity V of the mass.

properties of a spring are such that, when compressed or stretched, the spring is anticipating its eventual return to its rest position. This physical property is called elastic reactance, and represents the storage of energy. As the spring reacts with the applied sinusoidal force, two important principles must be kept in mind. First, the elastic reactance vector of the spring precedes the force vector by +90 degrees. Second, the amount of elastic reactance decreases as the frequency of the applied sinusoidal force increases. In other words, at lower frequencies, the amount of elastic reactance will be greater than at higher frequencies. This can be expressed mathematically as

$$X_E = \frac{S}{2\pi f}$$

where X_E is the elastic reactance, f is the frequency of the applied force, and S represents the elasticity or stiffness of the spring. Consider the relative values of X_E when: 1) f increases, or 2) when S increases. In the first instance X_E will decrease with increasing frequency. In the second instance X_E will increase as the spring increases in stiffness.

Mass has the physical property of inertia. In other words, during sinusoidal motion, as the velocity of the force slows down and reverses direction, the mass reactance will oppose this change somewhat like a reluctant horse. The inertia of the mass reacts with the force, and two important principles

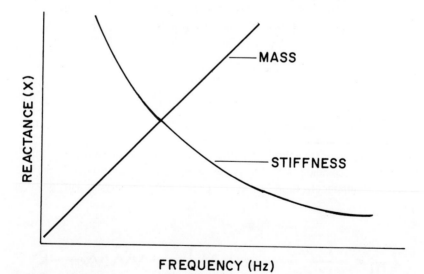

Figure 4. The interaction of mass and stiffness reactances are illustrated. The total reactance X is the algebraic summation of the mass (positive) reactance and the stiffness-elastic (negative) reactance. The intersection of the reactances represents resonance.

must be understood. First, the mass reactance vector will lag the force vector by −90 degrees. Second, the amount of mass reactance will increase as the frequency of the applied sinusoidal force increases. At lower frequencies mass reactance is minimal, but at higher frequencies the mass reactance predominates. This can be expressed mathematically as

$$X_M = 2\pi f M$$

where X_M is the mass reactance, f is again the frequency of the applied force, and M represents the physical mass or weight of the vibrating object-mass. Consider the relative values of X_M when: 1) f increases and 2) when M increases. In both instances X_M will also increase.

The interaction of the two imaginary reactive components of impedance is illustrated in Figure 4. Where the two reactances intersect, resonance of the system is represented since: 1) the reactive frequencies are identical (forced vibration); 2) the relative amplitude of the reactances are equal; and 3) the two reactances are 180 degrees out of phase. The latter is true because the mass reactance is always −90 degrees and the elastic reactance is always +90 degrees relative to the applied force. Therefore, the reactance will be minimal, resulting in resonance of the system. It should be noted, however, that some relatively constant resistive component will remain. The vector solution, as adapted from Møller (1964), is illustrated for this situation in Figure 5.

Imagine that the force F in the simple mass-spring system in Figure 3 is now represented in Figure 5 as the larger horizontal vector F plotted on the real (X) axis, to the right. For reference, call this 0 degrees. Furthermore, imagine that the force vector is rotating clockwise (through the quadrant order I, IV, III, II, I, etc.) at a constant velocity $2\pi f$. As the force vector rotates, the mass reactance lags behind by −90 degrees and is therefore plotted upward on the imaginary (Y) axis. The stiffness vector (elastic reactance) is plotted downward on the imaginary axis since it precedes the force vector by +90 degrees. Assume that the frequency of the force is relatively low, and therefore the stiffness vector will be greater than the mass vector (recall Figure 4). These two vectors will then sum algebraically as the imaginary X vector pointing downward in Figure 5. This vector by itself is +90 degrees relative to the force because stiffness controls the system at the assumed low frequency.

The remaining component to consider is the frictional resistance, R_m. Recall that this component is in phase with the applied force and therefore, in effect, merely shortens the force vector directly. The solution vector (Z) is the impedance of the system. It must be obtained by vector analysis based on geometric principles. Rusk (1960) states the rule for this procedure as the parallelogram law. Applying this law to vector analysis, Rusk states: "the resultant of two or more forces is that single force which would have the

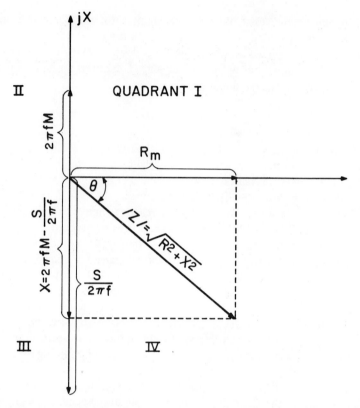

Figure 5. Mechanical impedance is illustrated in rectangular form. The magnitude Z and phase angle θ of the impedance vector results from the interaction in the mechanical system of mass M, stiffness S, and friction R_m to the sinusoidal force. The real axis is horizontal. The imaginary axis jX is vertical. In this instance the system is stiffness controlled, causing the impedance vector to be in quadrant IV. Adapted from Møller (1964).

same effect as the individual forces acting together, if it replaces them." Thus the vector solution for impedance (Z) will have two important characteristics: 1) a magnitude equal to the Pythagorian solution of $Z = \sqrt{R^2 + jX^2}$; and 2) a phase quantity representing the deflection of the resultant Z vector in quadrant IV. The relationship between the mechanical impedance concept described above and the acoustic impedance at the tympanic membrane is expressed as

$$Z_a = Z_m / A^2$$

where Z_a is the acoustic impedance, Z_m is the mechanical impedance, and A represents the effective area of the tympanic membrane (Metz, 1946; Møller, 1964; and Zwislocki, 1963). The basic unit of measurement of acoustic impedance is the acoustic ohm as defined by the American National Standard document (1960).

Acoustic Ohm (CGS). An acoustic resistance, reactance, or impedance has a magnitude of one acoustic (cgs) ohm when a sound pressure of 1 microbar produces a volume velocity of 1 cubic centimeter per second. (American National Standard document, 1960, p. 23)

Definition of Acoustic Admittance

If, rather than considering opposition to the flow of acoustic energy, we consider actual flow of energy, we will be measuring admittance (Y) of the system. Admittance is the reciprocal of impedance. The analogous terms of admittance are acoustic susceptance (B_A), the counterpart of reactance, and acoustic conductance (G_A), the counterpart of resistance (Newman and Fanger, 1973). The concept of acoustic admittance is illustrated in Figure 6.

Definition of Tympanometry

Tympanometry is the measurement of an acoustic parameter (impedance, reactance, resistance, compliance, admittance, susceptance, conductance,

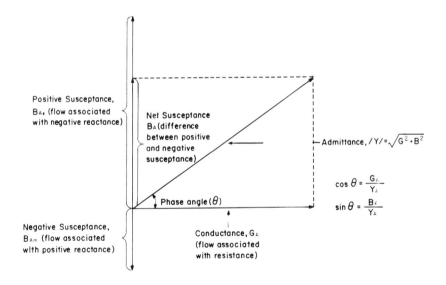

Figure 6. The concept of acoustic admittance is shown. The magnitude Y and phase angle θ of the admittance vector results from the interaction of the acoustic susceptance B and the acoustic conductance G. In this instance the mechanical system is stiffness controlled (below resonance) with the positive susceptance B_{As} dominating the negative susceptance B_{Am}. The net acoustic susceptance B_A and the acoustic conductance are resolved by the admittance vector being in quadrant I. The sine function of θ allows for the solution of susceptance $(B_A = \sin \theta \cdot Y_A)$ and the cosine function of θ resolves the conductance $(G_A = \cos \theta \cdot Y_A)$. Adapted from Newman and Fanger (1973).

etc.) while simultaneously varying the pressure in the sealed external auditory meatus of the measured ear. The studies of Van Dishoeck (1938) might be considered a basis for clinical tympanometry. He had patients simply report when a tone was "loudest" as he varied manometric pressure in the sealed ear canal. The point of maximal loudness corresponded to the measured middle ear pressure. Thomsen (1955) actually measured a parameter of acoustic impedance (percentage of absorption) with the Metz bridge as he increased ear canal pressure (0 to 400 mm H_2O). This represents, in effect, the positive side of a tympanogram, described later in this chapter. Tympanometry, as we know it presently, resulted from the electroacoustic instrument of Terkildsen and Nielsen (1960). Results with this instrument were first published by Terkildsen and Thomsen (1959).

MEASUREMENT OF ACOUSTIC IMPEDANCE, ACOUSTIC ADMITTANCE, AND TYMPANOMETRY

Current procedures and instrumentation for the measurement of middle ear acoustic impedance or admittance employ the previously described principles. The instruments used to obtain these measures are either mechanical-acoustic (Metz bridge, Zwislocki acoustic bridge) or electroacoustic (Madsen acoustic bridges, American Electromedics impedance audiometers, Peters acoustic bridges, Grason-Stadler otoadmittance meter[1]). Of the instruments in current use, only the Zwislocki acoustic bridge and the Grason-Stadler otoadmittance measure both the real and imaginary components of acoustic impedance or admittance. All of the instruments, with the exception of the Metz and Zwislocki instruments, are capable of providing tympanometric measurements. It is advisable not to refer to any of these measurements as "impedance audiometry" because no audiometric measures are involved in the actual procedures of tympanometry, acoustic impedance, and admittance.

Mechanical Acoustic Impedance Bridges

An acoustic bridge constructed specifically for acoustic impedance measurements of the human ear was developed by Metz (1946). His device was based on the acoustic bridge of Schuster (1934), which was designed to determine the acoustic properties of various materials. Metz utilized his acoustic bridge in the study of normal and pathological ears. He concluded that this instrument could be useful in the diagnosis of hearing impairments, especially for the determination of a conductive hearing loss associated with otosclerosis. The Metz apparatus was not generally accepted by other experimenters,

[1] Madsen Electronics, Branford, Canada; American Electromedics, Dobbs Ferry, N.Y.; Peters Electronics, Sheffield, England; Grason-Stadler, Co., Concord, Mass.

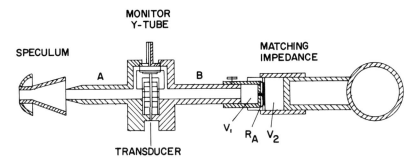

Figure 7. Schematic cross section drawing of the Zwislocki acoustic bridge. The speculum inserts into the subject's ear. The transducer produces sound waves of opposite phase in tube A and tube B. The volume of the subject's ear canal is set at V_1. The experimenter monitors the phase and amplitude relationship between tubes A and B while adjusting the matching impedance. R_1 is resistance and V_2 is the compliance volume. See text for additional explanation. Adapted from Zwislocki (1963).

probably because of its awkwardness and the calculations that were essential in order to interpret the data.

Zwislocki (1957a, 1957b, 1963) described the development and uses of a mechanical acoustic impedance bridge that is a refined version of the Metz device. This instrument is commercially available (Grason-Stadler, Zwislocki acoustic bridge, model 3), and is schematically represented in Figure 7.

As described by Zwislocki (1963), a symmetrical electroacoustic transducer is situated between two main tubes, A and B, having equal dimensions except for the variable impedance-matching section of tube B. The accurately measured volume of the subject's ear canal is added to volume (V_1) of tube B. This adjustment cancels the effect of the ear canal volume during the impedance measures. A pure tone between 125 and 1,500 Hz drives the transducer, establishing a separate continual sound wave within each of the two tubes. These two standing waves have the same amplitude and frequency, but are opposite in phase by 180 degrees *only when the impedances within the two tubes are identical.* The observer accomplishes this relationship by adjusting the variable impedance matching section of tube B until the impedance of a subject's ear is determined. The impedance equality (matching) can be detected by monitoring tubes A and B simultaneously with a Y tube until cancellation is obtained, indicating that the two sound pressures are of equal frequency and amplitude, but opposite in phase by 180 degrees. This is designated as a null point.

Resultant measures obtained by adjusting the matching impedance of the Zwislocki bridge are compliance, in equivalent volume ranging from 0.1 cc to a maximum of 5 cc, and arbitrary resistance units, from 0 to 60 on early models or in acoustic ohms of resistance on later models. Compliance can

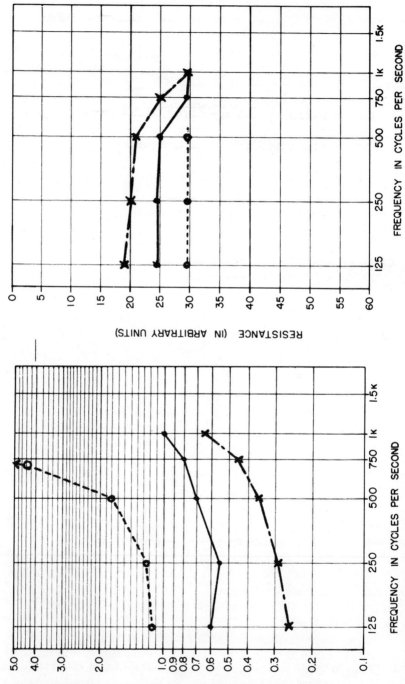

Figure 8. Comparative impedance measures for one ear without an incus (o——o——o), one normal ear (●–●–●), and one ear diagnosed as otosclerosis (x—–x). The imaginary component of impedance, compliance, is expressed in equivalent cc volume of air. The real component of impedance resistance, is expressed in arbitrary units. (Reprinted from Feldman, 1964, courtesy of S. Karger AG, Basel.)

then be converted to acoustic reactance (ohms), and arbitrary resistance can be converted to acoustic resistance (ohms).

Investigations with the Zwislocki acoustic bridge have been reported by several authors. Zwislocki (1963) described the impedance measures obtained from normal subjects, otosclerotic subjects, and a subject with a prosthesis replacement for the stapes. Among other things, he indicated that subjects could be differentiated best on the basis of impedance measures at lower frequencies (125, 250, and 500 Hz).

Feldman (1963, 1964) advocated the routine use of impedance measures in the diagnosis of hearing disorders. Figure 8 shows impedance measures that he reported for three individual subjects: one without an incus, one with a normal middle ear, and one with otosclerosis. He stated that these were typical examples demonstrating that measures obtained from a normal middle ear usually are intermediate in magnitude to the two pathological types of measures.

Tillman, Dallos, and Kuruvilla (1964) studied the reliability of measures obtained with the Zwislocki bridge. They measured 10 normal hearing subjects and concluded that compliance measures were more reliable than resistance measures. In addition, they also cautioned that compliance values at 1,000 Hz should be evaluated carefully because of the resonance of the middle ear.

The reliability of measures obtained with the Zwislocki bridge in a "typical clinical situation" was reported by Nixon and Glorig (1964). They stated that impedance measures showed greater variability as frequency increased. In addition to resonance of the ear, they attributed this variability to the possibility of a "measurement artifact." Consequently, they excluded data obtained at 1,200 and 1,500 Hz from their data analysis because the variability seemed to make these particular data meaningless.

The Zwislocki bridge also has been used in the study of the middle ear acoustic reflex (Dallos, 1964; Durrant and Shallop, 1969; Deutsch, 1972; Feldman, 1967; Feldman and Zwislocki, 1965; Lilly and Shepard, 1964; Shallop, 1965). These authors all verify the ease and usefulness of this instrument for detecting an acoustic reflex.

Considerable normative data and measurements of pathological ears are available for the Zwislocki acoustic bridge, with Zwislocki and Feldman (1970) being a primary source. Lilly et al. (1967) caution against the use of arbitrary resistance and equivalent compliance values being reported for this instrument. They suggest that absolute physical values should be reported in order to make these measurements more useful.

Table 1 is a presentation of some normative results (Shallop, 1965; Zwislocki and Feldman, 1970) obtained with the Zwislocki instrument. The results are converted to absolute physical measurements as recommended by Lilly (1972). Results for otosclerotic and poststapedectomized ears are pre-

Table 1. Medians and 80% ranges of acoustic impedance measures obtained at the tympanic membranes of normal ears with the Zwislocki acoustic bridge (Lilly, 1972, 1973; Shallop, 1965)

Frequency (Hz)	Range	Lilly (1972) (N = 24)[a,b]		Shallop (1965) (N = 40)[b]	
		$R_A - jX_A$	$Z_{TM} \angle\theta$	$R_A - jX_A$	$Z_{TM} \angle\theta$
250	90th percentile	$630 - j1,961$	$2,060 \angle-72.2°$	$600 - j2,277$	$2,354 \angle-75.2°$
250	Median	$420 - j1,471$	$1,530 \angle-74.1°$	$430 - j1,751$	$1,803 \angle-76.2°$
250	10th percentile	$280 - j1,038$	$1,075 \angle-74.9°$	$330 - j1,138$	$1,185 \angle-73.8°$
500	90th percentile	$510 - j882$	$1,019 \angle-60.0°$	$500 - j1,136$	$1,241 \angle-66.2°$
500	Median	$330 - j679$	$755 \angle-64.1°$	$390 - j669$	$774 \angle-59.8°$
500	10th percentile	$230 - j441$	$497 \angle-62.5°$	$260 - j479$	$545 \angle-61.5°$
750	90th percentile	$630 - j490$	$798 \angle-37.9°$	$500 - j607$	$786 \angle-50.5°$
750	Median	$390 - j346$	$521 \angle-41.6°$	$280 - j357$	$454 \angle-51.9°$
750	10th percentile	$230 - j235$	$329 \angle-45.6°$	$225 - j144$	$267 \angle-32.6°$
1,000	90th percentile	$630 - j368$	$730 \angle-30.3°$	$500 - j506$	$711 \angle-45.3°$
1,000	Median	$410 - j232$	$471 \angle-29.5°$	$280 - j144$	$314 \angle-27.2°$
1,000	10th percentile	$250 - j63$	$258 \angle-14.1°$	$225 - j144$	$241 \angle-21.6°$

[a]Data computed by Lilly from Zwislocki and Feldman (1970).
[b]R_A is resistance in acoustic ohms and $-jX_A$ is reactance in acoustic ohms. Z_{TM} is the computed impedance vector magnitude and phase solved by trigonometry, rectangular to polar conversion.

Table 2. Medians and 80% ranges of acoustic impedance measures obtained at the tympanic membranes of otosclerotic ears with the Zwislocki acoustic bridge (Shallop, 1965; Lilly, 1972, 1973)

Frequency (Hz)	Range	Lilly (1972) (N = 24)[a,b]		Shallop (1965) (N = 13)[b]	
		$R_A - jX_A$	$Z_{TM} \angle\theta$	$T_A - jX_A$	$Z_{TM} \angle\theta$
250	90th percentile	$1{,}190 - j5{,}883$	$6{,}002 \angle -78.6°$[c]	$2{,}000 - j6{,}832$	$7{,}118 \angle -73.7°$
250	Median	$520 - j3{,}530$	$3{,}568 \angle -81.6°$[c]	$550 - j3{,}036$	$3{,}085 \angle -79.7°$
250	10th percentile	$322 - j2{,}332$	$2{,}354 \angle -82.1°$	$350 - j2{,}280$	$2{,}307 \angle -81.3°$
500	90th percentile	$622 - j2{,}647$	$2{,}719 \angle -76.8°$	$675 - j3{,}415$	$3{,}481 \angle -78.8°$
500	Median	$380 - j1{,}471$	$1{,}519 \angle -75.5°$	$400 - j1{,}518$	$1{,}570 \angle -75.2°$
500	10th percentile	$230 - j1{,}103$	$1{,}127 \angle -78.2°$	$225 - j1{,}136$	$1{,}158 \angle -78.8°$
750	90th percentile	$646 - j1{,}471$	$1{,}607 \angle -66.3°$	$700 - j1{,}366$	$1{,}534 \angle -62.9°$
750	Median	$295 - j980$	$1{,}023 \angle -73.2°$	$243 - j885$	$918 \angle -74.6°$
750	10th percentile	$218 - j614$	$652 \angle -70.4°$	$188 - j467$	$503 \angle -68.1°$
1,000	90th percentile	$566 - j735$	$928 \angle -52.4°$	$350 - j759$	$836 \angle -65.2°$
1,000	Median	$280 - j421$	$506 \angle -56.4°$	$190 - j455$	$493 \angle -67.3°$
1,000	10th percentile	$209 - j250$	$326 \angle -50.1°$	$150 - j268$	$307 \angle -60.8°$

[a] Data computed by Lilly from Feldman (1971).
[b] R_A is resistance in acoustic ohms and $-jX_A$ is reactance in acoustic ohms. Z_{TM} is the computed impedance vector magnitude and phase solved by trigonometry, rectangular to polar conversion.

Table 3. Medians and 80% ranges of acoustic impedance measures obtained at the tympanic membranes of 40 poststapedectomized ears with the Zwislocki acoustic bridge (Shallop, 1965)

Frequency (Hz)	Range	$R_A - jX_A$ [a]	$Z_{TM} \angle\theta$ [b]
250	90th percentile	$450 - j2,277$	$2,321 \angle-78.8°$
250	Median	$225 - j850$	$879 \angle-75.2°$
250	10th percentile	$130 - j479$	$496 \angle-74.8°$
500	90th percentile	$330 - j911$	$968 \angle-70.1°$
500	Median	$185 - j303$	$355 \angle-58.6°$
500	10th percentile	$95 - j111$	$146 \angle-49.4°$
750	90th percentile	$400 - j434$	$590 \angle-47.3°$
750	Median	$225 - j63$	$234 \angle-15.6°$
750	10th percentile	$50 - jH60$	$161 \angle-21.8°$
1,000	90th percentile	$500 - j228$	$550 \angle-24.5°$
1,000	Median	$300 - j46$	$303 \angle-8.7°$
1,000	10th percentile	$210 - j\lessgtr46$	$215 \angle-12.4°$

[a] R_A is resistance in acoustic ohms and $-jX_A$ is reactance in acoustic ohms.
[b] Z_{TM} is the computed impedance vector magnitude and phase solved by trigonometry, rectangular to polar conversion.

sented in Tables 2 and 3, respectively. These results can be visualized by plotting them in rectangular form, e.g., Lilly (1972, p. 453).

Although measures with the Zwislocki bridge may not be as easy to obtain as with some of the electroacoustic instrumentation, its use for research and clinical value should not be overlooked. It also provides an excellent pedogogical technique for learning the concept of acoustic impedance by using various known and unknown test cavities.

Electroacoustic Instruments

Møller (1958) has described an electroacoustic impedance bridge similar in principle to a mechanical acoustic impedance bridge. Møller's instrument can be firmly secured to the head, allowing the subject to move without altering the placement of the bridge. The phase and amplitude adjustments, essential for determining impedance, involve electronic as compared to mechanical procedures. In two subsequent reports, Møller (1960, 1961) furnished detailed descriptions of his apparatus used in development of an electrical analog of the middle ear.

The bilateral simultaneous responses of the middle ear muscles were reported by Møller (1962) in a comprehensive article. Using several types of acoustic stimuli at various intensity levels, he demonstrated concisely that an electroacoustic bridge was effective in detecting bilateral impedances. In another publication Møller (1964) adapted his apparatus to animal studies on the middle ear muscles.

Another electroacoustic bridge was developed by Terkildsen and Nielsen (1960). They utilized their device in several diagnostic procedures. This bridge yields relative measures, preferably dynamic acoustic impedance (Pinto and Dallos, 1968), of impedance vector phase and magnitude. A fixed frequency of 220 Hz is the carrier frequency, since these investigators are of the opinion that only one frequency is needed to obtain adequate measures. Terkildsen (1964) reported that compliance measures between 0.05 and 0.60 cc indicated high impedance such as may be found in persons with otosclerosis. Normal measures were about 0.65 cc and low impedance was indicated by volumes between 1.05 and 3.5+ cc. The Terkildsen and Nielsen instrument was first produced commercially as the Madsen Z061. Subsequent instruments based on this design include the Madsen Z070, Z072, and the American Electromedics series. A similar instrument, the Peters acoustic bridge, AP61 (Brooks, 1973) is also available. All of these instruments are capable of tympanometry, described later in this chapter.

As Lilly et al. (1967) have pointed out, acoustic impedance or admittance measurements should be reported in absolute physical values. This requires that the instrument be capable of isolating the real and imaginary components of measurement. The only commercially available electroacoustic instruments which provide this capability are the Grason-Stadler otoadmittance meters (e.g., Model 1720), illustrated in Figure 9. Any future refinements or modifications of this instrument presumably will continue to have this

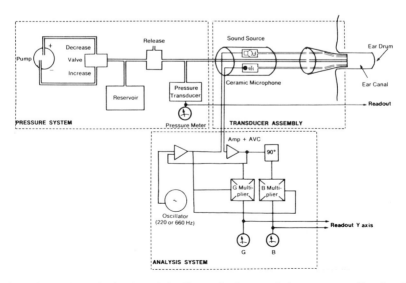

Figure 9. A schematic drawing of the Grason-Stadler otoadmittance meter. (Reprinted with permission: Newman and Fanger, 1973.)

feature as well as tympanometry. This instrument provides direct calibrated measures of acoustic susceptance and conductance (Newman and Fanger, 1973). It differs from the electroacoustic impedance instruments in three essential ways. First, the measurements are in acoustic admittance, the measure of energy flow, and as such the obtained millimho values can be added and subtracted without conversions. Second, the acoustic susceptance and conductance values can be observed or recorded simultaneously if desired. Third, two-measurement frequencies (220 and 660 Hz) are provided. The last two points make this instrument very useful in the measurement of middle ear function by tympanometry. In the future, instruments other than those mentioned probably will become commercially available.

All factors considered, it would seem more appropriate if acoustic admittance measurements rather than acoustic impedance measurements were utilized. However, whichever measure is used, it is essential that these electroacoustic devices have the capability to isolate the in-phase and the out-of-phase components. This will also make it possible to provide other means of graphically presenting results as proposed by Lilly (1972). Conversion of admittance values to impedance values or vice versa is not a difficult task (Rose, 1972), since impedance = 1/admittance.

Tympanometry

Most of us have experienced the changes in loudness associated with varying environmental ambient pressures. As we travel up a mountain, the air density decreases; normally we can equalize this decreased ambient rpessure by swallowing and affecting the primary function of the Eustachian tube, ventilation of the middle ear. Ascent and descent in elevation represent stress upon the mechanics of the middle ear. Von Békésy (1960) made a study of threshold changes in air conduction versus bone conduction signals under increased air pressures on the tympanic membrane. He identified an increase of sound pressure in the closed external meatus accompanied by increases of static pressure in the closed external meatus accompanied by increases of static pressure resulting from the increased impedance of the middle ear. He estimated a 30% increase of impedance at +600 mm H_2O.

Tympanometric measures of middle ear function are accomplished by varying the static air pressure in the sealed ear canal and simultaneously measuring a parameter of impedance or energy flow. When the ear canal static pressure is below or above ambient air pressure, acoustic impedance increases (admittance therefore decreases) for the normal middle ear. A hypothetical plotting of these parameters, called a tympanogram, is presented in Figure 10. It illustrates the variation of acoustic susceptance at 220 Hz with pressure changes. Conventionally, admittance and compliance values are plotted with increasing magnitude upward on a tympanogram, whereas increased impedance magnitude is plotted downward.

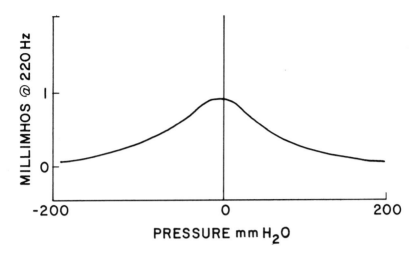

Figure 10. A tympanogram of hypothetical normal middle ear. Admittance in millimhos is maximal at ambient atmospheric pressure.

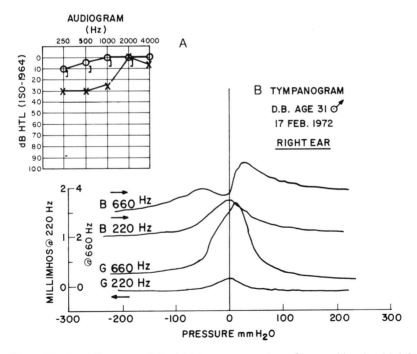

Figure 11. A, audiogram, and B, right tympanogram for a 31-year-old male with left Eustachian tube dysfunction. The atypical tympanogram tracings for conductance (G) and susceptance (B) at 660 Hz are probably the result of scar tissue noted on his tympanic membrane in the posterior-superior quadrant.

Clinically, Thomsen (1955, 1958) suggested the use of the Metz acoustic bridge in a pressure chamber as a procedure for studying middle ear and Eustachian tube functioning. The method was not practical, and subsequently, instruments like the one developed by Terkildsen and Nielsen (1960) were utilized clinically for the detection of middle ear pathology.

A detailed description of tympanograms is available (Feldman, in press); however, some examples of tympanograms will be presented here.

Compere (1972) inadequately questioned the value of impedance measurements and tympanometry while Bluestone, Berry, and Paradise (1973) suggested tympanometry to be "the most physiologic method available" for determining middle ear pressure. The latter represents the predominance of opinion regarding these measurements.

An example of the value of tympanometry is illustrated in the following case. A 30-year-old male with an unresolved unilateral conductive hearing loss was referred for audiological evaluation. The otologist's tentative diagnosis was otosclerosis, but he wanted further support for his opinion. Our audio-

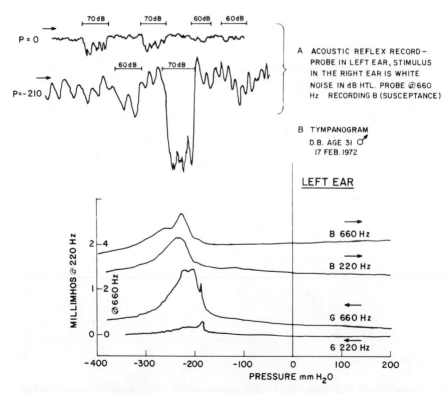

Figure 12. A, acoustic reflex tracings as detected with the probe in the left ear at ambient pressure and −210 mm H_2O. Stimulus to the right ear is 60 and 70 dB HTL of white noise. B, left tympanogram of D.B., age 31. All four tracings demonstrate the negative middle ear pressure resulting from Eustachian tube dysfunction.

gram shown in Figure 11A was consistent with previous audiograms for the previous year. The masked bone conduction thresholds did not suggest stapes fixation, i.e., no "Carhart notch." Tympanic membranes appeared within normal limits to the otologist, except for scarring of the right tympanic membrane. No retraction was evident in either tympanic membrane.

Tympanometry with the Grason-Stadler 1720 otoadmittance meter revealed an interesting tympanogram (arrows indicate the direction of pressure change) for the right ear (Figure 11B). The notching of the susceptance at 660 Hz is typical for tympanic scarring (Feldman, 1974). The tympanogram for the left ear (Figure 12B) demonstrates the presence of negative middle ear pressure, which was resolved by otological treatment. Hearing thresholds for the left ear returned to normal following treatment. Figure 12A illustrates the presence of an acoustic reflex in the left ear and the importance of detecting the reflex at the actual middle ear pressure, in this instance, about -210 mm H_2O.

Probe Frequency

There is controversy regarding the probe frequency needed for clinical tympanometric measurements. Recall that the mechanical acoustic impedance instruments can use a wide range of frequencies. However, electroacoustic instruments must be specifically calibrated for their probe frequencies. Lidén, Harford, and Hallen (1974) advocated 800 Hz. Alberti and Jerger (1974) concluded that only 220 Hz is necessary: "There does not seem to be a substantial clinical value in executing tympanometry at probe frequencies higher than 220 Hz" (Alberti and Jerger, 1974, p. 210). Feldman (1974) reported the value of a combined approach. He used 220 Hz and 660 Hz and pointed out that 660 Hz identified tympanic abnormalities better than 220 Hz. When tympanic abnormality is indicated by the notching of a 660 Hz tympanogram, caution must be used in the interpretation of static admittance/impedance measures. Even at 220 Hz, median impedance for persons with tympanic scarring was found to be 30% (600 acoustic ohms) of the median impedance (1,800 acoustic ohms) for the normal population without tympanic scarring.

Feldman's combined approach seems to be more plausible in view of the current evidence. It should be pointed out that his results were obtained with instrumentation capable of isolating the resistive and elastic components of impedance. Actually, conductance and susceptance were measured to determine total acoustic admittance, which was then converted to acoustic impedance.

Tympanometry with Neonates and Children

Tympanometry has been used successfully with neonates (Keith, 1973) and young children (Jerger, 1970; Jerger et al., 1974a,b). The findings confirm

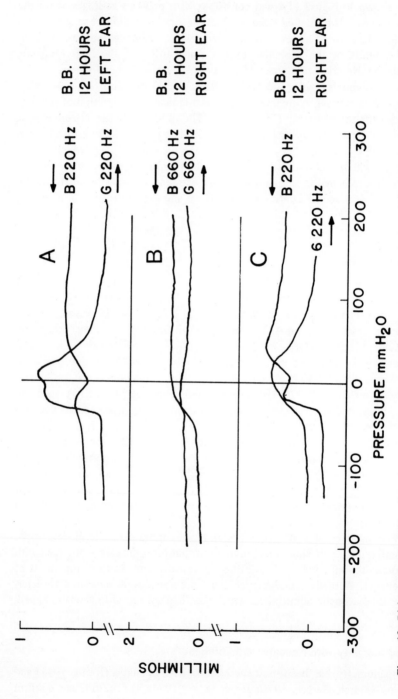

Figure 13. Right ear tympanogram for a neonate 12 hr old. Note the notching of the tracings primarily at 220 Hz and in the susceptance (B) tracings. G, conductance.

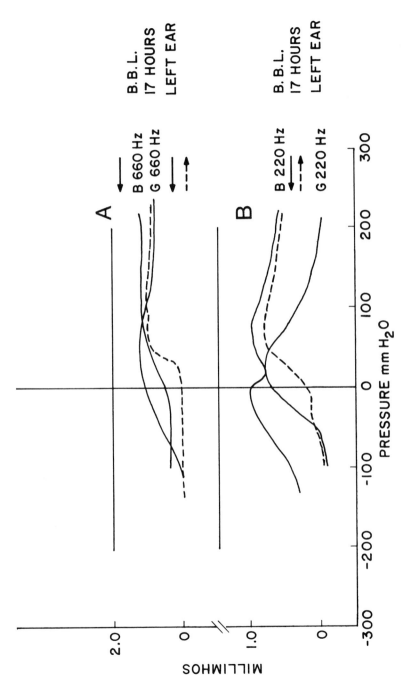

Figure 14. Left ear tympanogram for a neonate 17 hr old. Note the notching of the 220-Hz B (susceptance) tracing. A pressure change directional effect (mechanical hysteresis) is also noted. G, conductance.

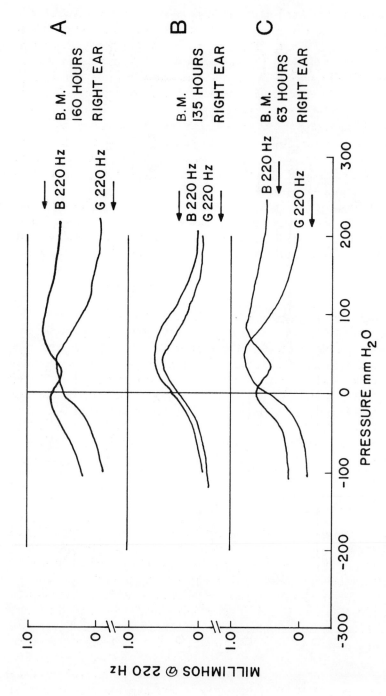

Figure 15. Right ear tympanograms (220 Hz) for a neonate. A, 160 hr after birth, B, 135 hr; and C, 63 hr.

the value of these measures relative to other audiometric results. Keith (1973) describes a W-shaped tympanogram that he observed in seven of 40 infants. This author has observed similar patterns with admittance tympanometric measurements (Shallop and Tom, unpublished data). Tympanogram notching was observed primarily at 220 Hz. At 660 Hz notching was seldom observed, and frequently the 660-Hz tympanograms had an unusual shape, as illustrated in Figure 13. The right ear tympanogram for a 12-hr-old infant at 220 Hz is seen in Figure 13C. Note the notching only of the susceptance (B) tracing. The pattern is similar for the left ear (Figure 13A) with notching of the susceptance and conductance (G) tracings. No notching is evident for the 660-Hz tympanogram of the right ear (Figure 13B). A 660-Hz tympanogram of the left ear was not obtained.

Tympanograms for another neonate (17 hr old) are presented in Figure 14. Again, notching is evident only at 220 Hz. Note also the effect of changing the direction of pressure. This effect, which we observed with several other neonates, seemed to be more prevalent for conductance than susceptance.

A third neonate's right ear tympanograms (220 Hz) are presented in Figure 15 (A, 160 hr; B, 135 hr; and C, 63 hr). One might consider the age at which these tympanograms no longer evidence notching.

From our results, we concur with Keith (1973) that tympanometry with neonates is not difficult to execute and that useful information about middle ear functioning of the neonate can be obtained. Some comments are appropriate. First, neonates can have ventilated middle ears within the 1st day of life. Second, neonates have a flaccid middle ear, which is noted by notching of the tympanogram at 220 Hz and by acoustic impedance which is less than the acoustic impedance of young children or adults. Third, the source of the notching tympanograms is probably not simply a flaccid tympanic membrane. Fourth, the notching is apparently primarily related to elastic sources rather than resistive elements.

Tympanogram Patterns

Jerger (1970) suggested three types of tympanograms: A, normal; B, otitis media; and C, negative middle ear pressures. Rock (1972) made some subcategories within Jerger's type A (A_S, A_D, and A_{DD}) to expand the number to six patterns. Lidén, Peterson, and Björkman (1970b) and Lidén, Harford, and Hallen (1974) identify five types (A–E) with their 800-Hz probe frequency instrument. Their A, B, and C types are essentially the same as those of Jerger. Type D is associated with hypermobility of the tympanic membrane and type E is associated with ossicular discontinuity. Feldman (in press) urges that tympanograms should not be typed, but that "each tympanogram can be interpreted with respect to a) *its peak pressure point,* b) *its peak amplitude* and c) *its shape.*" He feels that these descriptions will provide a better indication of the middle ear pathology when it is observed by tympanometry. In spite of Feldman's advice, it seems that tympanogram typing will still be used, at least until we can convince one another that it is not a simpler and better method than Feldman's procedure.

Mass Screening with Tympanometry

Two major problems are generally present in mass hearing screening programs of school age children: 1) children with a true hearing problem, who are not detected by audiometry, and 2) children without a true hearing problem, who are identified as having a hearing loss, i.e. overreferral. We might also consider those children with a transient middle ear pathology that is not detected by audiometry. One method to help identify middle ear pathology and sensorineural function that may be overlooked in mass screening programs is the use of tympanometry and acoustic reflex threshold detection (Brooks, 1968, 1969).

Three examples of the use of tympanometry and acoustic reflexes are reported by Brooks (1973), Renvall et al. (1973), and Harker and Van Wagoner (1974). These studies recommend the use of audiometry to identify high frequency hearing loss and the use of tympanometry to detect middle ear pathology. Audiometry may be insensitive to subtle middle ear problems and/or ambient noise may prevent the determination of adequate low frequency auditory thresholds. This is certain to be an area of future study (Naples, 1974).

Tympanometry is one of the most useful clinical tools yet devised for the diagnosis of middle ear pathology. Its usage probably will be applied to screening procedures because it is such a good measurement technique.

Eustachian Tube Function

There are many techniques for assessing Eustachian tube function and there are many theories regarding the mechanics of Eustachian tube function. Tympanometry probably will continue to provide a simple method for evaluating this important function (Bluestone, Berry, and Andrus, 1974). The understanding and solution of problems of Eustachian tube function probably will lead to considerable advancement in the treatment of middle ear pathologies.

MEASUREMENT OF THE FUNCTION OF THE MIDDLE EAR MUSCLES

The two muscles of the middle ear of man and most animals receive their primary neural innervation from two cranial nerves. The tensor tympani muscle is innervated by cranial nerve V and the stapedius muscle is innervated by cranial nerve VII. Secondary innervation of the middle ear muscles has been demonstrated (Blevins, 1963; Lawrence, 1962), especially some fibers of cranial nerve X to the stapedius muscle (Blevins, 1964). Both muscles create an increase of tension on the ossicular chain. However, the effect of the increased tension has a differential effect on the transmission of acoustic energy to the inner ear (Djupesland, 1967; Møller, 1965; Wever and Vernon, 1956).

The morphology of the ossicles and the middle ear muscles is such that a tensor tympani contraction pulls inward on the malleus and a stapedius contraction rocks the stapes posteriorly in the oval window. The acoustic responses of the muscles are considered to be graded to increasing stimulus intensity. By their morphology, these muscles may be considered antagonists, but whether they can be physiologically considered as truly synergistic has been questioned by Solomon (1967).

Reflexes of the middle ear muscles can be elicited by acoustic and nonacoustic (e.g., tactile and electrical) stimuli. Central factors may also influence their contraction. Clinically, the contractions of the middle ear muscles are important in the assessment of middle ear function. Before this point is discussed, theories of the functions and responses of middle ear muscles to acoustic stimulation are reviewed.

Theories of Middle Ear Muscle Function

There is numerous literature on this point, and the reader is referred to Jepsen (1963), Simmons (1959; 1964), and Dallos (1973). Dallos (1973) suggests that a combination of the following ideas may better represent the true nature of middle ear function.

Protection Theory This theory suggests that the acoustic middle ear reflex can serve as a means of protecting the inner ear from intense acoustic stimulation. This can be accomplished by alteration of the impedance and transmission characteristics of the middle ear as well as by mechanical decoupling of the stapes by the stapedius contraction. The onset of the acoustic reflex clearly does not allow for protection against intense, impulsive, and impact signals. (See Nixon's chapter in this book for further discussion on this point.)

Fixation Theory This theory suggests that both muscles add tension to secure the ossicular chain and to aid in the mechanical efficiency of the middle ear, especially at high sound pressures of high frequencies (von Békésy, 1936). When the middle ear is subjected to stress by alteration of static pressure across the tympanic membrane, differential effects are observed (Møller, 1965; Peterson and Lidén, 1970) for positive versus negative pressure changes. These effects are not in agreement with a strict fixation theory.

Accommodation Theory This theory assumes that the middle ear muscles serve to facilitate the transmission of energy to the cochlea. The theory is supported by the research of Simmons (1964), who suggests that there is continual adjustment of middle ear transmission by varying tension of the musculature of the middle ear. One would tend to think that an accommodation theory would be more appropriate in the design of a middle ear system, and that a protection theory requires intense sound pressures for support. The environmental noises we experience today may not have been anticipated in the original design. At present, the accommodation to control the signal-to-noise ratio of auditory input during various activities, as proposed by Simmons (1964) and further described by Dallos (1973), seems most plausible. One needs only to observe the auricular control demonstrated by animals such as horses, dogs, or cats to postulate such movements as a part of control mechanisms for improving signal transmission. The topic of the role of acoustic middle ear reflexes as a means of sensory control has been thoroughly described by Borg (1972).

Ventilation Theory Another speculative idea concerning the tensor tympani muscle might be labeled the ventilation theory. Ingelstedt and Jonson (1966) proposed that the tensor tympani muscle may serve to ventilate the middle ear by regulation of tympanic membrane tension. This creates positive pressure in the middle ear, possibly aiding Eustachian tube function spontaneously and during some skeletal muscle movements such as belching, chewing, and yawning. The importance of adequate middle ear ventilation and Eustachian tube mechanics has been modeled recently by Bluestone, Berry, and Andrus (1974).

Responses of the Tensor Tympani and Stapedius Muscles

The stapedius muscle is generally acknowledged to respond consistently to acoustic stimulation in man and animals. However, the tensor tympani muscle seems to repond consistently to acoustic stimulation in some animals and inconsistently in man.

Luscher (1929) observed an acoustic reflex of the stapedius muscle through a perforated tympanic membrane. Galambos and Rupert (1959) studied the acoustic reflex in cats. They showed that acoustic stimulation resulted in a response mainly from the stapedius muscle with an ipsilateral and contralateral latency of 10 msec. The tensor tympani muscle contracted also with a latency of 50 msec.

Terkildsen (1960) created interest in the role of the tensor tympani muscle when he reported a significant number of tensor tympani acoustic responses in man.

Concerning whether or not the human tensor tympani responds to acoustic stimulation, Perlman (1962) stated: "Acoustic contraction of the human tensor tympani muscle has not been observed directly or indirectly through acoustic impedance measurements. When the stapedius tendon is cut, no impedance change can be induced by acoustic stimuli in man."

Klockhoff (1961) stated that the tensor tympani does not respond to acoustic stimulation and demonstrated that this muscle will respond to tactile stimulation (an abrupt airstream directed at the eye independently of the person's ability to hear).

Djupesland (1962) obtained results similar to those of Klockhoff by stimulating the opposite pinna with an airstream. These responses to tactile stimulation were obtained in part from persons who did not respond reflexively to acoustic stimuli. Djupesland also reported "small impedance changes" in response to acoustic stimuli for two persons after stapedectomy, even though in a later report (1965) he stated that only the stapedius muscle contracted in response to sound. In this same article he indicated that the tensor tympani muscle responded only in conjunction with a startle response that included the contraction of the periorbital muscles.

A procedure for determining the function of the middle ear muscles was described by Weiss et al. (1962), who used a manometer to detect a change of air pressure in the ear canal. The responses were averaged by a computer of average transients. Weiss and his colleagues hypothesized that a negative pressure would indicate an inward movement of the eardrum whereas a positive pressure change would indicate an outward movement. From morphological and anatomic evidence, an inward movement of the eardrum could be associated with a contraction of the tensor tympani muscle whereas an outward displacement might indicate a contraction of the stapedius muscle.

Results indicated that both muscles contributed to the acoustic reflex in most subjects. As the duration of the stimulus signal increased, with intensity held constant, the responses of the subjects varied. A typical response demonstrated a positive pressure change, whereas other subjects demonstrated a negative pressure change. The latter responses are difficult to explain on the basis of only one middle ear muscle responding as advocated by Klockhoff (1961).

Holst, Ingelstedt, and Örtegren (1963) reported several results concerning the movement of the eardrum after stimulating the middle ear muscles by various procedures: 1) stimulation of the eye with a small blast of air caused the eardrum to move inward; 2) blowing air against the opposite auricle caused the eardrum to move outward; and 3) acoustic stimulation (500 Hz) of the opposite ear at an intensity of 127 dB SPL resulted in a biphasic movement of the eardrum, outward initially followed by an inward movement, representing a response of both middle ear muscles. Their results were obtained with a manometric system similar to the apparatus used by Weiss et al. (1962).

Feldman (1967) concluded that the tensor tympani muscle does not respond to acoustic stimulation; rather it is mediated by motor activity. He utilized the Zwislocki acoustic bridge for his studies. Lidén, Peterson, and Harford (1970) reported tensor tympani responses to acoustic stimulation in 13% of normal subjects. They used a more extensive measurement system than Feldman did. Also, it should be noted that when the tensor tympani responses did occur, it was only at sound pressures higher (100–110 dB HTL) than normally required for a stapedius muscle acoustic reflex (80–85 dB HTL). Thus, one would wonder if the few tensor tympani responses observed might not be mediated motor responses resulting from antagonistic action of the tensor tympani muscle as observed in some animal experiments.

Utilizing measurements of acoustic impedance and cochlear microphonic potentials, Møller (1964) studied the movements of the tympanic membrane in cats and rabbits. He concluded that, in contrast to the stapedius muscle, the tensor tympani moves the eardrum inward, creating a negative pressure within the ear canal. In other instances the stapedius muscle created a negative pressure and, in combination, the two muscles also created a negative pressure change. The combined effect of the middle ear muscles caused more impedance change than did contraction of either muscle alone. Møller concluded that even though the middle ear muscles are anatomically antagonistic, they are probably synergistic in their physiological function of controlling the "mobility and transmission property" of the middle ear.

Central Factors

Djupesland (1965) reported that the impedance of the ear changes 40–450 msec before the onset of phonation and continues for as long as 300 msec after the cessation of phonation. Expectation of a loud noise (a toy pistol pointed at the opposite ear) also caused contraction of both middle ear muscles, suggesting central control of these muscles.

The influence of central factors on the middle ear muscles was also demonstrated in a study by Fletcher and Riopelle (1960). They conditioned the acoustic reflex with a brief tone just prior to a rifle noise. This procedure decreased the temporary threshold shift as determined by audiometric procedures.

Lidén, Peterson, and Harford (1970) reported a few subjects who were able to contract voluntarily the middle ear musculature. They felt they were able to differentiate between stapedius and tensor tympani responses. Reger (1960) reported the low frequency hearing threshold changes associated with these voluntary contractions.

Recruitment

Metz (1952) employed measures of the acoustic reflex as an objective indication of recruitment. Ewertsen (1973) suggested the use of simple symbols for recording these thresholds on an audiogram. Simply place an arrow on the audiogram (→ for right and ← for left) to indicate the threshold.

Lidén (1970) reported extensive clinical and experimental results on recruitment indicated by decreased dynamic range between pure tone and acoustic reflex thresholds. He concluded that this test indicates a cochlear lesion. Shallop (1973) reported the relationship among speech reception, the intensity range of intelligible speech, and the recruitment indicated by the acoustic reflex. The conclusion was that severity of recruitment indicated in this manner is correlated with decreased dynamic range for intelligible speech, suggesting the need for amplification limiting. Reflex growth rate above acoustic reflex threshold has also been suggested to be diagnostically valuable in sensorineural hearing loss (Peterson and Lidén, 1970). The term conductive recruitment has been proposed in certain cases by Anderson and Barr (1966). Relaxation of the acoustic reflex in response to pulsed stimuli has been shown to identify sensorineural (cochlear) lesions (Norris, Stelmachowicz, and Taylor, 1974).

Retrocochlear Lesions

Amplitude decay of the acoustic reflex has been proposed by Anderson, Barr, and Wedenberg (1970a, 1970b) as a test to evaluate lesions of the auditory nerve. Jerger et al. (1974c) have reported findings consistent with Anderson et al. Peterson and Liden (1970) report abnormal growth of the acoustic reflex with increasing intensity as a symptom of cortical lesions. Other authors have reported results of abnormal acoustic reflexes in brainstem lesions (Giacomelli and Mozzo, 1965; Greisen and Rasmussen, 1970; Steinberg and Lenhardt, 1972). The use of acoustic reflex is also helpful in the diagnosis of facial nerve lesions (Alford et al. 1973).

Acoustic Reflex as Predictor of Hearing Loss

It is a simple concept that the presence of an acoustic reflex indicates two functions: 1) sensorineural function in the stimulus ear, and 2) conductive function in the probe or reflex detection ear. Without residual hearing, an acoustic reflex cannot be elicited. However, a tactile reflex can be elicited provided that middle ear dysfunction is absent or minimal.

The acoustic reflex is known to have a lower SPL threshold for broadband noise than for pure tone stimulation (Djupesland, Flottorp, and Winther, 1967; Peterson and Lidén, 1970). Acoustic reflex thresholds and amount of impedance changes were also more affected by equal intensity low frequency pure tone versus high frequency pure tones.

Niemeyer and Sesterhenn (1972, 1974) described a procedure that utilizes the preceding evidence as a method to predict hearing loss magnitude and audiogram slope. Jerger et al. (1974a) described their experience with this procedure and reported that it was an accurate method of predicting hearing loss. This procedure can have an extremely valuable function in the determination of hearing ability in persons difficult to evaluate (e.g., babies, young children, and the mentally retarded). Terkildsen, Osterhammel, and Nielsen (1970) pointed out the importance of knowing the exact sound pressure level of the probe frequency when the acoustic reflex is being detected.

Temporal Summation of the Acoustic Reflex

Various time constants seem to be present in the auditory system; e.g., the duration of a tone can influence behavioral thresholds. Djupesland and Zwislocki (1971) reported the temporal summation characteristics of the acoustic reflex for 5–3,000 msec 2,000-Hz tone bursts. The threshold of the acoustic reflex became asymptotic at 500–1,000 msec. They attributed this fact of temporal summation of the acoustic reflex to brainstem function, specifically no higher than the superior olivary complex. Woodford et al. (1974) have studied this effect for subjects with normal versus sensorineural (cochlear) lesions. They reported that cochlear lesions had a reduced range of intensity-temporal summation functions. They discussed the possible clinical uses of these measurements.

Diphasic Acoustic Reflex

The normal pattern of the acoustic reflex in man is a monophasic increase of impedance that has a more rapid onset than decay (Møller, 1962). The probability of detecting an acoustic reflex is decreased when a conductive lesion is present in the middle ear. Terkildsen (1964) reported that he observed a reduced strength, decreased impedance, on-off acoustic reflex in some patients with otosclerosis. The two diphasic points of the reflex were in synchrony with the onset and cessation of the reflex stimulus. Flottrop and Djupesland (1970) and Terkildsen, Osterhammel, and Bretlau (1973) reported a combined total of over 200 ears in which they have observed these diphasic responses. The measurement of these responses represents not only a clinical sign of otosclerosis but a challenge to our understanding of middle ear function. Some questions raised include: 1) why impedance decreases during this reflex, 2) how the reflex is transmitted to the tympanic membrane, and 3) why the response is diphasic. The authors mentioned in this section have proposed some hypotheses worth the reader's consideration.

SUMMARY

This chapter has attempted to acquaint the reader with the historical aspects, the various measurements, and the present as well as future applications of middle ear function. In many ways the middle ear is well understood as a sound transducer and vibratory transmission system. Interestingly, however, we are in the midst of developing the use of measures of middle ear function as a method to assess sensorineural auditory function.

Future research on the measurement of middle ear function probably will continue to develop new information that will benefit persons with hearing loss and also will advance our knowledge of auditory function. Technology will enable new and improved measurement instruments that will be quickly outdated, but the principles of middle ear function will remain relevant.

REFERENCES

Alberti, P. W., and J. F. Jerger. 1974. Probe-tone frequency and the diagnostic value of tympanometry. Arch. Otolaryngol. 99: 206–210.

Alford, B. R., J. F. Jerger, A. C. Coates, C. R. Peterson, and S. C. Weber. 1973. Neurophysiology of facial nerve testing. Arch. Otolaryngol. 97: 214–219.

Anderson, H., and B. Barr. 1966. Conductive recruitment. Acta Otolaryngol. 62: 171–184.

Anderson, H., B. Barr, and E. Wedenberg. 1970a. Early diagnosis of VIIIth-nerve tumours by acoustic reflex tests. Acta Otolaryngol. 263(suppl.): 232–237.

Anderson, H., B. Barr, and E. Wedenberg. 1970b. The early detection of acoustic tumours by the stapedius reflex test. In G. E. W. Wolstenholme and J. Knight (eds.), Sensorineural Hearing Loss, pp. 275–289. J. & A. Churchill, London.

American National Standard document. ASA S1.1. 1960. American standard acoustical terminology. American National Standard Institute, New York.

Beatty, R. T. 1932. Hearing in Man and Animals. G. Bell and Sons, London. 227 p.

von Békésy, G. 1936. Zur physik des mittelohres und uber das horen bei fehlerhaftem trommelfell. Akust. Z. 1: 13–23.

von Békésy, G. 1941. Uber die messung der schwingungsamplitude der gehorknochelchen mittels einer kapazitiven sonde. Akust. Z. 6: 16.

von Békésy, G. 1960. Experiments in Hearing. McGraw-Hill, New York. 745p.

von Békésy, G., and W. Rosenblith. 1948. The early history of hearing: Observations and theories. J. Acoust. Soc. Amer. 20: 727–748.

Berengario da Carpi, J. (Work not seen; quoted by Fallopius and Schelhammer.) As cited by Wever, (1949).

Blevins, C. E. 1963. Innervation of the tensor tympani muscle of the cat. Amer. J. Anat. 113: 287–301.

Blevins, C. E. 1964. Studies on the innervation of the stapedius muscle of the cat. Anat. Rec. 149: 157–172.

Bluestone, C. D., Q. C. Berry, and J. L. Paradise. 1973. Audiometry and tympanometry in relation to middle ear effusions in children. Laryngoscope 83: 594–604.

Bluestone, C. D., Q. C. Berry, and W. S. Andrus. 1974. Mechanics of the eustachian tube as it influences susceptibility to and persistence of middle ear effusions in children. Ann. Otol. Rhinol. Laryngol. 83 (suppl. II): 1–8.

Borg, E. 1972. Acoustic middle ear reflexes: A sensory-control system. Acta Otolaryngol. 304 (suppl.): 5–34.

Brooks, D. N. 1968. An objective method of detecting fluid in the middle ear. Int. Audiol. 7: 280–286.

Brooks, D. N. 1969. The use of the electro-acoustic impedance bridge in the assessment of middle ear function. Int. Audiol. 8: 563–569.

Brooks, D. N. 1973. Hearing screening: A comparative study of an impedance method and pure tone screening. Scand. Audiol. 2: 67–72.

Carhart, R. 1962. Effect of stapes fixation on bone conduction. In H. F. Schuknecht (ed.), International Symposium on Otosclerosis, pp. 153–158. Little, Brown, Boston.

Compere, W. E. 1972. Diagnosis: Radiology and audiology. In A. Glorig and K. S. Gerwin (eds.), Otitis Media, pp. 185–189. Charles C Thomas, Springfield, Ill.

Cotugno, D. 1774. De Aquaeductibut Auris Humanae Internae. Viennae. As cited by Wever (1949).

Dallos, P. J. 1964. Dynamics of the acoustic reflexes: phenomenological aspects. J. Acoust. Soc. Amer. 36: 2175–2183.

Dallos, P. 1973. The Auditory Periphery. Academic Press, New York. 548 p.

Deutsch, L. J. 1972. The threshold of the stapedius reflex for pure tone and noise stimuli. Acta Otolaryngol. 74: 248–251.

DeWeese, D. D., and W. H. Saunders. 1960. Textbook of Otolaryngology. C. V. Mosby, St. Louis. 464 p.

Djupesland, G. 1962. Intra-aural muscular reflexes elicited by air current stimulation of the external ear. Acta Otolaryngol. 54: 143–153.

Djupesland, G. 1965. Electromyography of the tympanic muscles in man. Int. Audiol. 4: 34–41.

Djupesland, G., G. Flottorp, and F. Ø. Winther. 1967. Size and duration of acoustically elicited impedance changes in man. Acta Otolaryngol. 224(suppl.): 220–228.

Djupesland, G., and J. J. Zwislocki. 1971. Effect of temporal summation on the human stapedius reflex. Acta Otolaryngol. 71: 262–265.

Dragsten, P. R., W. W. Webb., J. A. Paton, and R. R. Capranica. 1974. Auditory membrane vibrations: Measurements at sub-Angstrom levels by optical hetrodyne spectrography. Science 185: 55–57.

Durrant, J. D., and J. K. Shallop. 1969. Effects of differing states of attention on acoustic reflex activity and temporary threshold shift. J. Acoust. Soc. Amer. 46: 907–913.

Duverney, G. J. c. 1683. A treatise of the organ of hearing. Translated into English by J. Marshall, 1737. Reprinted 1973 by AMS Press, New York. 145 p.

Eustachio, B. 1564. Opuscula anatomica. Venetius, pp. 148–164. As cited by Wever (1949).

Ewertsen, H. W. 1973. Audiogram interpretation. Standardisation of symbols for stapedius reflexes. Scand. Audiol. 2: 61–63.

Fallopius, G., Observationes anatomicae, ad Petrum Mannam, Venetiis (work not seen), as cited by Wever (1949).

Feldman, A. S. 1963. Impedance measurements at the eardrum as an aid to diagnosis. J. Speech Hear. Res. 6: 315–327.

Feldman, A. S. 1964. Acoustic impedance measurement as a clinical procedure. Int. Audiol. 3: 156–166.

Feldman, A. S. 1967. A report of further impedance studies of the acoustic reflex. J. Speech Hear. Res. 10: 616–622.

Feldman, A. S. 1971. Raw, acoustic-impedance data for 24 patients with clinical otosclerosis, and for 7 patients with ossicular discontinuity. Personal communication. As cited by Lilly, 1972.

Feldman, A. S. 1974. Eardrum abnormality and the measurement of middle ear function. Arch. Otolaryngol. 99: 211–217.

Feldman, A. S. Acoustic impedance/admittance measurement. In Physiological Measures of the Audio-Vestibular System, chap. 5. Academic Press, New York. In press.

Feldman, A. S., and J. Zwislocki. 1965. Effect of the acoustic reflex on the impedance at the eardrum. J. Speech Hear. Res. 8: 213–222.

Fischler, H., E. H. Frei, D. Spira, and M. Rubinstein. 1967. Dynamic response of middle-ear structures. J. Acoust. Soc. Amer. 41: 1220–1231.

Fletcher, J. L., and A. J. Riopelle. 1960. Protective effect of the acoustic reflex for impulsive noises. J. Acoust. Soc. Amer. 32: 401–404.

Flottorp, G., and G. Djupesland. 1970. Diphasic impedance change and its applicability in clinical work. Acta. Otolaryngol. 263(suppl.): 200–204.

Fournier, J. E. 1959. Bone conduction: Testing. *In* H. G. Kobrak (ed.), The Middle Ear, pp. 92–108. The University of Chicago Press, Chicago.

Galambos, R., and A. Rupert. 1959. Action of the middle ear muscles in normal cats. J. Acoust. Soc. Amer. 31: 349–355.

Giacomelli, F., and W. Mozzo. 1965. An experimental and clinical study on the influence of the brainstem reticular formation on the stapedial reflex. Int. Audiol. 4: 42–44.

Gilad, P., S. Shtrikman, P. Hillman, M. Rubinstein, and A. Eviatar. 1967. Application of the Mössbauer method to ear vibrations. J. Acoust. Soc. Amer. 41: 1232–126.

Greisen, O., and P. E. Rasmussen. 1970. Stapedius muscle reflexes and oto-neurological examinations in brain-stem tumors. Acta Otolaryngol. 70: 366–370.

Guinan, J. J., Jr., and W. T. Peake. 1967. Middle-ear characteristics of anesthetized cats. J. Acoust. Soc. Amer. 41: 1237–1261.

Gulick, W. L. 1971. Hearing: Physiology and Psychophysics. Oxford University Press, New York. p. 33.

Harker, L. A., and R. Van Wagoner. 1974. Application of impedance audiometry as a screening instrument. Acta Otolaryngol. 77: 198–201.

Harford, E. R. 1973. Tympanometry for eustachian tube evaluation. Arch. Otolaryngol. 97: 17–20.

Helmholtz, H. L. F. 1885. On the Sensations of Tone. Translated by A. J. Ellis. Reprinted 1954 by Dover, New York.

Holst, H. E., S. Ingelstedt, and U. Örtegren. 1963. Ear drum movements following stimulation of the middle ear muscles. Acta Otolaryngol. 182(suppl.): 73–83.

Ingelstedt, S., and B. Jonson. 1966. Mechanisms of the gas exchange in the normal human middle ear. Acta Otolaryngol. 224(suppl.): 452–461.

Ingrassia, G. F. c. 1546. (Work not seen; quoted by Schelhammer.) As cited by Wever (1949).

Jepsen, O. 1963. Middle-ear muscle reflexes in man. *In* J. Jerger (ed.), Modern Developments in Audiology, pp. 193–239. Academic Press, New York.

Jerger, J. 1970. Clinical experience with impedance audiometry. Arch. Otolaryngol. 92: 311–324.

Jerger, J., S. Jerger, and L. Mauldin. 1972. Studies in impedance audiometry. Arch. Otolaryngol. 96: 513–523.

Jerger, J., P. Burney, L. Mauldin, and B. Crump. 1974a. Predicting hearing loss from the acoustic reflex. J. Speech Hear. Disord. 39: 11–22.

Jerger, J., L. Anthony, S. Jerger, and L. Mauldin. 1974b. Studies in impedance audiometry. Arch. Otolaryngol. 99: 165–171.

Jerger, J., E. Harford, J. Clemis, and B. Alford. 1974c. The acoustic reflex in eighth nerve disorders. Arch. Otolaryngol. 99: 409–413.

Johnstone, B. M., and A. J. F. Boyle. 1967. Basilar membrane vibration examined with the Mössbauer technique. Science 158: 389–390.

Johnstone, B. M., K. J. Taylor, and A. J. Boyle. 1970. Mechanics of the guinea pig cochlea. J. Acoust. Soc. Amer. 47: 504–509.

Keith, R. W. 1973. Impedance audiometry with neonates. Arch. Otolaryngol. 97: 465–467.

Khanna, S. M., and J. Tonndorf. 1971. The vibratory pattern of the round window in cats. J. Acoust. Soc. Amer. 50: 1475–1483.

Khanna, S. M., and J. Tonndorf. 1972. Tympanic membrane vibrations in cats studied by time-averaged holography. J. Acoust. Soc. Amer. 51: 1904—1920.

Klockhoff, I. 1961. Middle ear muscle reflexes in man. Acta Otolaryngol. 164(suppl.): 8—92.

Kobrak, H. G. 1959. The Middle Ear. The University of Chicago Press, Chicago. 254 p.

Lawrence, M. F. 1962. Middle-ear mechanics and surgery for deafness. J. Acoust. Soc. Amer. 34: 1509—1513.

Lidén, G. 1970. The stapedius muscle reflex used as an objective recruitment test: A clinical and experimental study. In G. E. W. Wolstenholme and J. Knight (eds.), Sensorineural Hearing Loss, pp. 295—308. J. & A. Churchill, London.

Lidén, G., E. Harford, and O. Hallen. 1974. Tympanometry for the diagnosis of ossicular disruption. Arch. Otolaryngol. 99: 23—29.

Lidén, G., J. L. Peterson, and G. Björkman. 1970a. Tympanometry: A method for analysis of middle-ear function. Acta Otolaryngol. 263(suppl.): 218—224.

Lidén, G., J. L. Peterson, and G. Björkman. 1970b. Tympanometry. Arch. Otolaryngol. 92: 248—257.

Lidén, G., J. L. Peterson, and E. R. Harford. 1970. Simultaneous recording of changes in relative impedance and air pressure during acoustic and non-acoustic elicitation of the middle-ear reflexes. Acta Otolaryngol. 263: 208—217.

Lilly, D. J. 1972. Acoustic impedance at the tympanic membrane. In J. Katz (ed.), Handbook of Clinical Audiology, pp. 434—469. Williams & Wilkins, Baltimore.

Lilly, D. J. 1973. Measurement of acoustic impedance at the tympanic membrane. In J. Jerger (ed.), Modern Developments in Audiology, pp. 345—406. Academic Press, New York.

Lilly, D. J., and D. C. Shepard. 1964. A rebalance technique for the measurement of absolute changes in acoustic impedance due to the acoustic reflex. ASHA 6: 381.

Lilly, D. J., D. Sherman, A. J. Compton, C. G. Fisher, and P. J. Carney. 1967. Annual review of JSHR research. J. Speech Hear. Disord. 33: 303—317.

Luscher, E. 1929. Die funktion des musculus stapedium beim menschen. Z. Hals-. Nasen-. Ohrenheilk. 23: 105. As cited by Perlman (1962).

Metz, O. 1946. The acoustic impedance measured on normal and pathological ears. Acta Otolaryngol. 63(suppl.): 11—254.

Metz, O. 1952. Threshold of reflex contractions of the muscles of the middle ear and recruitment of loudness. Arch. Otolaryngol. 55: 536—543.

Møller, A. R. 1958. Intra-aural muscle contraction in man, examined by measuring acoustic impedance of the ear. Laryngoscope 68: 48—62.

Møller, A. R. 1960. Improved technique for detailed measurements of the middle ear impedance. J. Acoust. Soc. Amer. 32: 250—257.

Moller, A. R. 1961. Network model of the middle ear. J. Acoust. Soc. Amer. 33: 168—176.

Møller, A. R. 1962. Acoustic reflex in man. J. Acoust. Soc. Amer. 34: 1524—1534.

Møller, A. R. 1964. The acoustic impedance in experimental studies on the middle ear. Int. Audiol. 3: 123—129.

Møller, A. R. 1965. An experimental study of the acoustic impedance of the middle ear and its transmission properties. Acta Otolaryngol. 60: 129—149.

Müller, J. 1840. Handbuch der physiologie des menschen. J. Holscher. Coblenz. As cited by Lawrence (1962).

Naples, G. M. 1974. A study of the relative effectiveness of tympanometry and five other identification techniques for detecting children with aural abnormalities. Unpublished masters thesis. Ohio University, Athens. 106 p.

Newman, B. T., and D. M. Fanger. 1973. Otoadmittance Handbook 2. Grason-Stadler, Concord, Mass. 38 p.

Niemeyer, W., and G. Sesterhenn. 1972. Calculating the hearing threshold from the stapedius reflex threshold for different sound stimuli. Paper presented at the 11th International Congress of Audiology, October 5, Budapest, Hungary.

Niemeyer, W., and G. Sesterhenn. 1974. Calculating the hearing threshold from the stapedius reflex threshold for different sound stimuli. Audiology 13: 421–427.

Nixon, J. C., and A. Glorig. 1964. Reliability of acoustic impedance measures of the eardrum. J. Aud. Res. 4: 261–276.

Norris, T. W., P. G. Stelmachowicz, and D. J. Taylor. 1974. Acoustic reflex relaxation to identify sensorineural hearing impairment. Arch. Otolaryngol. 99: 194–197.

Onchi, Y. 1961. Mechanism of the middle ear. J. Acoust. Soc. Amer. 33: 794–805.

Perlman, H. B. 1962. Physiology of the middle ear muscles in man. In H. Schuknecht (ed.), Otosclerosis. Little, Brown, Boston.

Perrault, C. c. 1680. Du bruit. In C. and P. Perrault (eds.), Oeuvres Diverses de Physique et de Mechanique. Aleide. As cited by Wever (1949).

Peterson, J. L., and G. Lidén. 1970. Tympanometry in human temporal bones. Arch. Otolaryngol. 92: 258–266.

Pinto, L. H., and P. J. Dallos. 1968. An acoustic bridge for measuring the static and dynamic impedance of the eardrum. IEEE Trans. Biomed. Eng. 15: 10–16.

Reger, S. N. 1960. Effects of middle ear muscle action on certain psychophysical measurements. Ann. Otol. Rhinol. Laryngol. 69: 1179.

Renvall, U., G. Lidén, S. Jungert, and E. Nilsson. 1973. Impedance audiometry as screening method in school children. Scand. Audiol. 2: 133–137.

Rhode, W. S. 1971. Observations of the vibration of the basilar membrane in squirrel monkeys using the Mössbauer technique. J. Acoust. Soc. Amer. 49: 1218–1231.

Rock, E. H. 1972. Electroacoustic impedance measurements (Madsen) in clinical otology. Impedance Newslett. 1: 1–42.

Rose, D. A. 1973. G-B to Y/Z conversion chart. In B. T. Newman and D. M. Fanger (eds.), Otoadmittance Handbook 2, appendix I, C.2. Grason-Stadler, Concord, Mass.

Rusk, R. D. 1960. Introduction to College Physics. Appleton-Century-Crofts, New York. 530 p.

Salomon, G. 1967. On the continuous control of the middle ear muscle activity in cat. Acta Otolaryngol. 224(suppl.): 218–219.

Schelhammer, G. C. 1684. De auditu, liber unus. As cited by Wever (1949).

Schuster, K. 1934. Eine methode zum vergleich akustirker impedangen. Phys. Z. 35: 408–409.

Shallop, J. K. 1965. A study of acoustic impedance and middle-ear function. Unpublished doctoral dissertation. Ohio State University, Columbus. 98 p.

Shallop, J. K. 1973. Some relationships among speech reception, the dynamic range of intelligible speech and the acoustic reflex. Scand. Audiol. 2: 119–122.

Simmons, F. B. 1959. Middle ear muscle activity at moderate sound levels. Ann. Otol. Rhinol. Laryngol. 68: 1126–1143.

Simmons, F. B. 1964. Variable nature of the middle ear muscle reflex. Int. Audiol. 3: 136–146.

Sivian, L. J., and S. D. White. 1933. On minimal audible sound field. J. Acoust. Soc. Amer. 4: 288–321.

Steinberg, D., and E. Lenhardt. 1972. Impedance findings in central hearing disorders. Laryngol. Rhinol. Otol. 51: 693–699.

Terkildsen, K. 1960. Acoustic reflexes of the human musculus tensor tympani. Acta Otolaryngol. 158(suppl.): 230–238.

Terkildsen, K. 1964. Clinical application of impedance measurements with a fixed frequency technique. Int. Audiol. 3: 147–154.

Terkildsen, K., and S. Nielsen. 1960. An electroacoustic impedance measuring bridge for clinical use. Arch. Otolaryngol. 72: 339–346.

Terkildsen, K., P. Osterhammel, and P. Bretlau. 1973. Acoustic middle ear muscle reflexes in patients with otosclerosis. Arch. Otolaryngol. 98: 152–155.

Terkildsen, K., P. Osterhammel, and S. Nielsen. 1970. Impedance measurements: Probe tone intensity and middle-ear reflexes. Acta Otolaryngol. 263(suppl.): 205–207.

Terkildsen, K., and K. A. Thomsen. 1959. The influence of pressure variations on the impedance of the human ear drum. J. Laryngol. Otol. 73: 409–418.

Thomsen, K. A. 1955. Eustachian tube function tested by employment of impedance measuring. Acta Otolaryngol. 45: 252–267.

Thomsen, K. A. 1958. Investigations on the tubal function and measurement of the middle ear pressure in pressure chamber. Acta Otolaryngol. 140(suppl.): 269–278.

Tillman, T. W., P. J. Dallos, and T. Kuruvilla. 1964. Reliability of measures obtained with the Zwislocki acoustic bridge. J. Acoust. Soc. Amer. 36: 582–588.

Tonndorf, J. 1966. Bone conduction: Studies in experimental animals. A collection of seven papers. Acta Otolaryngol. 213(suppl.): 132.

Tonndorf, J., and S. M. Khanna. 1968. Submicroscopic displacement amplitudes of the tympanic membrane (cat) measured by a laser interferometer. J. Acoust. Soc. Amer. 44: 1546–1554.

Valsalva, A. M. c. 1700. De aure humana tractatus, Rehnum. As cited by Wever (1949).

Van Dishoeck, H. E. A. 1938. Das pneumophon. Arch. Ohren-. Nasen-. Kehlk. 53: 144.

Varolius, C. c. 1591. Anatomiae sive de resolutione corporis humani, libri IIII, Francofurti. As cited by Wever (1949).

Vesalius, A., De humani corporis fabrica, libri septum, Basileae (work not seen), as cited by Wever (1949).

Webster, A. G. 1919. Acoustical impedance, and the theory of horns and of the phonograph. Proc. Natl. Acad. Sci. 5: 275–282.

Weiss, H. S., J. R. Mundie, Jr., J. L. Cashin, and E. W. Shinabarger. 1962. The normal human intra-aural muscle reflex in response to sound. Acta Otolaryngol. 55: 505–515.

Wever, E. G. 1949. Theory of Hearing. John Wiley & Sons, New York. 484 p.

Wever, E. G. 1962. The transmission of sound in the ear. *In* H. Schuknecht (ed.), Otosclerosis. Little, Brown, Boston.

Wever, E. G., and M. Lawrence. 1950. The transmission properties of the middle ear. Ann. Otol. Rhinol. Laryngol. 59: 5−18.

Wever, E. G., and J. A. Vernon. 1956. The effects of the tympanic muscle reflexes upon sound transmission. Acta Otolaryngol. 45: 433−439.

Wilska, A. 1959. A direct method for determining threshold amplitudes of the eardrum at various frequencies. *In* H. G. Kobrak (ed.), The Middle Ear, pp. 76−79.

Woodford, C., D. Henderson, R. Hamernik, and A. Feldman. 1974. The threshold-duration function of the acoustic reflex in man. In preparation.

Yearsley, J. 1863. Deafness. John Churchill and Sons, London. 301 p.

Zwislocki, J. 1957a. Some measurements of the impedance at the eardrum. J. Acoust. Soc. Amer. 29: 349−356.

Zwislocki, J. 1957b. Some impedance measurements on normal and pathological ears. J. Acoust. Soc. Amer. 29: 1312−1317.

Zwislocki, J. 1963. An acoustic method for clinical examination of the ear. J. Speech Hear. Res. 6: 303−314.

Zwislocki, J., and A. Feldman. 1970. Acoustic impedance of pathological ears. ASHA Monogr. No. 15.

The Measurement
of Hearing by Computer

Robert B. Mahaffey, Ph.D.
Associate Professor
Institute of Speech and Hearing Sciences
The University of North Carolina at Chapel Hill

CONTENTS

INTRODUCTION

The purpose of this chapter is to portray the digital computer along with peripheral devices as essential systems in the measurement of hearing. To achieve this purpose, the emphasis of the chapter is on techniques rather than on the goals or the findings of the research discussed. The techniques cited emphasize interfacing and examples of various interfacing configurations rather than the computer, with the assumptions that most readers are familiar with the basic operations of digital computers, and that most digital computers function somewhat alike.

The measurement of hearing, whether with or without the aid of a computer, can be discussed in terms of stimulus-response paradigms. That is, if a known signal is presented to the auditory system, and if the response can be accurately and meaningfully measured, some knowledge can be gained about the operations of the intervening auditory system. The complicating factors are that the majority of the auditory system is embedded in the cranium and not available for direct observation and that the auditory system consists of thousands of sensory cells and millions of neurons. Furthermore, if the subject's response is a conditioned or voluntary one, there is a multitude of intervening behavioral variables, not psychoacoustic, that are

323

introduced between the stimulus and the response In this chapter, measurement is discussed in terms of the quantification of the stimuli, the quantification of behavioral responses, the quantification of physiological responses, and finally, the clinical procedures that can be used to quantify pathological hearing functions. In addition to the direct measurement of hearing functions, the construction of models of the auditory system on the computer is discussed as a means of guiding and formulating theoretical and empirical research into the measurement of hearing.

THE COMPUTER AND ITS INTERFACE

Although the computer by itself may serve the researcher as a means of processing data in statistical analyses, storing and retrieving information, and in mathematical model formulation, its true value in auditory function laboratories comes from its ability to control peripheral equipment for the generation of stimuli, its ability to consume large amounts of data from numerous sources simultaneously, and its ability to make real time decisions on the data acquired. The interfacing of a computer to data acquisition systems and to control units is analagous to hooking eyes, ears, arms, and hands to the brain. The interfacing and the associated peripheral devices permit the computers to sense the state of the outside world directly, make decisions, and then to do some thing about it.

A fully equipped computer system can provide the following services for the scientist in his laboratory: 1) it can store, manipulate, and retrieve large amounts of data at very rapid speeds concurrent with other essential processes; 2) it can perform data reductions and statistical analyses on the stored data according to programmed rules; 3) it can provide means for model simulations and the integration of known functions and data with theoretical functions for the testing of hypothetical models; 4) it can provide on-line data acquisition and control for the laboratory with intervening analysis of data for contingent operations; and 5) in some instances it can serve as a data communications link between distant laboratories or between local laboratory computers and large data processing centers.

Laboratory computers come in two basic sizes, large and small. The large computers are capable of handling enormous quantities of data and many simultaneous functions. These systems are often faster and more powerful than one laboratory can justify and are therefore "time shared" or multiplexed to a number of laboratories that more or less share the power and the storage capabilities. In keeping with their capabilities, these systems are also expensive and must maintain a high use ratio to justify their operating costs. The small computer, or minicomputer, is more suited to the dedicated applications where "number crunching" or the handling of large volumes of data is not a major application, but where economy and ease of interfacing and adaptation are essential to the research at hand. A marriage of the two can result in the minicomputer serving as a "front end" to a larger computer. Often, it is economical for a number of small computers to interact simultaneously with a large computer located at a general operations center. A computer-based laboratory has many alternative configurations, and the advantages and disadvantages of each alternative must be weighed on the basis of cost, application, and other services that are available. The large system is efficient, easy to program, powerful, and expensive to operate. On the other hand, the minicomputer is more difficult to program, far less powerful, and far less expensive. However, a small computer can "belong" to a laboratory, and the advantages of being independent from a large scale computer operation and its associated politics and restrictions are considerable.

INTERFACING THE COMPUTER

Because digital computers use binary logic or the "bit" approach to handling and manipulating data, a computer—large or small—may be viewed as a complex series of switches and logic circuits that operate with each switch or logic circuit being either in the "on" position or in the "off" position at any given time. When using a computer as a number handling device, the groups of switches or bits can be viewed as numerical entities represented in binary arithmetic. On the other hand, to the scientist utilizing a computer in the laboratory, the many switches function as an array of remotely controlled switching lines for peripheral units and for getting data from the outside world into the computer's processor. The interface serves as a means of getting information out of and in to the computer to and from the outside world via the computer's data lines. Furthermore, such a computer system is highly versatile and can be readily changed from one experimental set-up to another merely by changing the program in the computer's memory.

The increasing use of the computer in the psychoacoustic laboratory and in the physiology laboratory is largely based on its ease of interacting with real-world devices such as graphic displays, servomotors, analog-to-digital converters, digital-to-analog converters, numerous transducers, electronic sensors, and an array of other digitally controllable signal-generating and regulating devices. The devices which serve input functions allow the computer to accept specific information from the outside world and to process it according to prescribed rules and formulas. This information may come from a subject depressing a switch, an electroencephalographic recording, an acoustic stimulus detected by a microphone, or from any source of information that can be electrically encoded. The interfaced devices which serve output functions allow the computer to specify the operating parameters of the hardware devices which generate stimuli, control tape recorders, drive servomotors, and generate visual displays, and to control practically any other device which may be controlled electrically. The precision of these peripheral devices in conjunction with the power of the computer and the accuracy of sensing devices has provided for data acquisition and experimental control in the auditory laboratory previously held to be technologically unmanageable.

The specific devices that make precision interfacing feasible are relatively few, but each has diversified applications that make it a general purpose device and versatile in the measurement of hearing. There are four basic interfacing devices.

1. The analog-to-digital (A/D) converter is a data acquisition device that has as its input a dc voltage of some significance to the experimenter. The converter acts as a rapid digital voltmeter and digitizes the incoming voltage by converting it to digital form. Even the most economical analog-to-digital converters are capable of making many thousands of conversions per second.

2. The digital-to-analog (D/A) converter is the converse of the A/D converter. It takes numerical values from the computer and converts them to voltages. The D/A converter, like the A/D converter, can make thousands of these conversions per second and can therefore re-create the analog signal that the A/D converter had originally converted to digital form. The D/A converter, paired with a second D/A converter, also can be used to drive the horizontal and vertical amplifiers of an oscilliscope to generate visual displays.

3. The buffered digital input is a device that interfaces directly to the computer's data lines and acts as a middle man between the computer and data coming from peripheral devices. The buffered input accepts data from the peripheral device and holds it until the computer is ready to process it. Because the computer operates at speeds many times faster than the peripheral devices, one computer can service several buffered peripherals. The buffered input may be used to accept data from response buttons (switches), counters, electronic triggers, and many other devices having digital outputs.

4. The buffered digital output is similar to the buffered input in that it acts as a middle man between the computer's data lines and the outside world; but with the buffered output, the information is flowing out of the computer rather than into it. These digital outputs are usually used as control lines to peripheral devices and may be used to gate on and off a tone or light, to set an attenuator, or to release a food pellet to an experimental animal in a conditioning experiment. As with the buffered input, the buffered output permits the fast operations of the computer to control simultaneously a number of slower peripheral devices.

Most of the other interfacing devices are elaborations or modifications of these four devices. Since the input and output of the computer are electrical, digital and analog inputs and outputs can handle most of the possible signal configurations. With these four interfacing devices in mind, it is possible to discuss a number of laboratory systems designed for data acquisition and control for the measurement of hearing.

QUANTIFICATION OF STIMULI

In considering the measurement of hearing as a stimulus-response paradigm, not only is the response relevant, the stimulus is equally important. Historically, one of the problems confronting researchers has been the elusiveness of the perfect stimulus. Stimuli are always a compromise between the experimentally ideal and the technologically feasible. To narrow this gap, the laboratory computer has become increasingly popular because of the versatility and precision that it introduces into stimulus generation. Its capabilities stem from its timing precision and its ease of programming. Even the lower cost computers have accuracy in the millionth-of-a-second range, a figure far more reliable than the accuracy previously available with conventional equipment. The stimulus can be altered at the experimenter's command via programming changes, and the computer can monitor the signal which it produces and modifies according to the original signal specifications.

Perhaps the simplest method of generating a signal under the computer's control is to use a buffered digital output as a gating voltage to an oscillator or function generator. With this interface, when the buffered output is in the "one" state or the "on" state, the oscillator produces a sine wave; on the other hand, when the buffered output is in the "zero" state or the "off" state, the oscillator ceases to produce the waveform. The computer's timing serves to determine the waveform's duration quite precisely. The generated signal then may be presented as a stimulus of known onset, duration, frequency, amplitude, and phase. Such an application may be useful in a study of short-tone perception or of interstimulus interval in perception. In the simple circuit described, most of the signal-generating chore is placed on the peripheral device, and such an application is restricted to studies that can rely on commonly defined waveforms, such as sine functions or rectangular functions, for which waveform generators are commercially available.

A modification of the configuration that would expand its versatility would be the use of an oscillator whose frequency could be digitally selected. These oscillators are available in a number of configurations and price ranges. The least complicated of these units has a number of pre-set frequencies that can be selected by digital switching. In effect, one of these selectable oscillators is comparable to an array of the single-frequency oscillators placed in tandem, except that the selectable frequency unit is more compact and efficient, in that many of the electronic components are common to all frequencies. A more involved frequency-selectable oscillator is the directly programmable function generator, which can be digitally controlled to oscillate at any discrete frequency within its range. These units are precision instruments and are quite versatile, though equally expensive (see Figure 1).

Another approach to controlling the frequency of a peripherally generated signal is to use a computer-controlled digital-to-analog converter or programmable voltage source to produce a dc voltage proportional to the

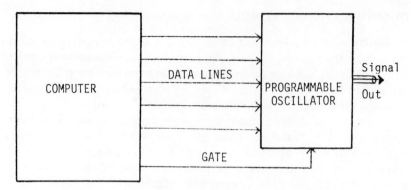

Figure 1. Computer control of programmable oscillator.

frequency to be produced. This voltage, in turn, may be used to regulate the output frequency of a voltage-controlled generator (VCG). These generators vary their output frequency as a function of an input dc voltage. Thus, the digital value transferred to the D/A converter varies the frequency produced by the generator. This circuitry (see Figure 2) permits the continuous varying of frequency as opposed to the discrete frequency steps available with the programmable oscillator. The resolution of the D/A-VCG system may be set so that fine increments are obtainable in a narrow frequency range, as would be required in frequency modulation studies in the measurement of hearing.

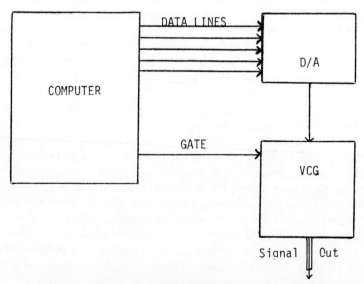

Figure 2. Computer control of variable frequency source.

The signal sources described above have one significant limitation in common: they are severely limited in the signal functions which they can produce. In essence, they are restricted to those signals for which simple function generators are available. Since the auditory system dedicates very little of its time to listening to pure tones, square waves, and saw-tooth waves, the measurement of the auditory system's performance also must include measurement with other, more realistic, signals of known characteristics. For example, the auditory system's processing of a speech wave is probably quite different from its processing of a sine wave or square wave simply because of the stochastic nature of speech signals. To meet the psychoacoustic laboratory's need for a multifactored analog signal, the digital-to-analog converter can be used directly to generate specified waveforms computed and stored in the computer's memory (see Figure 3). To generate these signals, sequential numerical values are transferred at equal time intervals to the D/A converter in rapid succession. The analog output from the converter is then amplified, filtered to minimize switching transients, and used as a signal source.

The D/A conversion process is particularly applicable to the study of the auditory system because, like other perceptual systems, it relies on changes and perceptual boundaries more than it does on the consistency of a signal for its information, and the D/A converter is a feasible means of generating signals with known amounts of change. With the direct synthesis approach, it will be possible to gain insight into the auditory system's methods of defining threshold limits, of establishing perceptual boundaries between phonemes, and of processing musical messages. These applications are truly in their primitive state at the current time and merely provide a means for future research.

To afford additional control of a signal being generated, the amplitude may be computer regulated. The most direct means of control can be

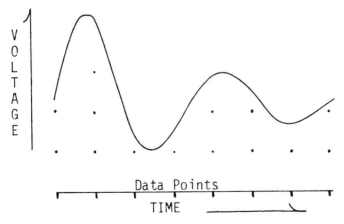

Figure 3. D/A converter generation of waveform.

achieved with a programmable attenuator in the signal line between the signal source and the sound transducer. The digitally programmable attenuator is available as a relay-driven unit or as a solid state unit and acts as a precision attenuator, with the amount of attenuation to be introduced into the signal line controlled by a digital buffered output from the computer. The most common programmable attenuators use eight logic lines. Each line controls one stage of attenuation, with the stages being accumulative. Figure 4 illustrates how the eight logic lines can control attenuation in 0.5-dB steps from 0 to 127.5 dB. The logic lines that are in the "one" state introduce their corresponding amounts of attenuation into the signal line with the sum of the amounts of attenuation being the total amount of attenuation in the line. In the example, if bits 2, 4, and 8 were all in the "one" state with all others being in the "zero" state, the total amount of attenuation would be 40.5 dB. If all eight bits were in the "one" state, the total amount of attenuation would be 127.5 dB. If all bits were in the "zero" state, there would be no attenuation introduced into the signal line.

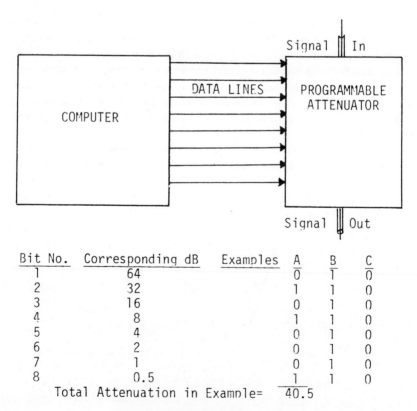

Bit No.	Corresponding dB	Examples	A	B	C
1	64		0	1	0
2	32		1	1	0
3	16		0	1	0
4	8		1	1	0
5	4		0	1	0
6	2		0	1	0
7	1		0	1	0
8	0.5		1	1	0
	Total Attenuation in Example=		40.5		

Figure 4. Digitally controlled attenuator.

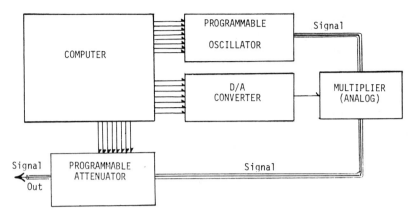

Figure 5. General purpose computer-controlled signal source.

In the programmable attenuator, the steps of attenuation are discrete, and the device therefore would be unsatisfactory for amplitude modulation studies. As with the frequency modulation circuit previously described, a digital-to-analog converter can be coupled to an amplitude modulation device or signal multiplier for fine control of amplitude. In general, the amplitude modulators do not have adequate dynamic range or sufficient signal-to-noise ratio for use as an attenuator. To achieve the maximal attenuation range with the greatest amplitude resolution, a D/A-controlled amplitude modulator coupled to the input side of a programmable attenuator affords the fine control of the modulator with the wide range of the attenuator. Figure 5 illustrates a general purpose signal source that incorporates a gated function generator with programmable frequency selection, a D/A converter-controlled analog multiplier, and a programmable attenuator. With such a configuration, the computer could direct the generation of a signal of known frequency, duration, and amplitude, all of which would be under program control.

The computer also can be utilized to control a variety of other devices such as tape recorders, servomotors, X-Y plotters, and most other devices that can be made electrically controllable. The range of applications and interfaces is limitless.

QUANTIFICATION OF BEHAVIORAL RESPONSES

In the stimulus-response paradigm for measuring hearing, it is necessary to identify the nature of the response being evoked and the information that is to be derived from that response. A subject's response to an auditory stimulus may be a psychological response or a physiological response. A psychological response may be a simple indication that a signal has been detected or it may be a more complex multiple choice indication in response to a discrimination task. A physiological response may be, for example, a cochlear microphonic potential, a single neuron's response, or an EEG signal from the scalp. In general, the psychological responses are conditioned responses whereas the physiological responses are measurements of the conductive and analytical processes of auditory pathway.

The simplest form of the psychological response for the computer to process is the subject's depressing of a response button, indicating to the computer that a response has been made by the subject. The response button, which in effect closes a switch contact, triggers one of the buffered input lines which the computer samples to see if a response has been made. The next step after the single response button is the panel of switches that might be used in a multiple choice discrimination task. Figure 6 illustrates how each of these buttons is connected to one of the buffered input lines which the computer samples as it did with the single response button. The computer can then be programmed to respond according to the button which is depressed. In place of the single push button any number of response detectors may be substituted to detect the occurrence of an event. Each of these detectors, however, is limited to the detection of discrete binary events.

A more interesting detector is the gauge which detects responses on a continuous scale. A potentiometer may be coupled to an A/D converter so that the degree of rotation in a method of adjustment study may be entered into the computer. A strain gauge may be attached to a finger to measure the amount of flexing in a magnitude estimation study. The output of a sound-level meter may be coupled to an A/D converter to measure the subject's vocal intensity in an auditory-vocal cybernetics study. Each of the above gauges measures psychological responses on a continuum and forwards the information to the computer.

In summary, the psychological indicators are those which can detect conditioned or voluntary responses from a subject and can direct the information to the computer for analysis. The measures are usually rather easy to define and to quantify. The problem remains, however, to identify to what extent a subject's conditioned response is actually a measure of his perception of an acoustic event.

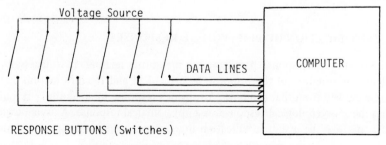

Figure 6. Multiple choice answer box interface.

QUANTIFICATION OF PHYSIOLOGICAL EVENTS

The physical and physiological measurement of hearing is more of a problem with transducers than with computers. In this chapter the term transducer is used to designate a device that performs the conversion of a physical or physiological event to an electrical signal that can be interfaced with a computer for the subsequent analysis of the electrical signal, or vice versa. This analysis is then interpreted as being indicative of the original physical or physiological event.

The purpose of using transducers in the measurement of hearing is to monitor the physical and physiological changes that occur in the peripheral and central hearing mechanisms as a function of stimulation. The events to be measured may be mechanical, as in basilar membrane motion; electrical, as in nervous system conduction; or chemical, as in metabolic change. Diverse experimental methods are employed to convert the events to electrical signals. Transducers function as the physiological events cause direct or indirect changes in the electrical properties of the sensing elements. The electrical qualities of the sensing elements may be made to vary as the events alter the capacitance, resistance, inductance, or piezoelectric or electromagnetic linkages of the transducer. The change in the electrical properties are then useful approximations of the amount of physical or physiological change that occurs concurrent with a stimulus.

A transducer is functionally the sense organ of the measurement system. It is, by definition, a highly specialized device which ideally responds to only one type of energy from a specified source. Its purpose is to represent faithfully in electrical form a physiological or physical event. A transducer should obey five criteria for the faithful measurement of an event: amplitude linearity, adequate frequency response, freedom from phase distortion, high validity, and nonreactivity.

The amplitude linearity of a transducer may be defined as the faithfulness with which changes in the strength of the event being measured are reflected in the amplitude of the electrical signal produced. For instance, if a strain gauge is being used to measure the tension of the tensor tympani muscle, the varying resistance in the gauge should coincide linearly with the change in the muscle's tension so that the amount of resistance change is truly representative of the muscle's contraction, and the accuracy of the measure should not vary as a function of the muscle's tension. Absolute linearity, unfortunately, has never been achieved, and small amounts of nonlinearity are inherent in most if not all physical and physiological measures.

The frequency response of a transducer is the range of frequencies that it will convert to electrical energy in a faithful manner. A transducer has physical properties that place limitations on its frequency range and on the sensitivity that it will have in measurements.

In experimental procedures where the concurrence of events is important, it is essential that a transducer follow the events that it is measuring without a

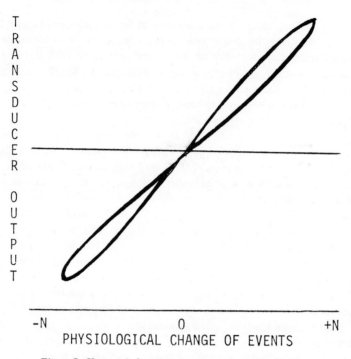

T
R
A
N
S
D
U
C
E
R

O
U
T
P
U
T

-N   0   +N
PHYSIOLOGICAL CHANGE OF EVENTS

Figure 7. Hysteresis function demonstrating lag in transducers.

time lag. Unfortunately, they are plagued by inertia, which creates an inherent phase lag in the events that they are tracking. Figure 7 illustrates the lag in response that can result from this inertia. As the mechanical or physiological event changes, the electrical output of the transducer lags slightly behind so that there is often a slight difference between the changes in the event and the change in the output of the transducer. This lag is called hysteresis and exists in all transducers, even those having no moving parts. The amount of hysteresis is also affected by the rate of change. If the hysteresis properties are known for a given transducer, the analyzing computer can be programmed to compensate for the phase distortions.

The validity of a transducer's measure is the extent to which it is measuring that and only that which the experimenter thinks it is measuring. Transducers are designed to measure specific types of energy changes, but they are subject to artifactual measurements. These artifacts are changes in conditions which are present but which are not the events that the experimenter wishes to measure. For example, in the measurement of EEG potentials, a subject that begins to perspire during the recording process produces variations in the EEG signals that are functions of the sweating rather than of the brain activity. The transducers are functioning as they should, but the presence of the perspiration creates conditions that distort the true EEG signals. In the case of sweat artifacts, they can be eliminated by environmental control. For those that cannot be eliminated, there must be means for accounting for the errors in the data analysis.

Irrespective of the physical or physiological event being measured, the transducer, insofar as possible, must not interfere with or alter the event being measured. However, the current state of most transducers is such that they require a coupling with the event that they are to measure, either directly or indirectly, and this coupling places a load on the system being measured. Although indirect measures place less of a loading on the system than do direct measures, the indirect measures are more subject to artifacts. The proper selection and application of transducers is truly a key to reliable and valid measurement of the hearing processes.

Equally important to the selection and application of transducers is the calibration of the measuring devices. If the measuring device is not calibrated accurately, the measures are relative or even meaningless. The methods of calibrating transducers should be examined critically to ensure the reliability and the validity of the data acquired from them. In general, the more efficient transducers (i.e., those with the strongest coupling to the system being measured) are the most precisely calibrated and require the least amount of electronic manipulation to couple the transducer's output to the computer interface. Those which cannot be directly calibrated with the physical or physiological events that they are to measure, are of time-domain interest only because of the relative nature of the measure with the passage of time. That is, the obtained measures are not absolute values but reflect approximate changes that take place over time. At best, calibration is an approximation of the accuracy of a measuring device, and with advanced technology in transducers will come significantly more refined and definitive measures of hearing.

MEASUREMENT OF HEARING

The measurement of hearing has historically followed three primary directions: 1) psychoacoustics, in which the subject's conditioned responses are studied as a means of measuring the perceptual parameters of hearing; 2) physiological acoustics, in which the mechanical and nervous components of the subject's auditory system are studied as a means of measuring the reception and conduction of acoustic stimuli; and 3) clinical procedures, which combine psychoacoustics with physiological acoustics to differentiate between pathological and normal auditory systems and to diagnose the probable etiologies of pathologies that exist. Virtually all aspects of these measurements have been subjected to computerization at one time or another with varying degrees of success and refinement. The following section of this chapter cites a few applications in each of these three categories to illustrate the applications and the techniques, and the works cited are in no way intended as an exhaustive review of all applications that have been made of the computer in the measurement of hearing.

PSYCHOACOUSTIC APPLICATIONS

Houtsma and Goldstein (1972) utilized a DEC PDP-4 computer and associated peripheral equipment to investigate subjects' perceptions of pitch of complex tones in melody patterns. Their experimental apparatus included the above mentioned computer, two programmable oscillators, a dual channel electronic switch under computer control, audiomixers and amplifiers, earphones, and a multiple choice answer box which indicated to the computer the subjects' responses. Figure 8 illustrates the configuration.

The experimental paradigm was designed to measure a subject's ability to identify the melody patterns of simple musical messages consisting of sequential tonal presentations. Each stimulus in the melody pattern consisted of the concurrent presentations of two upper harmonics of a tone, minus the fundamental frequency. Therefore, the task required that the subjects perceive a fundamental that was not actually present for each stimulus in the pattern and to determine the melody of the perceived fundamentals. The instrumentation permitted either the monaural presentation of both harmonics to one ear or the dichotic presentation, in which one of the upper harmonics went to the left ear and the other harmonic to the right ear. The results implied that a central processor combined the input from both ears for pitch perception of the missing fundamental.

A second psychoacoustic application of the computer to the measurement of hearing is Parameter Estimation by Sequential Testing (PEST). In this procedure devised by Taylor and Creelman (1967) and in subsequent applications, psychoacoustic measurements are derived on the basis of ongoing probabilities computation and specified rules. The procedure is particularly applicable to situations where a given threshold is to be determined by the sequential presentation of tones, as in an audiological test. As the subject responds to some tonal presentations and not to others, the computer performs a running tally of the responses and no-responses. In the PEST procedure, predetermined rules for threshold estimation are set for the type of measure to be obtained. These rules govern four parameters of the threshold tracking procedure: 1) when to change stimulus levels, 2) what level of stimulation to try next, 3) when to end the procedure, and 4) how to compute the level that will be taken as the derived psychoacoustic function. In the case of audiometric applications of PEST, this derived function might be the threshold of hearing for a given frequency.

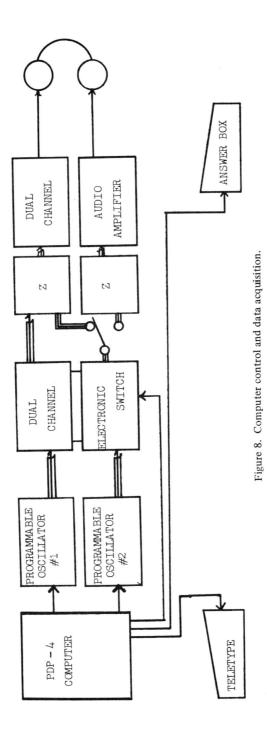

Figure 8. Computer control and data acquisition.

The rules for when to change levels are based on a target probability of response. For example, a target probability might be set at 60% correct of the total number of stimuli presented. This definition of threshold is really a probability statement rather than an absolute value of where hearing begins. In PEST's computation of a threshold, the system presents a series of stimuli to the subject and waits for his response. If he responds, the response is tallied; if he does not respond, the procedure advances to the next presentation and the process is repeated. After each trial, the computer determines if the ratio of the number of correct responses divided by the total number of trials is within the range of the target probability set by the experimenter. If the obtained ratio is considerably higher than the target probability, the stimulus level is taken as being too high, and a change of level in the downward direction is indicated. If the obtained ratio is considerably lower than the target probability, an upward change is indicated.

Included as a part of the target probability is a specified, acceptable deviation limit. This limit determines the permissible amount of tolerance or deviation from the target for determining that a ratio is within the target's range. For instance, if the 60% correct target were set, a ±10% deviation limit may be set so that any probability ratios between 50% and 70% would be accepted as "on target." The amount of tolerated deviation actually specifies the resolution and also the speed of the test procedure. If the target probability is a broad one, the test will be quick but not high in resolution because a large amount of error is tolerated. However, if the allowable deviation from the target is a narrow one, more trials will be necessary to determine the threshold, and the test will require more time.

The amount of change in a step is also specified by a set of rules based on the contingency of the subject's responses. Likewise, the tolerance rules specified by the experimenter determine when to stop varying parameters and when to calculate the threshold level.

The two primary advantages of the PEST procedure are that: 1) because of its efficiency it saves considerably more time than conventional threshold determination methods; and 2) the procedure is specifically defined, reproducible, and lacking in subjectivity. Because the procedure is such a complex one, dependent on a considerable amount of statistical computation, it is one well suited to the speed and capabilities of the digital computer.

The two examples of psychoacoustic applications of the computer have demonstrated that not only is the computer's controlling capability significant for the experimenter, but that the computer's logical and computational capabilities make possible experiments that have successive steps contingent upon the subject's responses to previous stimuli. Furthermore, the explicitly defined rules programmed into the computer operation minimize the subjectivity of the measurements, thus increasing the validity of the measure.

PHYSIOLOGICAL APPLICATIONS

An interim solution to the study of cochlear motion is the development of mathematical models based on empirical measurements and on derived functions. Peterson and Bogert (1950) proposed equations to describe basilar membrane motion as a function of stimulation and the distance along the membrane. Geisler and Hubbard (1971) applied these equations to a computerized simulation of the cochlea to permit manipulation of the parameters of the model. The model treats the cochlea as 31 interactive analog sections, with each section corresponding to approximatly 1 mm of the distance along the basilar membrane. Each successive section approximates the function of the corresponding portion of the basilar membrane upon receiving physical stimulation from the previous section. Each of the 31 sections has five variable parameters that correspond to the dynamic properties of that section. The actual model is instrumented on an analog computer that contains 31 sections. With the five controls per section, the manipulation of the model requires the setting of 155 individual potentiometers. These settings are managed by servomotors coupled to the potentiometer. The servomotors, in turn, are coupled to the buffered outputs of a digital computer. Therefore, in effect, the digital computer manages the parameters of the model, which is actually effected through an analog computer. Although the model could be totally hard-wired, the manipulation of the model would be practically unmanageable.

In direct physiological measurement the digital computer can accept large amounts of information derived from the nervous system and store it in its proper perspective. Sachs (1971) utilized the computer to investigate "two tone inhibition" in auditory nerve fibers. The research design provided for the placement of an electrode in the auditory nerve bundle, ideally terminating on one or two individual nerve fibers. The stimulus frequency which produced the maximal output from that fiber was then determined. This frequency was called the "critical frequency" for that fiber. The purpose of the study was to determine the effects that other frequencies would have on the nerve's output when presented concurrently with the critical frequency. Each pulse from the auditory nerve was stored in the computer's memory along with the frequency and temporal information about the critical frequency tone burst and the competing tone burst. As the competing stimulus was systematically varied in frequency, the nerve fibers' output was stored. After the effects of a range of frequencies had been measured, the results were displayed on a cathode ray tube dot matrix. From this display, it was possible to demonstrate that competing stimuli inhibited nerve output when the critical frequency and competing stimuli were presented concurrently.

Results such as these emphasize the need for further research into the function of the auditory pathway, and an even greater need for research into the physiological correlates of perception. Obviously, the findings from single nerve recordings demonstrate that nerves are not just data lines conducting in the way that telephone lines do. The encoded information on these pathways is very interactive with other pathways, which conduct information encoded according to different formats. Likewise, recordings from the dorsal and ventral cochlear nucleus, the superior olivary complex, and the entire auditory pathway up to the cortex demonstrate the presence of patterns, but they also all demonstrate many exceptions to the patterns, suggesting that exceptions are as common as the patterns.

In order for researchers to continue their investigations into the physiology of perception, new techniques that account for many events simultaneously will be necessary. With these techniques will come an increasing dependency on the power and the data handling capability of the computer. Likewise, computer-simulated models will become increasingly important as a means of creating theories for empirical testing. Because the nervous system seems to be very generalized in some of its functions and very specific in others, future models of the auditory pathways will of necessity have many parameters based on the specific function measures of today. Many physiological measures of today, such as EEG, may fall by the wayside in the future as more specific and exact means of physiological measurement and analysis become available.

Perception is a many dimensioned entity which avoids being measured directly. Perhaps in the next 10 years, the use of the computer along with expanded technology in data acquisition and analysis will afford new insights into the true understanding of perception.

CLINICAL APPLICATIONS

Wood, Mahaffey, and Peters (1973) have adopted the minicomputer to the testing of hearing for industrial hearing conservation programs. Their system is capable of obtaining pure tone thresholds on six subjects simultaneously, following the manual testing paradigm. In this system, the computer controls the frequency, intensity, and duration of the tone bursts and processes the subjects' responses. The procedure is one based on probabilities and is somewhat like the PEST procedure described earlier. In addition to the usual stimulus-response pattern, a contingent stimulus is added to the test. Each subject views a small light which is presented along with each tonal presentation and at times without the tone. The subject is instructed to respond only when he hears the tone, and that the tone will be present during a "light-on" condition. This procedure allows for the probabilistic computation of false responses. The principle advantage of the computer is that it performs limited interpretations in addition to the actual testing. The computer compares the derived thresholds with presbycusic curves for the age of each subject being tested. The system also records the results directly on magnetic tape for data processing.

A second clinical application was made by Wood, Goshorn, and Peters (1974) to test for functional hearing loss. The procedure utilizes the response time of the subject as an index of his certainty of response. With functional patients, a longer response time is required than with normal patients at threshold level. The computer serves the function of presenting the stimuli, processing the response, and computing the probability that the threshold is in fact a contrived one.

SUMMARY

This chapter has dealt with computer applications in the measurement of hearing, via psychoacoustic, physiological, and clinical procedures. The purpose of the examples has been to demonstrate that the capability of the computer for these applications is just beginning to be realized. As technology in transducers and laboratory procedures increases, the measurements will improve. The numerical processing capabilities of the computer in conjunction with its speech, precision, and interfacing possibilities will enable the computer to become the most essential piece of auditory measurement equipment.

REFERENCES

Geisler, C. D., and A. E. Hubbard. 1971. A hybrid-computer model of the cochlea. *In* M. B. Sachs (ed.), Physiology of the Auditory System, pp. 39–44. National Educational Consultants, Baltimore.

Houtsma, A. J. M., and J. L. Goldstein. 1972. The central origin of the pitch of complex tones: evidence from musical interval recognition. J. Acoust. Soc. Amer. 51: 520–529.

Peterson, L. C., and B. P. Bogert. 1950. A dynamical theory of the cochlea. J. Acoust. Soc. Amer. 22: 369–381.

Sachs, M. B. 1971. Quantitative studies of the responses of auditory-nerve fibers to two-tone stimuli. *In* M. B. Sachs (ed.), Physiology of the Auditory System, pp. 113–123. National Educational Consultants, Baltimore.

Taylor, M. M., and C. D. Creelman. 1967. PEST: efficient estimates on probability functions. J. Acoust. Soc. Amer. 41: 782–787.

Wood, T. J., E. Goshorn, and R. W. Peters. 1974. Auditory reaction times as an index of functional hearing loss. J. Acoust. Soc. Amer. 55S: 40.

Wood, T. J., R. B. Mahaffey, and R. W. Peters. 1973. A six-man computerized audiometer. J. Acoust. Soc. Amer. 54: 338.

Wood, T. J., W. W. Wittich, and R. B. Mahaffey. 1973. Computerized pure-tone audiometric procedures. J. Speech Hear. Res. 16: 676–684.

PRODUCTION—
ACOUSTICS

Experimental Physiology of the Larynx

Malcolm H. Hast, Ph.D.
Professor and Director of Research
Department of Otolaryngology and Maxillofacial Surgery
The Medical School, Northwestern University

CONTENTS

Introduction
Historical perspective
Some current techniques
Experiments by the author
  First experiment
  Second experiment
  Third experiment
Thoughts on the future
References

> *Pigmaei gigantum humeris impositi*
> *plusquam pisi gigantes vident.*
> Lucan

INTRODUCTION

This chapter describes methods of studying the physiology of the larynx and mechanisms of phonation in man and animals, from antiquity to the present. Greater emphasis, of course, is placed on modern methods and tools of measurement. No attempt has been made to survey the literature on the physiology of the larynx or to describe the mechanism of function or phonation; these topics have been well treated elsewhere (Kirchner, 1970; Kirchner, 1973). The description of past and current research is selective. A detailed outline of some procedures and instrumentation used by this author in his experiments on animals also is presented; this should enable other investigators or students to employ this chapter as a basic text or laboratory manual.

HISTORICAL PERSPECTIVE

Faced today with his armamentarium of polygraphs, oscilloscopes, amplifiers, computers, physiological transducers, waveform generators, and other wonderful "black boxes" and magnificent libraries, the budding scientist may wonder how his forebears were able to discover anything of scientific value. I'll tell you the how and the why that men with limited access to knowledge and crude instruments became the scientific giants of western civilization. They used their creative instincts and imagination, while devising their own methods and tools to discover and understand the secrets of nature.

One of these scientific giants, and the first to interest us, was Galen of Pergamon (130–200 A.D.). He was one of the great comparative anatomists, and also has been rightly named "the father of experimental physiology." In the study of the gross anatomy and experimental physiology of the larynx, Galen was "genesis;" his writings should be required reading (Lyons and Tower, 1962). Galen distinguished the intrinsic and extrinsic laryngeal muscles, dividing them into those which open and those which close the larynx. He described the cartilages as numbering three: the cricoid, thyroid, and arytenoid; he described the ventricles of the larynx and the vocal cords, the membranous lining of the larynx, the lubricating of the vocal cords by mucus and the superior and recurrent laryngeal nerves. He believed that the larynx was the instrument of voice, that the membranous glottis resisted the flow of air from the chest, and that voluntary contraction of the laryngeal muscles was controlled by the laryngeal nerves which derived from the brain. He also described several forms of laryngeal paralysis in which the laryngeal nerves were sectioned. Galen's most important contribution to the science of neurophysiology was his discovery that the brain, not the heart, controlled the muscles of the body and the voice. He demonstrated this hypothesis by cutting the laryngeal nerves of an unanesthetized squealing pig. The pig immediately became mute, thereby disproving the then current thought that the center of intelligence was located in the chest, and that the only purpose of the brain was to cool the blood.

Except for the few later theories on phonation proposed by Heinrici, Fabricius, and Dodart in the late 17th and early 18th centuries, no important work on laryngeal physiology was done until the middle of the 18th century. The 17th century work of Julius Casserius was a landmark in the comparative anatomy of the larynx, but in the physiology he followed the teachings of Galen (Hast and Holtzmark, 1969). The history of research on the experimental physiology of the larynx resumes with the investigations of the surgeon Antoine Ferrein (1741).

In 1741, Ferrein presented his experiments on the excised dog larynx before L'Academie Royal des Sciences in Paris. By approximating the glottis (compressing the larynx) and blowing air through the trachea, Ferrein disproved the belief that a dead vocal organ could not produce sound. He compared the laryngeal lips with the strings of the aeolian harp that are set into vibration by air flow; he termed these lips *cordes vocales*. He demonstrated that the pitch of the voice followed the law of strings, rising when the vocal cords were stretched or shortened and under increased tension. Ferrein incorrectly assumed that the phonatory sound was directly caused by vocal cord vibration alone, like that of a string without attached resonator. He also described the rise in pitch resulting from the approximation of the cricoid and thyroid cartilages. Ferrein repeated his experiments with a human cadaveric larynx. Much later, Helmholtz (1863) stated that the primary source of sound was caused by periodical puffs of air escaping through the glottis.

The 19th century was a turning point in the history of physiology. Before this period, scientists defined specific functions of a muscle by sectioning of nerves and anatomic dissection. By 1838, John Reid used electrical stimulation, in addition to nerve sectioning and anatomic dissection, to define the innervation of the laryngeal muscles. Using cats and dogs for in vivo experiments, he observed that the internal superior laryngeal nerve was purely sensory, and that the recurrent laryngeal was a motor nerve supplying all the muscles of the larynx except the cricothyroid, which was supplied by the external superior laryngeal nerve. In 1841, Professor Longet of the University of Paris confirmed, by physiological experiments, the mechanical theories proposed in 1829 by the Reverend Robert Willis (1833) on the action of the intrinsic laryngeal muscles. Longet stimulated individual branches of the recurrent nerve that innervate each of the intrinsic muscles of the larynx. Longet also substantiated Magendi's observation that the cricothyroid muscle lifts the cricoid cartilage up to the thyroid cartilage. He also demonstrated that the bulbar root of the spinal accessory nerve contains motor filaments which innervate the laryngeal muscles.

From Paris, our historical perspective must turn to Berlin and to one of the two greatest physiologists of the 19th century, Johannes Müller. The findings of his experiments formed the basis of the myoelastic-aerodynamic theory of the vibration of the vocal folds and of phonation. In the late 1830's, Professor Müller (1840) suspended an excised human cadaveric larynx in a frame to measure changes in length, tension, position, and vibration of the vocal folds, as well as differences brought about by various air pressures. With this experimental model, Müller was able to formulate, quantitatively, rules for the changes in vocal pitch and to validate Ferrein's theory that the voice originates by vibrations of the vocal folds.

Another of the truly significant events in the history of laryngeal science took place in 1854. Manuel Garcia (1855) invented the laryngeal mirror. This simple but powerful instrument enabled the scientist and physician, for the first time, to observe the living human larynx during phonation. Not many years later, Czermak (1861) published findings of the first attempt at laryngeal photography. His results were only fair, and it was not until 1883 that the process of laryngeal photography was perfected by Dr. T. R. French of New York. Although we use a head mirror and an electric bulb or fiberoptic light source today, the basic technique of the laryngoscope has not changed in over 100 years. Later, Ortel (1878) applied the stroboscopic principle to study, via the laryngeal mirror, laryngeal vibrations.

At the turn of the century, a major neurophysiological and neuroanatomic study on the larynx was published by Semon and Horsely (1890). Cortical stimulation in the monkey, cat, and dog showed that adductory movements of the vocal folds were represented principally in the cortex whereas abductory movements were located subcortically. In the macaque, the focal area for adduction was located in the foot of the ascending frontal gyrus between the anterior subcentral sulcus (dimple) and the inferior limb of the arcuate sulcus. This area was in contrast to the focus for extrinsic laryngeal movement located between the lower limb of the precentral gyrus and the anterior subcentral sulcus (dimple). The experiments of Leyton and Sherrington (1917) confirmed this separation of laryngeal representation in the gorilla and chimpanzee. Thus, there was early evidence that there existed two distinct foci on the motor cortex for the larynx, one for the movement of the intrinsic musculature and another for the extrinsic movement of the larynx as a whole, as in swallowing. Later, in 1938, Penfield explored the human cerebral cortex during neurosurgery and determined that vocalization in man is cortically represented. The text by Penfield and Roberts (1959) is well worth the student's time.

Two of the more important publications to appear in the first half of this century were Sir Victor Negus' (1929) text on the comparative anatomy and physiology of the larynx and Farnsworth's (1940) report on the development of a camera which could take high speed motion pictures of the vocal folds.

For Negus, a practicing otolaryngologist, what started as a masters thesis developed into the most extensive reference on the comparative morphology and function of the laryngeal organ to be written in this century. Although he engaged in little experimental work, his descriptions and illustrations of the larynges of most of the known animals have made this text a kind of "Bible" for scientists in the field of laryngology. Twenty-one years later, he revised his *Mechanism of the Larynx* (1929) and published his studies under the new title *The Comparative Anatomy and Physiology of the Larynx* (1949). Ownership of this later edition is a "must" for the personal library of the speech scientist or laryngeal physiologist.

With the development of the high speed motion picture camera by Bell Laboratories in 1940, experimental measurement of the motion of the human vocal folds became a reality. The camera has of course, improved; pictures are now in color, sound has been added and new models of the camera can achieve speeds of 6,000 frames/sec. By viewing the developed film at standard speeds of 16 or 24 frames/sec and with frame-by-frame analysis, the speech scientist can gain much information on both normal and abnormal laryngeal function (Koike and Hirano, 1973; Moore and von Leden, 1958).

SOME CURRENT TECHNIQUES

Although there are many techniques to study the mechanism of laryngeal function, they share a common empiricism with all science. The scientist will use observation, one or several methods of experimentation, and logic and intuitive reasoning to solve his problem. If his approach is one of "dissection and analysis" (Ingle, 1958), he may employ surgical, chemical, or physical methods in an effort to reduce the whole to its parts, and to study the behavior and the properties of these parts in isolated systems. With the realization of the fact that the whole is the reality and its division into parts may create artifacts that do not exist naturally in life, the researcher may study a system at multiple levels of disorganization, and when possible, test upon the whole system concepts based on isolated pieces of information about its parts; this is the method of "synthesis" (Ingle, 1958). This author has used both methods—of dissection and analysis, and synthesis—in his research on the neuromuscular properties and neurophysiology of the larynx, examples of which are illustrated later.

A good example of the method of dissection and analysis is in the series of experiments performed by van den Berg and Tan (1959) on excised human larynges. As illustrated in Figure 1, van den Berg and Tan reported and expanded the work of Müller by mounting freshly excised human cadaveric larynges on a rigid bar. With this method, both the modern techniques of

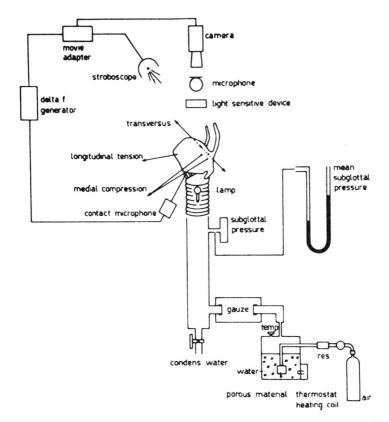

Figure 1. Method for experiments with human larynxes. (From van den Berg and Tan, 1959; reprinted by permission of the authors and S. Karger AG, Basel.)

stroboscopy and/or high speed sound motion picture photography can be used to analyze the motion of the vocal folds and phonation. Although this type of experimentation follows more closely the design of dissection and analysis, the examination of organ function as a system could lend itself to the criterion of synthesis.

Another method of experimentation is the "controlled experiment." In this method, certain conditions of the experiment are systematically altered, with changes in results noted, while all other conditions are kept constant or randomized. The objective is to determine the effect of the independent variable (Ingle, 1958). Examples of this type of laryngeal research are studies of changes in vocal length, pitch, and/or loudness in human phonation as measured by electromyography or the photoelectric methods of photoglotto-gram, electroglottogram, and roentgenography (see van den Berg, 1970 for a discussion of these methods). It should be noted that the photoelectric methods are useful only if one wishes to obtain information on differences within or between voices; other methods must be employed to describe physiological relationships.

The electromyograph (EMG) is one of the more practical and easy-to-use techniques in experimental physiology of the larynx. In 1929, Adrian and Bronk used concentric needle electrodes to study the physiology of muscle in the human and cat. The EMG was first employed as an instrument of recording and measurement of both normal and abnormal human laryngeal muscle function by Weddell, Feinstein, and Pattle in 1944. The technique of implanting wire electrodes into the laryngeal muscles continues to be widely used today in both animal experiments (Dedo and Hall, 1969; Murakami and Kirchner, 1972) and in the study of laryngeal nerve conduction and muscle function in humans (Atkins, 1973; Faaborg-Anderson, 1965; Gay et al., 1972). The EMG does, of course, have its limitations. In the "controlled method," in which we hope to study or manipulate an independent variable, say, the effect of a change in pitch on vocal fold movement, the implanted electrodes themselves can become an unwanted and uncontrolled variable. Electrodes, unlike the light of a photoelectric transducer (Hast, 1961; Sonesson, 1960), have a mechanical load that can interfere with vocal fold vibration, contaminating our measurements. An implanted electrode, regardless of size, can also produce a foreign body reaction. This is not to negate the value of the EMG technique but only to point out one of the important limitations of which the investigator should be aware. For a more complete discussion of the EMG, the reader should consult Basmajian (1967).

The production of voice requires a coordination of a number of factors: contraction of laryngeal muscles, vibrating mass and stiffness of the vocal fold, glottal air flow, subglottic air pressure, glottal resistance, the Bernouilli effect, and the acoustic coupling of the cavities above and below the glottis. To study and understand the mechanism of these variables, techniques have been developed to measure, either separately or in combination, each factor in the living animal model. Microphones, force transducers, pressure transducers, pneumotachometers, and other transducers are used in combination with oscilloscopes, tape recorders, inkwriters, and computers to monitor and measure the above parameters in the larynx. Examples of those procedures in which either or both the methods of dissection and/or synthesis have been used are found in works of Takenouchi et al. (1968), Koyama and his colleagues (1969, 1971), Hast (1969a, 1969b), and Hast et al. (1974). Details of some of these procedures are also given in the next section of this chapter.

A fairly recent technique that has been developed to study the vibratory vocal folds employs the principle of the ultrasonic echo (Hertz, Lindström, and Sonesson, 1970). An ultrasound transducer is positioned at the thyroid lamina about 1 cm below and lateral to thyroid prominence. With the probe focused on the vocal fold, an echo trace recording is obtained of the continuous vibration of the vocal fold with no interference from movements of the tongue or mandible and no discomfort to the patient. This procedure offers a good example of the controlled experiment.

Most of the techniques referred to above are primarily employed to study the physiology of the larynx on the peripheral level. There are, of course, special techniques designed to study the physiology of the larynx on the level of the central nervous system. An example of this area of research is described in the section to follow.

EXPERIMENTS BY THE AUTHOR

In this section, a few experiments are described in which the author studied physiological mechanisms of the larynx, both peripherally and centrally. Sufficient details of the rationale and methods are given so that the experiments can be repeated by others.

Before the procedures of specific experiments are presented, I would like to expand some of my thoughts on experimental science expressed in the previous section. What I propose is a few concepts that may assist the novice (and even the "scholar") in biological research. These thoughts should be accepted as guides, not as words of authority, for there is no authoritarianism in science; there is only observation, experience, facts, logic, and intuitive reasoning. If you bind your thinking and research to the authority of textbooks and journals, you will be doomed to a life of mediocrity. You must constantly doubt what you and others are saying and doing. Question your hypotheses, methods, and instrumentation (after all, you are a physical part of them); question your observations and conclusions—all are conceptions of human thought and design, possessing inherent defects. As a start, I shall point out the first inherent flaw in most physiological experiments. Any interference in the homeostasis of the experimental animal model, as a result of violating the *milieu intérieur* by drugs and/or surgery, which cannot be accounted for or measured, can be a source of error. Unfortunately, we will have to live with this error indefinitely, since all scientific research is subject to the principle of limited determinacy (Heisenberg's uncertainty principle).

In order to carry out successfully the three experiments described below, the student needs an animal surgery, surgical instruments and supplies, and some physiological instruments for nerve-muscle stimulation, measurement, and recording (refer to author's studies). The student also should refer to Markowitz, Archibald, and Downie (1964) for techniques and instruments needed for work in experimental surgery, and to a standard text for principles of general and special surgery (Higgins, 1968). He also should seek the advice of a trained surgeon.

First Experiment

The purpose of this experiment is to measure changes in and the relationships between subglottic air pressure and fundamental frequency of phonation as a function of a neural stimulation. The study is performed with a mongrel dog as the animal model.

The animal is anesthetized with phenobarbital sodium, 25–30 mg/kg intravenously. With the animal in a supine position, a vertical midline incision is made from the level of the hyoid to the superior border of the manubrium

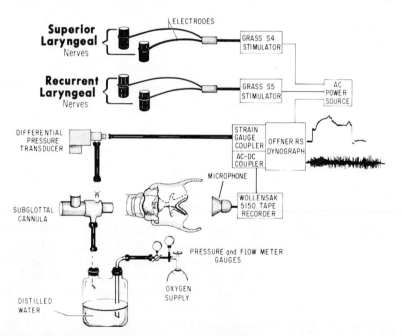

Figure 2. Method for measuring and recording subglottic air pressure and phonation in an animal. (From Hast, 1969b; reprinted by permission.)

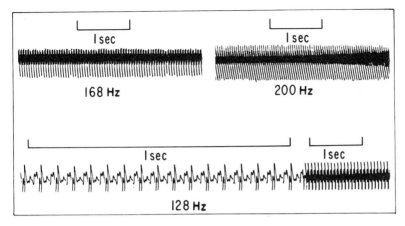

Figure 3. Fundamental frequency of phonation from recordings of a dog; total peaks of the waveform X 8. (From Hast, 1968; reprinted by permission.)

of the sternum. The pretracheal muscles are separated and carried laterally, exposing the trachea and larynx. Tracheotomy is performed, inferiorly, and a cannula is inserted to maintain an airway. A second cannula, constructed to accept an air-line and a differential air pressure transducer, is inserted into the trachea just inferior to the cricoid cartilage. The recurrent laryngeal nerves are then freed, approximately 2 cm distally, and tagged with 4-0 silk. The extrinsic branches of the superior laryngeal nerves are also isolated and tagged. The dog's mouth is held open by a clamp and a microphone is placed to the side.

As illustrated in Figure 2, a pressure transducer and air hose are connected to the subglottal cannula, and the nerves are placed on bipolar shielded electrodes bathed in a pool of warm oil. Air is delivered at a flow rate of 10 m/min, and the nerves are stimulated with a train of monophasic pulses. Since the degree of contraction of a muscle fiber is dependent on the amplitude and frequency of the current, the nerves should be stimulated at amplitudes of 0.3–1.3 v, pulse duration of 0.1–1.0 msec, and a stimulus train of 30–120 Hz. By varying the amplitude and frequency of the stimulus artifact, various changes in vocal pitch, intensity, and subglottal air pressure may be observed. Interesting changes in pitch can also be recorded by varying, independently, parameters of the stimulus to the superior nerves.

A simple method of recording and analyzing the fundamental frequency of phonation is to use a multispeed tape recorder. The animal's vocalization is recorded at 7.5 inches/sec and played back into an inkwriter at 15/16 inch/sec (1/8 speed), as illustrated in Figure 3. Changes in subglottal air pressure are easily calibrated by a mercury manometer, and the response of the transducer recorded by an inkwriter or oscilloscope. There is another point the student should keep in mind. Since the larynx is functionally and primarily a respiratory organ, the trains of electrical shocks should be presented only between respirations (approximately 1–5 sec in length). In addition, airflow, a constant in this experiment, can be varied if one wishes to add an additional variable to this experiment. For a more detailed discussion on the application of the above method to experimental surgery, the student should see Hast (1968, 1969b).

Second Experiment

The purpose of this second exercise is to measure the mechanical properties of the cricothyroid and the thyroarytenoid muscles in an animal. Knowledge of the contractile properties of the laryngeal muscles contributes to our understanding of the mechanism of action and function of the laryngeal organ.

The most suitable laboratory animal for this experiment is the dog. The subhuman primate is, of course, the best animal model to study. There are two problems, though, with using monkeys: cost and operative procedures. The operative procedures on these small animals require the aid of an operation microscope, microsurgical instruments, and surgical experience. For a detailed discussion of comparative physiological studies on the larynx by the author, the reader should refer to Hast (1966a, 1966b, 1967a, 1967b, 1969a) and Hast and Golbus (1971).

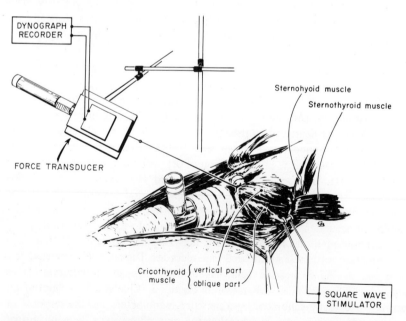

Figure 4. Method of recording mechanical properties of the cricothyroid muscle. (From Hast, 1966a; reprinted by permission.)

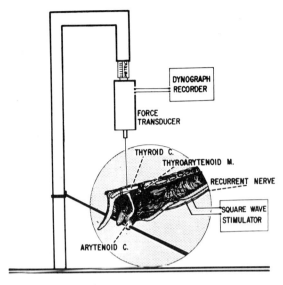

Figure 5.   Method for recording mechanical properties of the thyroarytenoid muscle. (From Hast, 1967a; reprinted by permission of S. Karger AG, Basel; first printed in Hast, 1966b, and reprinted here by permission.)

In this experiment, as in the first, animals are anesthetized with phenobarbital sodium, 25–30 mg/kg intravenously.

The animals are placed in a supine position, tracheotomy is performed to maintain a free airway, and the larynx is exposed from the hyoid bone to the second or third tracheal ring. The recurrent laryngeal and extrinsic branch of the superior laryngeal nerves are freed unilaterally and tagged.

A ventromedian incision is then made through the larynx from the hyoid to the first tracheal ring. This is followed by two mediolateral incisions of the thyroid cartilage, one superior and one inferior to the vocal fold. The origin of the thyroarytenoid muscle is finally freed by sectioning the thyroid cartilage perpendicular to and between the mediolateral incisions. A length of silk is tied into the cricoid attachment of the cricothyroid muscle and another into the thyroid attachment of the thyroarytenoid muscle. To further isolate the thyroarytenoid muscle from the interaction of other intrinsic muscles, the arytenoid cartilage is sutured to the thyroid cartilage or fixed by a clamp to a rigid stand; ties are made with 3-0 surgical suture.

The free end of each piece of silk is tied to a force displacement transducer (Figures 4 and 5) attached to a heavy stand. The output signal of the transducer is amplified and recorded by a high speed inkwriter or oscilloscope. Isometric recordings are made of each muscle separately. Measurements of the mechanical properties of contraction time, one half relaxation time, tetanus, and tetanus to twitch tension ratio are taken at the in situ resting length of each muscle. Since the speed of muscle contraction has a high temperature coefficient (Q_{10} = 1.53), temperature should be maintained at 37°C (±0.2°) by the heat of an electric lamp and monitored by a thermistor probe connected to the circuit of a calibrated electrical thermometer. The preparation is bathed by a physiological irrigating solution. It also should be noted that the in situ resting length must be maintained since the progressive lengthening of a muscle would increase the contraction time of the twitch.

The laryngeal nerves are attached to shielded bipolar platinum electrodes and bathed in a pool of warm mineral oil. After the threshold of muscle contraction is established, the amplitude of the electrical stimulus is increased to a supramaximal voltage of 1–2 v. The nerves are stimulated with square wave pulses of a duration of 0.1 msec at a frequency of 1–150/sec. Trains of stimuli are limited to 2 sec, and an interval of 10 sec is maintained between successive tentani to allow for dissipation of post-tetanic potentiation of muscle twitches. An example of a recording of mechanical properties of an isometrically contracting cricothyroid muscle is shown in Figure 6.

A comparison of measurements of the mechanical properties of intrinsic laryngeal muscles to other striated muscles of the body will reveal that the cricothyroid muscle is a "fast" muscle, and that the thyroarytenoid is one of the "fastest" contracting of the voluntary muscles.

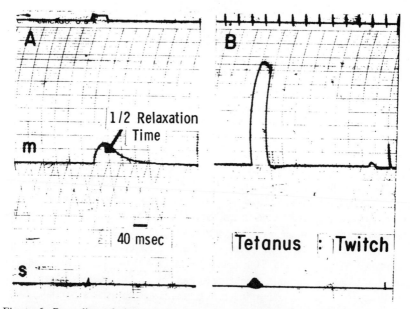

Figure 6. Recording of three mechanical properties of the cricothyroid muscle. A, contraction and half relaxation times; B, muscle tetanus and twitch tension. m, muscle; s, stimulus. (From Hast, 1966a; reprinted by permission.)

Third Experiment

This third experiment in special physiology also involves animal surgery; but in this experiment, the techniques of neurosurgery are added. The purpose of this experiment is to localize the cortical motor area(s) of an animal brain that control the vocal folds and muscles of the larynx, and to measure the laryngeal response time and contractile properties via central stimulation.

If one wishes to relate his findings to human function, the best animal model for this type of study is the subhuman primate. The author has used both the squirrel monkey (Hast, 1966b) and the rhesus monkey (*Macaca mulatta*) in his work (Hast et al., 1974). The method given below employs the adult male rhesus monkey as the experimental subject. The procedure will be described in three parts: anesthesia, surgery and recording, and stimulation and exploration.

Anesthesia A tranquilizer (Sernylan 1 mg/kg) is administered before the animal is removed from its home squeeze-cage. Surgery is initiated under a minimal dosage (0.25 ml) of a barbiturate (Diabutal 60 mg/ml), given intraperiotoneally, and is supplanted by α-chloralose (70 mg/kg) once a continuous intravenous drip of 5% dextrose in lactated Ringer's solution is initiated. Approximately 2 ml/hr of a 3.5% solution of α-chloralose, dissolved in polyethylene glycol-200, is necessary to maintain a level of anesthesia which suppresses movement and reflexes while allowing normal laryngeal and pharyngeal reflexes to remain after induction.

Surgery and Recording The head is secured in a heavy metal holder. The scalp is opened by an incision that extends from the zygomatic arch, along the orbital ridge, to the midline, and from the midline caudally to the occipital pole. When a bilateral experiment is planned, two such L-shaped flaps are taken on either side of the head. The temporal muscle is dissected free from the skull on one or both sides down to the zygomatic arch and retracted caudally. The calvarium is opened with a trephine and the bone is rongeured away from an area directly above the zygoma. This area is bounded posteriorly by the external auditory canal and anteriorly by the orbital ridge. The resulting craniectomy is somewhat rectangular in shape, about 2×4 cm in size, and allows exposure of the inferolateral aspect of the frontal cortex. The exposed dura is left unopened. The area is loosely packed with saline-soaked Webril (Kendall), and the flap is closed with wound clips. The head is removed from the holder, and the animal is respositioned for tracheostomy.

With the animal in a supine position, a tracheostomy is performed to maintain a free air passage, and the larynx is exposed from the hyoid bone to the second or third tracheal ring. All operative procedures are performed with the aid of an operation microscope and microsurgical instruments. Either one of two methods can be used to record the muscle response. For localization of "mapping procedures," the technique of electromyography can be employed, using the bipolar indwelling electrode as described in Basmajian

(1967). For measuring the contractile properties of laryngeal muscles, the procedures are similar to those described in the second experiment.

After the surgical procedures are completed in the neck, the wound clips are removed from the scalp, the flap is reopened, and the dura is incised in stellate fashion. The exposed cortex should constantly be irrigated with warm saline solution or covered with saline solution-saturated Webril when not being stimulated.

Stimulation and Exploration The cortex is stimulated with a monopolar electrode, 0.25 mm in diameter, covered with an insulator to within 0.5 mm of the tip. The electrode is applied lightly but firmly to the cortical surface. The indifferent electrode is connected to the moist cotton packing in wide contact with the dura, skull, and skin. The cortex is stimulated with a 100/sec biphasic train of pulses, controlled from a waveform generator and produced by a physiological stimulator. The stimulus pulse is led through a stimulus isolation unit and constant current unit to the monopolar electrode. Animals are stimulated at intervals of 2 min and always between inspiratory-expiratory periods of respiration. The duration of the stimulus train is limited to 100 msec and the stimulus pulse duration to 5 msec.

The area of the cortex to be explored is bounded anteriorly by the inferior ramus of the arcuate sulcus and posteriorly by the lower limb of the central sulcus. By careful exploration, stimulating each square millimeter, points can be localized which yield, at lowest current values, isolated contractions of the cricothyroid and thyroarytenoid muscles. It will be found that current thresholds usually vary from point to point and with different animals; the range is from 0.155 mA to 1.55 mA. In addition to recording muscle contractions electrically, responses can be verified visually through an operation microscope.

THOUGHTS ON THE FUTURE

Future research in experimental physiology of the larynx will probably be determined by at least three factors common to all research: the intellect and imagination of the investigator, the working hypotheses of the community of scholars in this area of science, and the discovery or development of new methods and instruments.

I will not dwell on the first factor, the scientist, for the very existence of the creative and productive scientist is probably more a matter of natural chance than of training and environment. The second factor, the working hypotheses of a scientific field, is of singular importance since it affects the course of the third factor, the development of new methods and instruments.

Where and when did the concept originate that the larynx is "the organ of voice," and that its structure and function in man were uniquely designed for communication? No matter; this has been the working hypothesis of too many investigators of laryngeal physiology. These researchers are either not aware or have forgotten that many species of animals who have a larynx never use it as a "vocal" organ. As Negus (1949) points out: "If a study of the organ be made with the premise that it was evolved for phonation, confusion will arise in interpreting its structure and function." The larynx is an organ of the respiratory system (Murakami and Kirchner, 1972). Its primary functions are to protect the airway, assist in adjusting intrinsic airway resistance during respiration, aid the lungs in air-mixing within the alveoli, and contribute to the regulation of frequency and depth of breathing. Vocalization is a secondary (probably learned) function. This biological premise has formed the basis of the author's research for over a decade, and until it becomes one of the primary working hypotheses of most investigators, new findings on laryngeal physiology will be limited. It is true that the larynx functions in communication and as a musical instrument, but one does not need a larynx to vocalize.

As the scientist is the progenitor of hypotheses and designs, laboratory methods and instruments are merely the offspring of the conception. Although new techniques and instruments can, in some circumstances, lead our experiments into new realms of exploration, these tools should not enslave our creative instincts from the formation of new constructs. The course of future research on the larynx already has been partly charted by present conception and experiment.

I believe that the recent work, by this author and others, on the morphology and physiology of the larynx, in the first half of this decade, will form the basis for future experiments. I refer in particular to the renewed interest in embryology (Hast, 1972), the examination of microstructure by histochemical techniques (Sahgal and Hast, 1974), and the physiological studies on the primate brain to define the cortical motor and sensory topography of the larynx (Hast et al., 1974; O'Brien, Pimpaneau, and Albe-Fessard, 1971). Where will these studies lead?

For this decade and probably the remainder of this century, increased work will be done with several species of subhuman primate. Work in descriptive embryology will continue, eventually giving way to studies in experimental embryology of the primate. The histochemistry and ultrastructure of the tissues of the larynx will be explored, using the latest techniques of electronmicroscopy and biochemistry. As our knowledge of developmental anatomy increases, and the morphology of the larynx is eventually defined on a histochemical and ultrastructural level, we will then be capable of describing physiological function in terms of structure.

Neurophysiological studies will proceed at a more rapid pace as surgical technique and recording instrumentation become more refined and discriminating. The larynx will be plotted discretely, by single cell recording, on the motor and sensory cortex of the subhuman primate. The neural pathways will be traced, by neuroanatomic and neurochemical techniques, to the peripheral laryngeal organ; and the cortical and subcortical connections of the central nervous system between the larynx, the heart (Kirchner, 1973), the motor speech areas, and the auditory system will be defined and mapped. In addition, the control and regulation of the larynx through the autonomic nervous system will be clarified. Later, monkeys will have implanted in their brains miniature automated telestimulation receivers (Maurus and Pruscha, 1972); with a bank of these receivers implanted throughout their brains, motor and sensory areas (and even cells) could be controlled by a radio transmitter linked to a computer. An unlimited amount of information would then be collected which could, eventually, be "written out" in the form of three dimensional schematics of the entire organization of the brain and its connections to the peripheral organ.

Experimental physiology will change from "destructive" to "nondestructive" research. Thereafter, the larynx will be studied structurally, chemically, and physiologically in the living human, with instruments that will neither come in contact with nor alter any tissues of the organ. The mechanism of action of the larynx will be understood.

With the further development of microsurgery, pharmacology, and electronic technology, laboratory findings will be directly applied to human function. Clinical problems involving the larynx, both peripherally and centrally, will be duplicated in the subhuman primate model. The data and solutions to these problems will then be incorporated into the medical diagnosis and treatment of the human patient. Finally, in centuries to come, scientists will devise new constructs of science to explore and eventually discover the physical basis of mind.

REFERENCES

Adrian, E. D., and D. W. Bronk. 1929. The discharge of impulses in motor nerve fibers. II. The frequency of discharge in reflex and voluntary contractions. J. Physiol. 67: 119–151.
Atkins, J. P. Jr. 1973. An electromyographic study of recurrent nerve conduction and its clinical applications. Laryngoscope 83: 796–807.
Basmajian, J. V. 1967. Muscles Alive: Their Functions Revealed by Electromyography. 2nd Ed. Williams & Wilkins, Baltimore.
van den Berg, J. 1970. Mechanism of the larynx and the laryngeal vibrations. In B. Malmberg (ed.), Manual of Phonetics, pp. 278–308. 2nd Ed. North-Holland, Amsterdam.
van den Berg, J., and T. S. Tan. 1959. Results of experiments with human larynxes. Pract. Otorhinolaryngol. 21: 425–450.
Czermak, J. 1861. De l'application de la photographie à la laryngoscopie et a la rhinoscopie. C.R. Acad. Sci. 53: 966–968.
Dedo, H. H., and W. H. Hall. 1969. Electrodes in laryngeal electromygraphy. Ann. Otol. Rhinol. Laryngol. 78: 172–180.
Faaborg-Andersen, K. 1965. Electromyography of laryngeal muscles in humans. Technics and results. In Current Problems in Phoniatrics and Logopedics, pp. 1–72. Vol. 3. S. Karger, Basel.

Farnsworth, D. W. 1940. High-speed motion pictures of the human vocal cords. Bell Lab. Rec. 18: 203–208.

Ferrein, A. 1741. De la formation de la voix. Mem. Acad. R. Sci. 409–432.

French, T. R. 1883. On photographing the larynx. Arch. Laryngol. 4: 235–243.

Garcia, M. 1855. Physiological observations on the human voice. Lond. Edinburgh Dub. Phil. Mag. 10: 218.

Gay, T., H. Hirose, M. Strome, and M. Swashima. 1972. Electromyography of the intrinsic laryngeal muscles during phonation. Ann. Otol. Rhinol. Laryngol. 81: 401–409.

Hast, M. H. 1961. Subglottic air pressure and neural stimulation in phonation. J. Appl. Physiol. 16: 1142–1146.

Hast, M. H. 1966a. Mechanical properties of the cricothyroid muscle. Laryngoscope 76: 537–548.

Hast, M. H. 1966b. Physiological mechanisms of phonation: tension of the vocal fold muscle. Acta Otolaryngol. 62: 309–318.

Hast, M. H. 1967a. Mechanical properties of the vocal fold muscle. Pract. Otorhinolaryngol. 29: 53–56.

Hast, M. H. 1967b. The respiratory muscle of the larynx. Ann. Otol. Rhinol. Laryngol. 76: 489–497.

Hast, M. H. 1968. Studies on the extrinsic laryngeal muscles. Arch. Otolaryngol. 88: 71–76.

Hast, M. H. 1969a. The primate larynx. Acta Otolaryngol. 67: 84–92.

Hast, M. H. 1969b. Transposition of laryngeal muscles for cricothyroid paralysis. Arch. Otolaryngol. 90: 93–97.

Hast, M. H. 1972. Early development of the human laryngeal muscles. Ann. Otol. Rhinol. Laryngol. 81: 524–531.

Hast, M. H., J. M. Fischer, A. B. Wetzel, and V. E. Thompson. 1974. Cortical motor representation of the laryngeal muscles in Macaca mulatta. Brain Res. 73: 229–240.

Hast, M. H., and S. Golbus. 1971. Physiology of the lateral cricoarytenoid muscle. Pract. Otorhinolaryngol. 33: 209–214.

Hast, M. H., and E. B. Holtzmark (trans.). 1969. The larynx, organ of voice by Julius Casserius. Acta Otolaryngol. 261(suppl.): 1–36.

Hast, M. H., and B. Milojevic. 1966. The response of the vocal folds to electrical stimulation of the inferior frontal cortex of the squirrel monkey. Acta Otolaryngol. 61: 196–204.

Helmholtz, H., von. 1863. Die Lehre von den Tonenempfindungen. Braunschweiger. Musik-Verlag, Braunschweig.

Hertz, C. H., K. Lindström, and B. Sonesson. 1970. Ultrasonic recording of the vibrating vocal folds. Acta Otolaryngol. 69: 223–230.

Higgins, G. A. 1968. Orr's Operations of General Surgery. 4th Ed. W. B. Saunders, Philadelphia.

Ingle, D. 1958. Principles of Research in Biology and Medicine. J. P. Lippincott, Philadelphia.

Kirchner, J. (ed.). 1970. Pressman and Kelemen's Physiology of the Larynx. 2nd Ed. American Academy of Ophthalmology and Otolaryngology, Rochester, N.Y.

Kirchner, J. 1973. Physiology of the larynx. In D. A. Shumrick and M. M. Paparella (eds.), Otolaryngology, pp. 371–379. Vol. 1. W. B. Saunders, Philadelphia.

Koike, Y., and M. Hirano. 1973. Glottal-area time function and subglottal-pressure variation. J. Acoust. Soc. Amer. 54: 1618–1627.

Koyama, T., J. E. Harvey, and J. H. Ogura. 1971. Mechanics of voice production, II. Regulation of pitch. Laryngoscope 81: 47–65.
Koyama, T., M. Kawaski, and J. H. Ogura. 1969. Mechanics of voice production. I. Regulation of vocal intensity. Laryngoscope 79: 337–354.
Leyton, A. S. F., and C. S. Sherrington. 1917. Observation on the excitable cortex of the chimpanzee, orangutan and gorilla. Q. J. Exp. Physiol. 11: 135–222.
Longet, F. A. 1841. Recherches Expérimentales sur les Functions des Nerfs des Muscles du Larynx. Bechet et Labe, Paris.
Lyons, M. C., and B. Towers (eds.). 1962. Galen on Anatomical Procedures: The Later Books, pp. 67–217. Translated by W. L. H. Duckworth. The University Press, Cambridge.
Markowitz, J., J. Archibald, and H. G. Downie. 1964. Experimental Surgery. 5th Ed. Williams & Wilkins, Baltimore.
Maurus, M., and H. Pruscha. 1972. Quantitative analyses of behavioral sequences elicited by automated telestimulation in squirrel monkeys. Exp. Brain Res. 14: 372–394.
Moore, P., and H. von Leden. 1958. Dynamic variations of the vibratory pattern in the normal larynx. Folia Phoniatr. 10: 205–238.
Müller, J. 1840. Von der Stimme und Sprache. In Handbuch der Physiologie des Menchen. Bd. 2, Buch. 4. Coblenz.
Murakami, Y., and J. A. Kirchner. 1972. Respiratory movements of the vocal cords. Laryngoscope 82: 454–467.
Negus, V. E. 1929. The Mechanism of the Larynx. C. V. Mosby, St. Louis.
Negus, V. E. 1949. The Comparative Anatomy and Physiology of the Larynx. William Heinemann Medical Books Ltd., London.
O'Brien, J. H., A. Pimpaneau, and D. Albe-Fessard. 1971. Evoked cortical responses to vagal, laryngeal and facial afferents in monkeys under chloralose anaesthesia. Electroenceph. Clin. Neurophysiol. 31: 7–20.
Ortel, M. 1878. Uber eine neue Laryngostroboskipische Untersuchungsmethode. Zentralbl. Med. Wiss. 16: 81–82.
Penfield, W. 1938. The cerebral cortex in man. I. The cerebral cortex and consciousness. Arch. Neurol. Psychiatr. 40: 417–442.
Penfield, W., and L. Robert. 1959. Speech and Brain Mechanisms. Princeton University Press, Princeton, N.J.
Reid, J. 1838. An experimental investigation into the functions of the eight pair of nerves. Edinburgh Med. Surg. J. p. 138.
Sahgal, V., and M. H. Hast. 1974. Histochemistry of primate laryngeal muscles. Acta Otolaryngol. 78: 277–281.
Semon, F., and V. Horsley. 1890. An experimental investigation of the central motor innervation of the larynx. Phil. Trans. R. Soc. Lond. B 181: 187–211.
Sonesson, B. 1960. On the anatomy and vibratory pattern of the human vocal folds. Acta Otolaryngol. 156(suppl.): 1–80.
Takenouchi, S., T. Koyama, M. Kawaski, and J. H. Ogura. 1968. Movements of the vocal cords. Acta Otolaryngol. 65: 33–50.
Weddle, G., B. Feinstein, and R. E. Pattle. 1944. The electrical activity of voluntary muscle in man under normal and pathological conditions. Brain 67: 178–257.
Willis, R. 1833. On the mechanism of the larynx. Trans. Camb. Phil. Soc. 4: 323–352.

Method of Acoustic Analysis of Intonation

Yukio Takefuta, Ph.D.
Associate Professor
Chiba University
Chiba, Japan;
Consultant, Ohio Department of Health

CONTENTS

Introduction
Experiment
Collection of sample intonations
Extraction of physical correlates
Relative efficiencies of the extracted physical correlates
Relative efficiencies of certain characteristics of
frequency variations
Normalization of frequency variation
Transformation of frequency variation
Information points in intonation
Feature extraction
Test of the analysis procedures
Summary
References

INTRODUCTION

Intonation creates a variety of linguistic contrast in speech and adds fine nuances that no words can express. In addition, it conveys the speaker's attitude toward the subject matter, expresses his emotional condition, and possibly increases the naturalness and intelligibility of speech. Therefore, it is an important speech signal, and a good understanding of this signal is very much needed. However, in spite of the common and persisting misunderstanding of some linguists and speech scientists that intonation is an easy, insignificant topic, it is a very difficult and challenging signal to analyze scientifically. Researchers Schubiger (1958), Crystal (1969), and Lehiste (1970) expressed their opinions as follows. "Intonation is much more diffi-

This research was supported in part by a contract between the Office of Naval Research and the Ohio State University Research Foundation, and in part by the 1972 Science Education Research Grant from the Ministry of Education, Japan. Computer time for developing programs was provided by the Instruction and Research Computer Center of the Ohio State University. This chapter was completed while the author was at the Ohio State University.

cult to describe than the articulation of sounds" (Schubiger, 1958, p. 1). "It is understandable that the study of intonation and related features should be in such a state, when one considers the difficulties involved in subjecting this aspect of language to analysis" (Crystal, 1969, p. 2). "They (prosodic features) seem more elusive than segmental features" (Lehiste, 1970, p. 1).

The present state of art in analyzing and describing intonation is extremely discouraging. Chomsky and Halle stated it convincingly as follows. "Our investigations of these (prosodic) features have not progressed to a point where a discussion in print would be useful" (Chomsky and Halle, 1968, p. 329). This state has not changed significantly in 1973. "Even though a number of investigators have attempted to specify the precise roles played by each of the suprasegmental parameters in oral communication, there is yet little definitive information to that end" (Minifie, 1973, p. 281).

When one looks further for the reasons why the study of intonation fell so much behind the studies of the other topics of linguistics and speech science, it soon becomes evident that the problem was not only the difficulty of the topic itself, but also the fact that there have been "no appropriate methodologies" available for the studies of intonation. "Recent intonational studies show such variety in technique and method that the results are difficult to compare" (Hadding-Koch, 1961, p. 7). "Again, the absence of any well-defined theory and procedures of analysis has resulted in distortions and vague conceptual terminology in many of the textbooks which purport to be introductions to intonation and related features in English" (Crystal, 1969, p. 2). More specifically, the most outstanding of the methodological problems for studying the structure of English intonation have been fourfold: 1) difficulty of classifying intonations, especially into pairs of minimal contrast; 2) low reliability of auditory analysis; 3) extreme difficulty of instrumentally extracting the fundamental frequency of speech; and 4) the lack of methodology to normalize and transform the extracted physical parameters for detecting the functional features of intonation.

Needless to say, if one wants to study a speech signal scientifically, the development of a reliable and valid method of analysis is essential. Therefore, in this chapter, one of the innovative experiments which was conducted to develop a comprehensive method for analyzing and describing intonation is discussed. Traditionally, there have been two schools in the study of intonation: instrumental analysis and auditory analysis. However, neither group could successfully analyze intonation. As it was mentioned in the preceding paragraph, the auditory analysis was found unreliable and the instrumental analysis was considered invalid.

The third and the most recent approach is the one in which the instrumentally extracted physical data (F_0) are processed until they match the auditory recognition of intonational contrast. This method requires a sophisticated use of an electronics computer, which seems to be the right direction to the successful analysis of this complex speech signal. As a matter of fact, a computer is not only an essential instrument for the complex processing in the analysis of instrumentally extracted data, but is also the only instrument that can extract the raw data of intonation (fundamental frequency) accurately. Nevertheless, since few researchers in linguistics or speech and hearing science are familiar with the applicability of the computer, analysis of intonation by a computer (data processing) has not been known to most researchers.

The objective of this chapter is to describe briefly the computer (digital) techniques developed at the phonetics laboratory of the Ohio State University (Columbus, Ohio) for a reliable and valid analysis of American intonation. The study is comprised of a series of nine experiments and includes the development of a method of collecting samples of intonation, methods of the data processing for the extraction (reception); normalization and transformation (perception) of physical parameters; and the detection (recognition) of intonation patterns.

EXPERIMENT

1. Collection of Sample Intonations

A female college student recorded 10 short, everyday sentences of American English. The list of sentences is presented in Table 1. Recording of the 10 sentences was made three times. In the first round of recording, each sentence was recorded twice in two different intonations, thus obtaining 10 pairs of contrastive intonations (not necessarily linguistic contrast). Each intonation was identified as 0011, 0112, 1011, 1112 . . . 9011, 9112, etc. In this system of identification, the first digit shows the sentence (0–9); the second digit, the type of intonation (0 and 1) (for example, advice (0) versus threat (1)); the third digit, the round of recording (1, 2, 3); and the last digit shows the order of recording for the same sentence (1 and 2). In the second round, each sentence was recorded twice again, but only with the intonation type (0) used for the sentence in the first round of recording, thus obtaining intonations 0021, 0022, 1021, 1022 . . . 9021, 9022, etc., for 10 "noncontrastive pairs." In the third round, the recording of each sentence was made twice, again with the intonation type (1) used in the first round of recording for that sentence. Thus, intonations 0131, 0132, 1131, 1132 . . . 9131, 9132, etc., were obtained for another set of 10 noncontrastive pairs. The complete list of samples of intonation obtained in this manner is also presented in Table 1.

Since any pairs of these samples of intonation which have the same digit in the first and second identifying position are intended to be all noncontrastive, 60 noncontrastive pairs should have been obtained from this recording. Any pairs of samples which have the same digit in the first position but a different digit in the second position were recorded to be samples of con-

Table 1. List of sentences used to produce samples of intonation, and list of 60 sample intonations produced by the speaker to obtain 110 pairs of contrastive and noncontrastive intonation

			Round of recording (3rd digit)	1		2		3	
			Order of recording (4th digit)	1	2	1	2	1	2
Type of intonation (2nd digit)									
Sentence (1st digit)									
My name is Bill.	0	0		0011		0021	0022		
		1		0112				0131	0132
I've been here five minutes.	1	0		1011		1021	1022		
		1		1112				1131	1132
Do you want coffee or milk?	2	0		2011		2021	2022		
		1		2112				2131	2132
You don't eat that.	3	0		3011		3021	3022		
		1		3112				3131	3132
I want to go home.	4	0		4011		4021	4022		
		1		4112				4131	4132
You'd better do it.	5	0		5011		5021	5022		
		1		5112				5131	5132
I won't tell.	6	0		6011		6021	6022		
		1		6112				6131	6132
That's all.	7	0		7011		7021	7022		
		1		7112				7131	7132
I never heard it before.	8	0		8011		8021	8022		
		1		8112				8131	8132
That's okay.	9	0		9011		9021	9022		
		1		9112				9131	9132

SENTENCE

INTONATION

trastive intonations. Thus, 50 pairs of contrastive pairs should have been obtained. Actually, however, when all 110 pairs of intonations were presented to a panel of listeners, it was found that the speaker failed in producing the intended intonations in more than a few cases. There were 39 pairs which were judged the "same" or noncontrastive by the listeners and 71 pairs which were judged "different" or contrastive.

2. Extraction of Physical Correlates

Physical correlates of speech sounds are generally said to be the following: intensity, duration, fundamental frequency, and spectrum structure. In this study, all correlates except the spectrum structure were extracted as possibly relevant physical signals of American intonation. The recorded samples of intonation were played back on an FM tape recorder, and its output was fed into an analog-to-digital converter for digitizing the continuous waveforms of the utterances. Once the voltage variations of the waveforms are obtained in digital values from the analog-to-digital converter, the intensity level can be computed by using the following formula:

$$dB = 20 \log_{10} \frac{E_2}{E_1}$$

where E represents the peak voltage on the waveform.

Computation of the duration of the signal is even easier. Since the rate of computing the intensity level (25/sec) is predetermined and known, the duration of the signal can be obtained simply by counting the number of intensity levels which exceeded the criterion value and by dividing it by 25.

Extraction of the fundamental frequency is not as easy as the measurement of overall intensity variation or the duration of the signal. Many different attempts were made by researchers to develop a pitch extraction program, and such techniques as "autocorrelation" or "cepstrum" were among the popular ones reported in professional journals. However, in this study, a modified autocorrelation technique was used to extract the fundamental frequency. This program, developed at the phonetics laboratory of the Ohio State University, was found to be relatively fast and still extremely accurate in its function. The detection of periodicity in the waveforms is made in this program by computing the coefficients of correlation between the two consecutive spans of data sets. The computation of correlation is started with each span of data slightly shorter than one wavelength and continued with successively expanded spans of data. The highest coefficient can be obtained when the two spans of data picked to compute the correlation match the two consecutive wavelengths. Then, since the rate of sampling by the analog-to-digital converter is known (5 kHz), the period of wave motion can be detected by comparing the sampling rate and the number of sampled data in the span which produced the highest coefficient. The economy of computing time was increased by setting an appropriate upper and lower limit for the range of scanning for the periodicity. The accuracy was assured by checking the detected frequency with the difference in the frequencies of first and second harmonics, second and third harmonics, etc., before the result of computation was finally accepted.

3. Relative Efficiencies of the Extracted Physical Correlates

The relative efficiencies of the extracted physical parameters as intonational signals were examined by computing the "index of signal detectability" for each parameter. The index (d') can be computed by the following formula (Swets, 1964):

$$d' = \frac{M_s - M_n}{\sigma_n}$$

where M_s is the mean of the magnitudes of the parameter in the signal; M_n is the mean of the magnitudes of the parameter in noise; and σ_n is the variance of the magnitudes of the parameter in noise.

This index essentially tells the following relationship between the signal and the parameter. If the physical correlate or parameter being tested is efficient as a signal, then the magnitudes of the parameter are greater in the signal (M_s), the magnitudes are smaller in the noise (M_n), and a high value of index will be obtained. On the other hand, if the magnitudes are random among the signal and the noise, then a lower value of index will be obtained. In order to use this formula in the present study, the parameter of the signal was defined as any difference found in contrastive pairs of intonation, and the parameter of the noise was defined as any difference found in noncontrastive pairs of intonation.

Table 2. Indexes of signal detectability computed for each of the three physical parameters as intonational signals

Physical correlate	Psychological sensation	Index of signal detectability
Frequency variation (Hz)	Overall pitch pattern	1.8
Intensity variation (dB)	Overall loudness pattern	1.0
Duration of signal (msec)	Length of signal	0.8

The measure of difference in duration was made by directly comparing the numbers of measured data. However, for the intensity and the fundamental frequency, similarity or dissimilarity of overall patterns of variation was measured by computing coefficients of correlation between the respective parameters in the paired intonations. When all the indexes of signal detectability were computed, fundamental frequency variation was found to be the most efficient physical correlate as an intonational signal. Intensity variation was the next, and duration was the least efficient. The summary of the indexes of the signal detectability for the three parameters is presented in Table 2.

4. Relative Efficiencies of Certain Characteristics of Frequency Variations

Since the pattern of frequency variation was the most efficient physical correlate among the three parameters tested in part 3 of the experiment, the relative efficiencies of some other characteristics of this parameter were examined. First, the mean and the standard deviation of the values of frequency variation were computed for each sample of intonation. They are assumed to be the physical parameters which elicit the listener's psychological sensation of the pitch level and the pitch range, respectively. Then the average difference in two consecutive values of fundamental frequency (upward and downward change separately) was computed. The average difference in two consecutive values is assumed to be the main physical correlate for the listeners' psychological sensation of the rate of pitch change. The relative efficiencies of these characteristics as intonational signals were examined by the same procedure used in part 3 of this experiment, i.e., by comparing the mean magnitudes of difference between the pairs of contrastive intonations and the pairs of noncontrastive intonations. The results of computing the indexes of signal detectability for the three additional characteristics of frequency variation are summarized in Table 3. Apparently, these characteristics are not significant as intonational signals.

Table 3. Indexes of signal detectability computed for each of the three characteristics of frequency variation as intonational signals

Characteristics of frequency variation	Psychological sensation	Index of signal detectability
Mean	Pitch level	0.5
Standard deviation	Pitch range	0.4
Rate of frequency change	Rate of pitch change	0.6

5. Normalization of Frequency Variation

In the study of speech signals, it is always important to delete the individual differences in the produced signal, in other words, to normalize the physical parameters. In the study of intonation, the normalization of the data (pattern of frequency variation) in terms of the range and duration seems to be necessary. This is obvious if we consider the results of the experiment in part 4 of this study, and also the following two facts: 1) men and women, or adults and children have different pitch levels and ranges, but they have about the same set of intonations and can communicate with each other, and 2) there are many fast talkers and slow talkers and they also have the same set of intonations.

Range normalization and time normalization can be easily done by a computer. For example, any set of data can be converted to a set of data ranging from 0 to 1 by using the following formula:

$$\text{Normalized data}_n = \frac{\text{Raw data}_n - \text{minimum}}{\text{maximum} - \text{minimum}}$$

Then, by multiplying a constant to the right of the formula, the range can be further modified to any desirable one (0–10, 0–100, etc.).

In this study, maximum and minimum were determined by measuring the highest and the lowest values of fundamental frequency registered in the speaker's entire 60 utterances, instead of the highest and the lowest values in each utterance. This method of determining maximum and minimum for normalization is advantageous, in the sense that a speaker's intentional use of different pitch level or range for a particular intonation is retained after normalization.

Time normalization can be accomplished by using the same formula to stretch out or compress the sampled data. However, if it is desired to obtain the same number of data after normalization, it can be done by the following method. First, fundamental frequencies between the consecutively sampled values are assumed to change linearly from one value to another. Then, any number of values needed can be read from the ordered set of straight lines connecting the sampled values. In this study, the range and the time were first normalized to 0–100 units.

6. Transformation of Frequency Variation

It is often said that the physical analysis of frequency variation is too detailed and that a listener's perception of pitch may not match the exact instrumental analysis of the variation of fundamental frequency. In order to test the validity of this statement several methods of transforming the data of frequency variation were attempted. They were: 1) conversion of frequency scale (Hz) to musical scale (tone), 2) reduction of the number of distinctive units on the frequency range, and 3) reduction of the sampling rate on the time scale.

The first transformation was accomplished by using the following formula (Fairbanks, 1966):

$$N \text{ tones} = 19.92 \log_{10} \frac{f_n}{f_0}$$

where f_0 is the criterion frequency and f_n is the fundamental frequency to be converted. No significant change in the signal detectability was found after this transformation.

Reduction of the number of units on the frequency range was made by dividing all normalized frequency values by an increasingly larger number (2, 3, 4, etc.), each time computing the index of signal detectability. The number of distinctive units becomes smaller as the frequency values are divided by a larger number, because the values below the decimal point are automatically discarded when an integer mode of computation is used. The index of signal detectability never went higher than when all 100 distinctive units were used, but the index did not decrease (efficiency was not reduced) by gradually decreasing the number of distinctive units until it became only 4 units.

Reduction of the sampling rate on the time scale was made by sampling the values of normalized frequency variation at increasingly lower rate. First, the data were sampled at every other value of 100 normalized values, then every second value, every third value, and so on. Again, the index never increased by reducing the number of values on the time scale. It decreased after the number of sampled values became 25 for an utterance.

The fourth method of transforming the frequency variation was made by fitting linear regression lines to the variation of the fundamental frequency. First, only one line was fitted to the entire curve of frequency variation, then two lines (one line for the first half of the curve and the other for the second half), three lines (one line for the initial one third of the curve, one line for the middle portion, and then another line for the last one third of the curve), and so on. The formula used to fit regression lines was (Ostle, 1963):

$$\hat{y} = b_0 + b_1 x,$$

where b_1 and b_0 are given by the following formula:

$$b_1 = \frac{\Sigma xy - (\Sigma x)(\Sigma y)/n}{\Sigma y^2 - (\Sigma x)^2/n}$$

$$b_0 = \bar{y} - b_1 \bar{x}$$

The transformed frequency variation by one linear regression line was understandably very low in efficiency. The efficiency was increased as the number of fitted regression lines increased to five. The efficiency went down gradually after the number of lines exceeded eight for each intonation. The pitch patterns obtained by fitting five, six, seven, or eight regression lines to the original pattern of normalized frequency variation were all slightly more efficient as intonational signals (higher indexes of signal detectability were obtained) than the original pattern.

7. Information Points in Intonation

Up to this part of the experiment, all the searches for the physical parameter or characteristics of intonation have been done with an implicit assumption that the significant intonational signal is evenly distributed along the entire span of the utterance. In this part of the experiment, the validity of this assumption was tested by comparing the frequency variations after deleting the first one third (head), the middle one third (body), and the final one third (tail) of the frequency variation, respectively. The magnitudes of difference between the partial frequency variations of the contrastive pairs of intonation and those of the noncontrastive pairs of intonation were used to compute the index of signal detectability. When the index was computed, it was found that the assumption of even distribution was false. The frequency variation in the tail portion was found to be the most important intonational signal. The head portion was the second and the middle portion was least efficient as an intonational signal.

8. Feature Extraction

From the result of part 7 of the experiment, it became obvious that simple statistical processing of physical parameters along the entire span of utterances does not work for the purpose of analyzing intonational signals. The next step to be tested was feature extraction, a more sophisticated processing of data in analyzing signals. In this part of the experiment, the results obtained in the preceding parts of the experiment were all used very effectively to determine how to extract the features. For example, from the results of the studies in parts 2 and 3, it was learned that the pattern of frequency variation should be the main physical parameter to be analyzed for the search of features. From part 6 of the study, it was learned that the range of pitch variation can be as small as 4 distinctive units. Also from part 6, it was learned that two or three segments are needed if a complex pitch pattern is considered for each segment. In addition, the fitting of linear regression lines to the curve of frequency variation was found very effective in the description and recognition of intonation patterns.

The first additional study concerned how to segment the utterances into two or three segments. For this purpose, four different methods were considered.

1. Division of the entire curve of frequency variation into two or three segments of equal duration
2. Segmentation of the utterance according to the word or phrase boundary (referring to the sound spectrogram of the utterance)
3. Use of pitch shifts (unvoiced portion of the utterance) as the boundary
4. Use of the intensity levels extracted in part 2 of the study as the reference for division

The first three methods did not work efficiently. The fourth method not only was convenient to use with the computer but also was found very effective in defining simple pitch patterns. After comparing all the pauses (low intensity levels) found in the utterance, two or three longest ones (one, if there is only one) were used to determine the limit of segments.

The patterns of normalized frequency variations segmented into shorter durations by this method were considerably simpler, and a combination of two or three straight lines could be easily fitted to each segment with little distortion of the original patterns. One advantage to using a linear regression analysis to describe pitch patterns is that the patterns of frequency variation could be represented by one number (the slope of a linear equation) per line. The frequency distribution of the slopes of all regression lines fitted to the segmented sections of normalized frequency variation is presented in Table 4. Then, by setting a number of appropriate criteria (1.1, 0.3, and −0.3) for classifying the values of the slopes, all the linear patterns could be classified either "fast rising" (+↗), "rising" (↗), "level" (→), or "falling" (↘). These linear patterns were tentatively termed as the fundamental pattern features.

The combination of two or three (depending upon the duration of the segment) fundamental pattern features read from each segment of the utterance was then called a pitch pattern. The intonation pattern of each utterance was in turn defined as a combination of pitch patterns. The structure of the intonation pattern is graphically represented in Figure 1.

Since pitch patterns are defined as the combination of two or three of the four possible fundamental pattern features, 80 different pitch patterns were to be expected. The 80 possible pitch patterns are presented in Table 5. In this preliminary study, the speaker used only 75% of the total 80 possible patterns.

9. Test of the Analysis Procedures

The best test for the validity and reliability of the procedure developed to analyze any speech sounds is to use the procedure and try to recognize the linguistic or other signal from natural speech samples. As recognition of a linguistic signal is fundamentally the identification of two speech samples which are linguistically noncontrastive as the "same," and the identification

Table 4. Frequency distribution of slopes of all regression lines fitted to the segmented sections of normalized frequency variation[a]

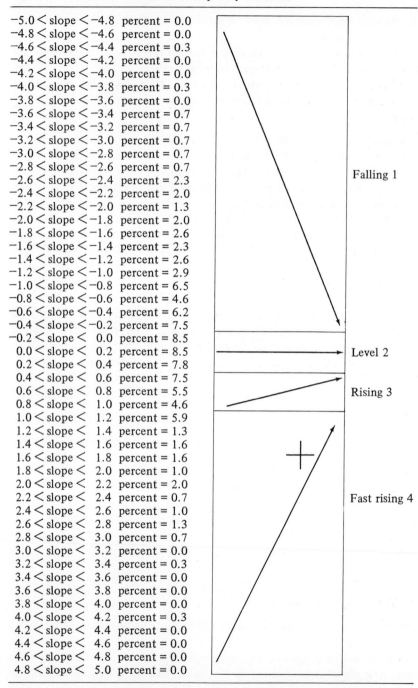

−5.0 < slope < −4.8	percent = 0.0	
−4.8 < slope < −4.6	percent = 0.0	
−4.6 < slope < −4.4	percent = 0.3	
−4.4 < slope < −4.2	percent = 0.0	
−4.2 < slope < −4.0	percent = 0.0	
−4.0 < slope < −3.8	percent = 0.3	
−3.8 < slope < −3.6	percent = 0.0	
−3.6 < slope < −3.4	percent = 0.7	
−3.4 < slope < −3.2	percent = 0.7	
−3.2 < slope < −3.0	percent = 0.7	
−3.0 < slope < −2.8	percent = 0.7	
−2.8 < slope < −2.6	percent = 0.7	Falling 1
−2.6 < slope < −2.4	percent = 2.3	
−2.4 < slope < −2.2	percent = 2.0	
−2.2 < slope < −2.0	percent = 1.3	
−2.0 < slope < −1.8	percent = 2.0	
−1.8 < slope < −1.6	percent = 2.6	
−1.6 < slope < −1.4	percent = 2.3	
−1.4 < slope < −1.2	percent = 2.6	
−1.2 < slope < −1.0	percent = 2.9	
−1.0 < slope < −0.8	percent = 6.5	
−0.8 < slope < −0.6	percent = 4.6	
−0.6 < slope < −0.4	percent = 6.2	
−0.4 < slope < −0.2	percent = 7.5	
−0.2 < slope < 0.0	percent = 8.5	
0.0 < slope < 0.2	percent = 8.5	Level 2
0.2 < slope < 0.4	percent = 7.8	
0.4 < slope < 0.6	percent = 7.5	
0.6 < slope < 0.8	percent = 5.5	Rising 3
0.8 < slope < 1.0	percent = 4.6	
1.0 < slope < 1.2	percent = 5.9	
1.2 < slope < 1.4	percent = 1.3	
1.4 < slope < 1.6	percent = 1.6	
1.6 < slope < 1.8	percent = 1.6	
1.8 < slope < 2.0	percent = 1.0	
2.0 < slope < 2.2	percent = 2.0	
2.2 < slope < 2.4	percent = 0.7	Fast rising 4
2.4 < slope < 2.6	percent = 1.0	
2.6 < slope < 2.8	percent = 1.3	
2.8 < slope < 3.0	percent = 0.7	
3.0 < slope < 3.2	percent = 0.0	
3.2 < slope < 3.4	percent = 0.3	
3.4 < slope < 3.6	percent = 0.0	
3.6 < slope < 3.8	percent = 0.0	
3.8 < slope < 4.0	percent = 0.0	
4.0 < slope < 4.2	percent = 0.3	
4.2 < slope < 4.4	percent = 0.0	
4.4 < slope < 4.6	percent = 0.0	
4.6 < slope < 4.8	percent = 0.0	
4.8 < slope < 5.0	percent = 0.0	

[a]The linear patterns having the slopes ranging from −4.6 to 4.2 are classified into four fundamental pattern features: falling 1, level 2, rising 3, and fast rising 4.

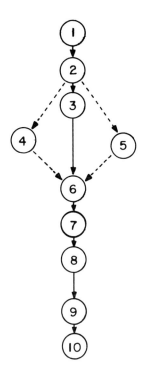

1. Recording of an utterance

2. A - D conversion

3. Extraction of F_O

4. Measurement of intensity

5. Measurement of duration

6. Normalization of frequency variation

7. Segmentation

8. Transformation

    (Extraction of pattern features and pitch patterns)

9. Detection of peak segment

10. Identification of intonation patterns.

Figure 1. A schematic representation of the process of simulating the perception of intonational signals.

Table 5. Pitch patterns defined as combinations of 2 or 3 of 4 fundamental pattern features

Fundamental pattern features	All possible pitch patterns			
1	11	111	211	311	411
	12	112	212	312	412
2	13	113	213	313	413
	14	114	214	314	414
3	21	121	221	321	421
	22	122	222	322	422
4	23	123	223	323	423
	24	124	224	324	424
	31	131	231	331	431
	32	132	232	332	432
	33	133	233	333	433
	34	134	234	334	434
	41	141	241	341	441
	42	142	242	342	442
	43	143	243	343	443
	44	144	244	344	444

Table 6. Cardinal and cognate pitch patterns in American intonation for the identification of the cardinal pitch patterns in the segment in which the frequency variation reaches the peak

Cardinal patterns	Cognate patterns						
Fast rising: 21	1	2	4	41	43	44	111
	211	212	311	312	411	412	
Rising: 31	3	24	31	32	33	34	141
	241	243	343	344			
Delayed rising: 23	13	121	123	131	223	231	233
	322	331	333				

of two speech samples which are linguistically contrastive as "different," the 110 original pairs of contrastive and noncontrastive pairs were used for the test.

It was found that the contrastive pairs of intonation did not always contain different pitch patterns, or intonation patterns, in the paired utterances. Furthermore, the noncontrastive pairs did not always contain the same pitch patterns. In order to solve these problems, the following two rules were added. First, the position of the highest frequency value in the entire span of the utterance is critically important, and if the highest frequency value is in different segments of the utterances, then the intonations are contrastive, even if the pitch patterns are the same. Second, the 80 pitch patterns mechanically obtained by reading the slopes of two or three regression lines fitted to the frequency variations in a segment have to be reorganized, so that

Table 7. Cardinal and cognate pitch patterns in American intonation for the identification of cardinal pitch patterns in the final segment of the utterance

Cardinal patterns	Cognate patterns					
Falling						
Type 1: 11	1	11	21	111	121	211
	221	311	411	421		
Type 2: 31	21	31	121	131	221	231
	341	421	431			
Level						
Type 1: 22	2	22	122	222		
Type 2: 12	12	212				
Rising						
Type 1: 34	24	34	134			
Type 2: 23	3	13	23	123		

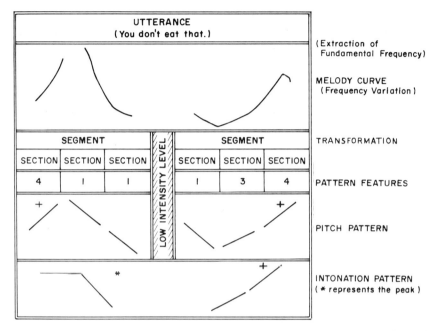

Figure 2. The structure of the intonation pattern defined on the basis of pitch patterns and fundamental pattern features.

some of them are "cardinal patterns" and others are "cognate" of the cardinal patterns. Furthermore, in deciding the cardinal and cognate patterns, it was found that a different set of rules had to be used for the segment where the normalized frequency variation reaches the highest frequency values in the utterance and for the final segment of the utterance. The cardinal patterns and the cognate patterns for both of these segments are presented in Tables 6 and 7.

After the adjustment in the identification of pitch patterns, the entire set of procedures was tested again by letting the computer separate the contrastive and noncontrastive pairs of intonation automatically. The result was very promising. There were only 39 noncontrastive pairs of intonation and 71 contrastive pairs tested in total. However, the computer could decide correctly in all cases whether the pair was contrastive or noncontrastive. The process of simulating the perception of intonational signals used in this study is schematically presented in Figure 2.

SUMMARY

Computer methods were described for extracting physical parameters, comparing the relative efficiency of the parameters as intonational signals, processing the extracted data, and extracting and identifying pitch patterns. Fundamental pattern features and cardinal pitch patterns were defined and proposed as constituents of intonation patterns. The result of using these methods in objective description of intonation patterns or automatic detection of intonational signals was very promising.

Since only one speaker supplied the samples of intonation in this study, the study reported here is only preliminary. However, various ways of normalizing or transforming the frequency variation have been incorporated to cancel out the possible individual difference, and this investigator hopes that a similar technique, possibly with slight modifications, will be used advantageously for more comprehensive and general study of American intonation. If the procedures used here are found valid for more varied inputs of speech samples, these algorithms may be used advantageously for designing a teaching aid for students of a second language or for persons with hearing loss; the computer programs may also be a useful tool for a linguistic research in the laboratories of experimental phonetics.

REFERENCES

Chomsky, N., and M. Halle. 1968. The Sound Pattern of English. Harper and Row, New York. p. 329.

Crystal, D. 1969. Prosodic Systems and Intonation in English. University Press, Cambridge. pp. 1 and 2.

Fairbanks, G. 1966. Experimental Phonetics. Selected Articles. University of Illinois Press, Urbana. p. 274.

Hadding-Koch, K. 1961. Acoustic-Phonetic Studies in the Intonation of Southern Swedish. Gleerup, Lund, Sweden. p. 7.

Lehiste, I. 1970. Suprasegmentals. MIT Press, Cambridge, Mass. p. 1.

Minifie, F. D. 1973. Normal Aspects of Speech, Hearing and Language. Prentice-Hall, Englewood Cliffs, N.J. p. 281.

Ostle, B. 1963. Statistics in Research. Iowa State University Press, Ames. p. 585.

Schubiger, M. 1958. English Intonation, Its Form and Function. Max Meimeyer Verlag, Tübingen, W. Germany. p. 1.

Swets, J. A. 1964. Signal Detection and Recognition by Human Observers. Contemporary Readings. John Wiley & Sons, New York. p. 702.

Measurements and Analysis of Visible Speech

Joseph G. Agnello, Ph.D.
Professor of Speech and Hearing Sciences
University of Cincinnati

CONTENTS

INTRODUCTION

Black's (1973) introductory essay in the reprint of Scripture's *The Elements of Experimental Phonetics*, first published in 1902, succinctly traces the origin of the term experimental phonetics. Both the origin and development of experimental phonetics are unavoidably related to the theory of measurement. Instrumental measurements have contributed decisively to the advancement of experimental phonetics. Most of these advancements have been in the form of assessing the subjective impressions of past phoneticians and linguists. Some of these subjective reports on phonetic events can be best appreciated through Ladefoged's (1972) historical viewpoints on the origin of the description and classification of the vowels. It is amazing that many students and teachers of phonetics still advocate that there is a reality about the "articulatory cardinal vowel diagram" when, in fact, these imaginary tongue positions may have little if anything to do with the acoustic and perceptual data. If one fixes his tongue in a relatively stable position and whispers each vowel, an approximation of the vowel's qualities can be realized. Ladefoged's (1972) specification of a cardinal vowel follows the classical psychometric procedure of instructing a trained observer to adhere to a specific criterion of the physical event under scrutiny. There is obvious merit in depending on the ear to make the final perceptual judgment of speech because there is no more sensitive analyzer of speech than the ear

379

itself. The human perceptual system evolved in order to achieve just that. Helmholtz (1887) and Smith (1947), depending solely on their aural abilities, estimated with a great deal of accuracy the formant (resonance) values of vowels of their own language.

The usual ambiguity found in research data pertaining to the relationships of articulatory, acoustic, and perceptual events of speech generally can be traced to two main sources: to speaker variance/listener variance, such as dialect, rate, stress, and other prosodic parameters; and to instrumental variance, such as task of the subjects, instruction to subjects, psychometric method, limitation of the measuring device, and method of scaling data that does not represent the dimension of the sensory modality. Measuring and assessing definite features of speech that significantly relate perception to acoustics is quite difficult. Perception of speech is a pattern recognition problem. Pattern recognition entails a complex research paradigm to relate the physical pattern to the psychological reality. The psychological reality is more than likely another way of specifying an individual's personal "grammar." The best research method for relating the acoustic signal to perception is in the manner of speech analysis by synthesis. The analysis is ambiguous if the analytic data of the measuring or synthesis device cannot portray the physical pattern with some proximity to the psychological reality.

In experimental phonetics research, it is not only the design that must adhere to "good" scientific methodology, but a great deal of attention must be addressed to the analytic system employed for data reduction or stimulus presentation. This may seem to be an obvious statement of fact. However, experimental phonetics is one of the few scientific disciplines that treats an aspect of language—speech—as both a stimulus and a response. The analytic systems used in speech perception or production studies attempt to define the parameters that contribute to production, perception, or both. The acoustic speech signal, once it is recorded, becomes the stimulus. While it was being recorded by a speaker it was the response. The problem is further complicated when language (or speech, or a "perceptual judgment") is employed to assess or create a dimension on some cognitive scale to express the parameter.

A speech synthesis device can be used as a highly sophisticated informant. Thus, an experimenter can create his own speech stimuli. In essence, if the experimenter has access to enough control parameters on the synthesizer, he can create a complex acoustic signal of his own choice. However, he must do all this by assumptions based on his own hearing impressions or by using a panel of competent phoneticians. There is yet to be developed a test to assess a listener's proficiency in judging speech quality. In teaching phonetics, it is apparent that every listener has his own linguistic bias. Training a listener to be free of his linguistic bias is no simple feat.

Alexander John Willis was the first acoustic phonetician. Willis (1829) concluded that each vowel had a unique pitch with its own resonance tone. He arrived at this conclusion by conducting what may have been the first analysis-by-synthesis experiment. Willis vibrated a reed at one end of a tube and was able to generate different vowel-like sounds.

The approach to speech as a pattern recognition problem was probably first advocated by A. M. Bell (1900) through his phonetic notation system, which he so appropriately designated "visible speech." A chapter in Bell's book suggests a "cure" for stammering. It is noteworthy that he advocated a good voice with proper control of the articulators. Based on this approach, a speech comparator to facilitate "fluency" is presented in another section of this chapter. This author has hypothesized that stuttering is a disorder of phonological transition (Agnello, 1971). Experimental phonetics provides data pertaining to an understanding of the normal speech process. This understanding eventually should lead to a more effective approach in treating deviant speech. Stuttering is essentially a timing disorder. Knowledge of the crucial timing features of specific articulatory events is essential for developing adequate techniques in the management of the disorder of stuttering.

Ellis (1954), who translated Helmholtz's vowel theory in *Sensation of Tones,* also praised A. M. Bell's visible speech notation system of 1900:

> I think, then, that Mr. Bell is justified in the somewhat bold title which he has assumed for his mode of writing—"Visible Speech". I only hope that, for the advantage of linguists, such an alphabet may be soon made accessible, and that, for the intercourse of nations, it may be adopted generally . . . Mr. Melville Bell and his sons have now been kind enough to devote several hours to explaining to me thoroughly the whole phonetic theory and plan of symbolization and to read the exhibit on paper before me examples of its use, sufficiently numerous to enable me to form a complete judgment of its powers and merits . . . My impressions in favor of Mr. Bell's scheme are so strong, that it is necessary for me to guard against any suspicion of being biased in giving them expression.

In 1879, the son of A. M. Bell, A. G. Bell, who personally taught Ellis to use his father's visible speech system, reported some resonance values for the vowels his father designated "cardinal vowels." Bell Laboratories (Crandall, 1925; Fletcher, 1929) began advocating the unique resonance patterns of each vowel. These early attempts are important to current thinking on the relationship between the acoustic events of speech and the perceptual qualities of speech.

The interdisciplinary elements of experimental phonetics can be best appreciated through the logical sequence of events from speaker to acoustic media (via articulatory processes) and from acoustic media to listener (via perceptual features of vowel quality, cognition, and psychological states). When the speaker acts as his own listener there are numerous feedback loops that can be inferred (Fairbanks, 1954), as illustrated in the diagram below.

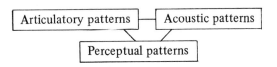

SOUND SPECTROGRAPH ANALYZER

It is impossible to discuss all of the approaches to measurement that have been developed through experimental phonetics. The sound spectrograph analyzer is discussed here because it is without doubt the instrument that has had the most influence on our understanding of the productive, acoustic, and perceptual aspects of speech.

Before 1940, many attempts, notably at Bell Laboratories, were devoted to the development of electronic systems that would visually transmit the complexity in the acoustic speech pattern. These systems were designed to display, graphically, multidimensional events, still in the tradition of Bell's "visible speech." However, most of these systems were time consuming, and their final outputs were inadequate visual representations of the complex speech signal. The early efforts to produce visible patterns of the acoustic waves of speech were dependent on numerous filters connected in parallel. However, many filters were needed in order to codify recognizable patterns of complex, visible speech signals. When the tuned circuit was conceived, it permitted a fairly efficient method for reconstructing the acoustic signal into a patterned visual display. The sound spectrographic analyzer is based on the tuned principle. It was developed just before World War II. It was not available for research until 1946 (Koenig, Dunn, and Lacy, 1946). The system was classified because of its potential in military usage.

Shown in Figure 1 is a schematic diagram of the essential components of one operation of the Kay Elemetrics (Pine Brook, N.J.) spectrographic

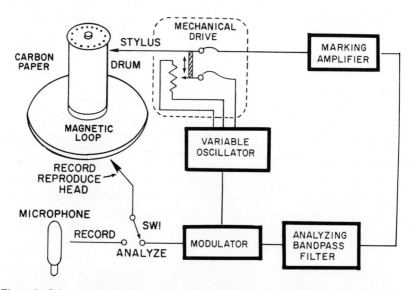

Figure 1. Schematic illustration of the sound spectrographic analyzer. (After Flanagan, 1972.)

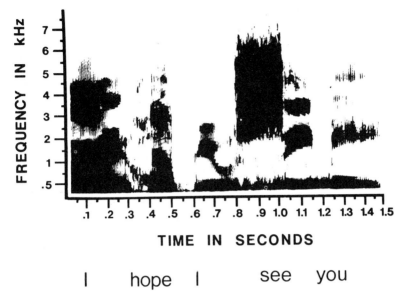

Figure 2. Typical wide-band spectrogram from the sound spectrographic analyzer.

analyzer. When the record switch is on, the speech signal from the microphone is recorded onto the magnetic loop. When the record switch is turned to reproduce, the signal is captured on the magnetic loop. An analysis of the speech sample is obtained by repeatedly passing the recorded sample through a series of fixed band-pass filters. Electronically, it is more convenient to use a fixed band-pass filter and gradually to pass the spectrum of the speech signal past the analyzing filter. This is accomplished by modulating a high frequency carrier with the speech signal past the fixed band-pass filters. By systematically varying the frequency of the carrier signal, the necessary conversion of the real frequency components are realized. The carrier frequency output is mechanically controlled by the magnetic loop. Consequently, the speech spectrum is systematically analyzed after a great number of repeated revolutions of the magnetic loop. The output voltage from the band-pass filter creates a varying spark on the stylus. This in turn burns an electrosensitive (carbon) paper set around the drum. The carbon on the paper is burned (darkened) in direct relationship to the magnitude of the electrical current. The amount of darkness (burning off of the carbon) approximates the logarithm of the current magnitude. The final graphic display is designated a spectrogram (Figure 2).

Typically, for speech, such spectrograms are usually specified as wide-band spectrograms; that is, a 300-Hz filter as opposed to narrow-band filter of 45 Hz. There are other types of output graphic dipslays that can be made with the sound spectrograph (Fant, 1968).

One of the early problems with the advent of the spectrographic analyzer was to instrumentally select filter bandwidths that would generate patterns that were assumed to be readable. It was believed that the visible pattern had to depict the impression of smooth continuity that the hearing modality received. Actually, before 1946, there were no data, nor are there any at present, that justify converting acoustic speech signals into visual symbols for readability. Possibly, it might be more advantageous to convert the acoustic signal into a display similar to that which occurs (traveling wave) on the basilar membrane. The most important relationship between the auditory modality and the visual modality is the temporal relationship. We are dealing with two multisensory modalities that, each in its own way, convert dimensions into meaningful cues. The weakness of the spectrographic analyzer is that the spectrograms display too much information for the visual modality. This became apparent in the early attempts to teach visible speech to the deaf. A more recent effort to overcome this problem is a system developed by Robson (1969) called "prosdynic print." The English alphabet was structured to instruct readers to speak in a specific prosodic manner.

The grammar of the visual language (printed script) is totally different from the grammar of the spoken language. This is evidenced by the lack of subvocalization noted among literate Japanese children whose written language contains, for the most part, no phonetic cues. This is in contrast to English, for example, where some children experience a reduced silent reading rate attributable to subvocalization.

The spectrographic analysis of speech has given us a tremendous wealth of data about the acoustic cues of speech and how these acoustic cues serve in the perception of speech, but to date it has failed as a "reading aid."

MEASUREMENT OF VOWEL FORMANTS THROUGH SPECTROGRAPHIC ANALYSIS

The inherent problems in measuring formant (F) values specific to cardinal vowels are best explained by Ladefoged (1972). It is absolutely necessary for anyone seriously interested in measuring F values to devote a great deal of attention to Ladefoged's cautions and recommendations. There is a great deal of ambiguity in measuring F values for specific vowels. As Lindblom (1962) has noted, some of this ambiguity is inherent in the speech wave and some is caused by the sonagraphic instrument. These sources of error are similar to those noted by Ladefoged. However, Ladefoged's approach is more extensive because of his attempt to relate source of error in formant measurements within the context of experimental methodology. Lindblom noted that:

1. The higher the fundamental frequency (above 175 Hz), the more difficult it is to ascertain F values. Thus, the voices of females and children create

difficulty, partially because of the reaction time of the filters and partially because of the tendency to obscure F_1 values.

2. The more asymmetrical a formant, the further the envelope peak may be from the strongest partial within the formant.

3. In lip narrow vowels only one slope may be noted, the second formant being relatively lower than the first.

4. The first two formants of back vowels are ambiguous because of their proximity to each other.

5. Close back vowels have low level energy in the upper formants.

6. Zeros, i.e., antiresonances, appear as spectral minima. They originate from the glottal signal or a superimposed nasalization. If there is a pole in the vicinity of such a zero, the frequency of the corresponding envelope peak may deviate considerably from that of the pole. Moreover, the existence of a zero may give rise to extra formants, i.e., "spurious" formants which do not belong to the F pattern proper.

Lindblom suggests three procedural steps in measuring F values for vowels.

1. Estimate the approximate location of the pole (frequency peak) by eye (use section-amplitude versus frequency).

2. Verify this pattern by comparing it to a standard section of a vowel of similar quality.

3. Enclose (trace in) the harmonics of the formant to be measured. Employ a transparent template with various section patterns of typical vowels that have been mathematically derived. Standard sections can be obtained by carefully recording various vowels of interest. Read off the frequency scale value for each peak.

Poles and zero values are based on the mathematical and the idealized value of vowels based, in turn, on the vocal tract configuration. The concept of the pole-zero measurement can be understood through Flanagan's description (1972). The application of pole-zero estimations are based on the ratio of the Fourier transform function on one periodic wave form. The transmission of the source signal (laryngeal tone) through the vocal tract creates peaks or maxima space along the frequency scale. These peaks are the formants which are the resonance feature of the vowels. The spacing of these peaks is a function of the vocal tract configuration. The valleys created by lowered peaks of specific harmonics are designated as zeros. When these so-called glottal zeros fall near the first two formants, they can create spurious reading in F_1 and F_2 values.

In essence, this method of employing idealized sections is similar to Ladefoged's (1972) use of Daniel Jones' "cardinal vowels" as an idealized model. Moving idealized template sections (step 3) until they match the formants of the talker is another means of correcting for differences in vocal tract dimensions of different speakers. The frequencies will vary across vowels and speakers, but the general patterns of the obtained sections will be similar.

However, deviation from the idealized sections is not solely attributable to physical differences in vocal tract dimensions across speakers but has been traced to excessive aspirational features, excessive nasalization (causing the nasal cavity to impose its resonance over oral cavity resonance), and distortions caused by laryngeal deviations. Other sources within the vocal tract that can create ambiguity in F measurements are: excessive intraoral air pressure that may in turn create source distortions, excessive muscular tension, and unusual lip postures.

Formant frequencies have been employed to estimate the vowel spectrum (Fant, 1956; Stevens and House, 1961). The relation between the location of the formant frequencies and the overall intensity level of the spectrum is that a lower shift of F_1 will cause the spectrum above F_1 to attenuate at a rate of 12 dB/octave shift. Articulatory constriction can cause a decrease in F_1. This is an extremely important rule of acoustic phonetics because articulatory behavior can mark the acoustic syllable division. Furthermore, the articulatory process (constriction) has a direct influence on the time variable of the formant transitional changes that are the acoustic cues for the consonants.

It should be mentioned that a great deal of research conducted on formant values concentrated on relatively simple utterances of each vowel within a fixed environment. In free running speech it is comparatively easy to perceive the formant movement patterns. The burst, the stop gaps, the formant transition into the vowel targets, the voicing features, and the acuteness and compactness of the higher frequency spectra are all readily recognized. For example, in the sample wide-band spectrogram of the sentence "I hope I see you" (Figure 2), there is no problem identifying the segments associated with each phonetic event. Some phoneticians will argue this point because there are more segments than phonetic units. However, those segments in excess are essentially transition segments. Some of these transitions are crucial for perception; others are the result of coarticulation, essential for ongoing speech. The spectrographer must hear the signal and see the pattern, or he must know the phonetic representation as noted in the sample shown. The ambiguity arises at the juncture boundaries or the transition regions between the open vocalic periods and the transient and/or burst segments. The open vocalic periods allow the productive and perceptual system ample time to ready itself for the variant transient acoustic cues of consonants. Vowels facilitate an ongoing process.

MEASUREMENT OF CONSONANT SPECTRA

The acoustic nature of vowels is that they are generally more steady state than consonants. It is reasonable to describe vowels as a static or steady state phenomena. However, Hollbrook and Fairbanks (1962) reported measurements that illustrate movement of F patterns of diphthongs. For relatively stable vowels (nondiphthongs), assessing F values at any point in time is equally representative of any other point in time. Most consonants are far more dynamic in their spectral changes. Consonantal perceptual features are dependent on transient acoustic cues. These transient acoustic cues escaped measurement from the early phoneticians. Only since the development of the Pattern-playback (Cooper, Liberman, and Borst, 1951) and other speech synthesizers (Borst, 1965; Flanagan, 1972) have researchers been able to determine the rapid spectral changes which affect perceptions of the transient or short consonantal segments, e.g., /p, b, t, d, k, g/. As shown in Figure 3, the Pattern-playback is somewhat the reverse process of the spectrographic analyzer. The experimenter "paints" his own F patterns on special paper, then passes the "painted" spectrogram over a series of photocells whose current activates a bank of resonant circuits that drives a loudspeaker. Figure 4 is an example of a painted spectrogram. The acoustic cues of burst, voice bar, formant, transition, and vowel F pattern are depicted on this stylized spectrogram. The Pattern-playback produces synthesized speech from these acoustic cues and vowel F patterns. Time and intensity as characteristics on these painted wide-band spectrograms are also considered.

There are means other than the Pattern-playback method to synthesize speech in order to control and determine which acoustic cues may facilitate perception. The acoustic cues that serve as a primary influence on the identification of specific consonants have been reported by Cooper, Liberman, and Borst (1951). For the voiceless plosive consonants, the frequency

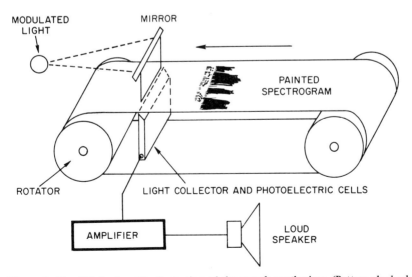

Figure 3. Simplified schematic illustration of the speech synthesizer. (Pattern-playback developed by Haskin Laboratories, New Haven, Conn.)

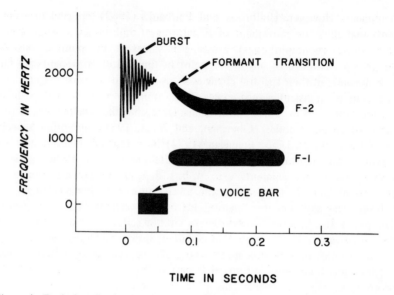

Figure 4. Typical stylized painted spectrogram used in the Pattern-playback system to generate speech-like sounds. Note the second formant downward transition shift into the second formant target of the vowel. These rapid formant transitions, e.g., 500 Hz/50 msec, are one acoustic cue to the perception of certain consonants.

regions of the noise burst seem to be adequate for the distinction of these consonants. The frequency regions for /t/ are well above 3 kHz regardless of the following vowel. The location of the burst is adequate to generate the perception of some plosively released consonants. However, for /p/ and /k/ the perceptibility is not only dependent on the frequency components of the burst (resultant from the articulatory release of built-up air pressure behind the point of closure), but also on the formant transition pattern of the neighboring vowel. If the frequency regions of the burst are in the vicinity of the second formant of the following vowel, the event is perceived as /k/. If the frequency components of the burst appear in the vicinity of F_1 or within any region other than F_2, then the event is perceived as a /p + vowel/ configuration.

Other noted acoustic cues that serve to distinguish the plosive consonants from each other are various formant transition patterns after the stop release that arise from specific frequency regions, e.g., /d/ has a second formant beginning at 1,800 Hz /b/ arising from 720 Hz (Delattre, Liberman, and Cooper, 1955). Liberman et al. (1957) data illustrated that the F_2 transition operated as a perceptual cue for the voiceless /p, t, k/. For example, after the silent interval the frequency region of the burst appeared at the second formant level. The F pattern transition leading into the following vowel formant target takes on numerous potentials. Each transition is crucially dependent on the second formant frequency region of the vowel following the release. Furthermore, the F_2 transition pattern serves to distinguish the voiced /b, d, g/ from /p, t, k/, with added cuing arising from the movement of the F_1 transition plus a secondary cue of the voice bar. Potter, Kopp, and Green (1947) referred to these F_2 transitions as "the hubs." More recently, Delattre et al. (1955) referred to F_2 as the "loci" of consonants.

Processes of acoustic and articulatory features have been reported to contribute to the distinction between the various stops and their respective voiced-voiceless cognates. These have included: 1) voice onset time and voice termination time, 2) formant transition patterns, 3) aspiration and spectra regions, 4) pharyngeal and lingual muscular tension, 5) general force of articulation [fortis-lenis], 6) lengthening, and 7) fundamental frequency of the voice. No single feature can contrast adequately the stop phonemes from the other phonemes. Also, prosodic features impose their influence over the phonemic features. There is considerable effort being made to determine the sets of features that contribute to the perceptual modalities. Furthermore, in neurological phonetics, there are still powerful questions that focus on how the human perceptual system is capable of segmenting and parcelling out these features.

Process of Segmentation

There are discrete and continuous segments observable within spectrograms of speech. Our hearing modality gives us the abstract notion that speech is a series of discrete events (phonemes). However, what we observe on spectrograms are various combinations of transient and continuous events. Discrete segments appear on spectrograms, but they have very little to do with our abstract concept of phonemes. The continuous events can be carefully divided into discrete segments. The segmentation process is the procedure in which the spectrographer first marks off the distinct boundaries that separate specific acoustic events and then attempts to relate those events to an articulatory process. These discrete segments can be readily noted in Figure 2. For example, a trained spectrographer will count a minimum of 15 definite segments within the spectrogram.

These segments can be attributed to various features pertaining to manner and/or place of articulation. Delattre (1951) related various F_1, F_2, and F_3 patterns to various articulatory gestures. Fant (1968) listed 20 acoustic events and related those events (segments) to specific articulation processes. Each acoustic segment is described according to the spectrum pattern of F_1, F_2, F_3, and F_4. Fant (1952) suggested the following procedures in reading spectrograms:

1. Visually determine each discrete segment.
2. Attempt to classify each segment to manner (nasal, plosive, fricative, glide, vowel, continuant).
3. Differentiate silence segments of pause from silent unvoiced gaps (>200 msec) (for plosives) or voiced gaps.

4. Determine minima for fundamental frequency of the voice; measure period between two glottal pulses; apply the formula $1/p = F_0$.)

5. Identify all vowels by parallel F_1 and F_2.

6. Average F_0 of each vowel through step 4.

7. Determine general place of articulation throughout the pattern.

8. Identify vowels and consonants not strongly influenced by coarticulation, e.g., fricatives (see Öhman, 1965).

9. Estimate the number of phonemes.

10. Identify the syllable nuclei (vowel).

11. Look for coarticulation and reduction of consonants.

12. Revise earlier assumptions.

13. Attempt narrow phonetic transcription below each segment.

14. Determine word boundaries.

15. Check each morpheme in a phonetic dictionary; also check against one's own spectrogram files.

16. Apply semantic rules.

A great number of inferences of articulatory behavior can be obtained via spectrograms. A degree of proficiency in reading spectrograms can be obtained by employing the 16-step procedure and applying Fant's (1968) and Delattre's (1951) observations of F patterns. A competence and knowledge of articulatory phonetics is required to read spectrograms.

Voice Onset and Voice Termination Measurements

Investigations by Lisker and Abramson (1964, 1967, 1971) on the voicing feature of sounds revealed that the presence or absence of voicing was *not* the most important cue in distinguishing between voiced and unvoiced stop consonants. Rather, it was the degree of voicing (voice murmur) with regard to the articulatory release. The perception of voicing is initiated (first glottal pulse observed on wide-band spectrograms) with regard to the articulatory release (spike feature or burst feature noted). This measure was designated as voice onset time (VOT) by Lisker et al. (1964).

A modified method of measuring VOT was reported by Agnello (1971) with the development of the Pressure Translator (Agnello, 1973). This instrument made possible the simultaneous portrayal of a wide-band spectrogram of speech and the physiological signal of intraoral air pressure represented on standard spectrographic paper. This system also can be adapted to portray ECG and EMG patterns onto standard spectrograms. The pressure translator (Kay Elemetrics) converted the intraoral air pressure pattern (dc signal) into an acoustic signal. The final output is illustrated in Figure 5. The modified VOT is measured at the point at which intraoral air pressure makes its greatest drop to zero base to the point in time of the first glottal pulse associated with the open vocalic period. This system of simultaneously portraying intraoral air pressure and wide-band spectrograms also made feasi-

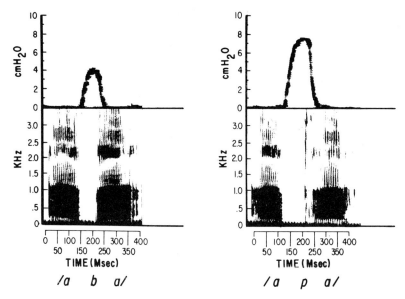

Figure 5. Sample spectrograms with intraoral air pressure simultaneously recorded during the production of /aba/ and /apa/. The Pressure Translator (model 6061A) is an accessory unit to the standard Kay Elemetrics spectrographic analyzer. The translator unit also can be adapted to convert EMG signals directly onto the spectrogram simultaneously with the speech signal.

ble the measurement of voice termination time (vowel + consonant). This is the time lapse from the last glottal pulse to maximal intraoral air pressure, or articulatory closure. This value is designated voice termination time (VTT). Agnello and McGlone (1972) reported that /p/ can be distinguished from /b/ through the temporal measures of VOT when intraoral air pressure release is used as a zero reference. Agnello, Wingate, and Wendell (1974) have reported VOT and VTT time as distinguishing /p/ from /b/ among 5- to 7-year-old children. VOT and VTT are significantly longer for children than for adults.

More recently, Stevens and Klatt (1974) have reported that voiced plosives in English normally have a VOT time of less than 25 msec and that they show significant formant transitions following voice onset. Voiceless plosives in prestressed syllables are characterized by VOT's exceeding 50 msec and the formant transitions are not as marked. Employing synthetic speech, they reported that the role of VOT and the presence or absence of the degree of formant transition following voicing onset are *the* cues for the voiced-voiceless distinction. There is a significant trading relationship between these cues. The presence or absence of rapid F transitions following voice onset produces changes in the magnitude of 15 msec in the location of the perceived phoneme boundary, measured in terms of absolute VOT. One can speculate that the auditory system may be predisposed to detect the presence of a rapid spectral change as a general property of the acoustic signal. The hypothesis that the acquisition of the voiced-voiceless distinction in infants as reported by Eimes (1971) may be conditioned initially by the presence or absence of these features.

VOT and VTT Measurements of Stutterers

Agnello (1971), Agnello and Wingate (1972), Agnello, Wingate, and Wendell (1974) further reported that VOT and VTT differences were noted between stutterers and nonstutterers while speaking fluently the syllables /pa, ap, ba, ab/. The means for VOT and VTT for children are presented in Figure 6. Adult VOT and VTT are shorter in temporal magnitude by approximately 50%. Adult stutterers differed significantly from adult nonstutterers in the VTT measures. Stuttering children differed significantly from nonstuttering children in the VOT measures. The results of these studies suggest that stuttering is a phonetic transition problem.

The previously mentioned VOT and VTT pertained to stutterers who uttered syllables in a fluent manner. Figure 7 is a nonfluent sample of a stuttered syllable. An adult stutterer attempted to produce the syllable /pa/ with the pressure trace shown above the acoustic trace. Note the attempt to drop the pressure (or release the articulatory labial closure). Yet the subject had to check the open vocalic period (silent interval) in an effort to approximate the idealized VOT for the prevocalic /p/. The attempts to drop the pressure (release labial closure) occurred when voicing was initiated too soon, thus generating the syllable /ba/, or during some attempts to initiate glottal activity.

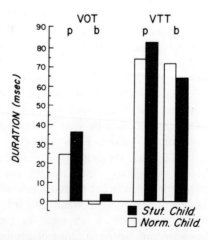

Figure 6. Mean VOT and VTT (in milliseconds) from 11 stutterers (stut.), 5–6 years old, and 11 nonstutterers (norm.), 5–6 years old. Adult VOT and VTT are one half the durational values shown for children.

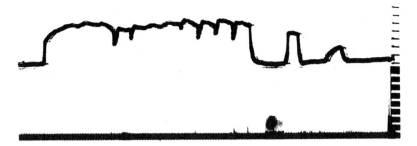

Figure 7. An adult stutterer attempting to produce the syllable three times /pa, pa, pa/. In his first efforts he had difficulty generating the appropriate VOT for /pa/ (15–20 msec). The last two pressure peaks (upper trace) show that he obtained plosive release, but because of extreme vocal tract constriction he had extremely weak harmonic signals.

Physiology of Articulatory Behavior

Lchiste (1967) has noted in her introduction in *Readings in Acoustic Phonetics* that "... we have reached a plateau ... in acoustic phonetics ... there is a renewed interest in articulatory phonetics, with electromyography as the most promising research technique and a resurgence ... in studies of perception when more becomes known of the function of the human brain." It should be mentioned that electromyography as employed by Kozhevnikov and Chistovich (1966) gives new insight to the timing patterns of specific muscle groups. Kozhevnikov and Chistovich make use of the concept of *syntagma*, which they define "... as a sentence or a part of a sentence distinguished by meaning. The syntagma is clearly connected with articulation and must ... be pronounced as one output." Syntagmas are distinguished from each other by pauses. A pause is the same kind of element in an articulatory program as all remaining complexes of articulatory movement accomplished during the extent of the syntagmas. If a pause is given in an utterance, there is no basis to expect that the fluctuations of the duration of the pause between syntagmas, in the case of repeated pronunciations of a phrase, will exceed the variance of the durations of the syntagmas. A pause more than likely reflects a stop in the operation of an automatic mechanism in connection with a change of articulatory programs. In this case, the duration of the pause between syntagmas has greater variance than the duration of the syntagmas themselves (intraphrasal pauses are greater than 200 msec).

The minimally noted pause is 200 msec. This is the length of pause that occurs between phrases (Agnello, 1963, 1974). Any syntagma constitutes a rhythmically organized sequence of movements bounded by pauses, usually exceeding 200 msec. A syntagma constitutes a character of this rhythmical pattern, which is further influenced by the position of the stress within the phrase. With electromyogrophy employed as a reference for specific timing elements of basic muscle groups, it is suggested that the elementary units of articulation may be so defined.

Defining the *basic units* of articulation may lead to an understanding of the speech perception-recognition process. Articulatory data and acoustic data eventually should be applied to speech and hearing disorders. Future research in experimental phonetics will have to examine larger units (syntagma-phrase).

A Comparator System for Stutterers

A speech comparator system was designed by Agnello and Nohr (in preparation) and a second prototype by Xetron Corporation (Cincinnati, Ohio). The comparator is used in speech therapy for stutterers and may have application for teaching speech to hearing-handicapped children. The general operations of the comparator are shown in Figure 8. Specific onset slope values of an envelope and F_1 and F_2 values can be set into the comparator at various selected time slots. At a predetermined time slot, the slope of an input signal is compared to a predetermined slope within the comparator. A logic system signals the speaker as to whether he was low, high, or matched the compara-

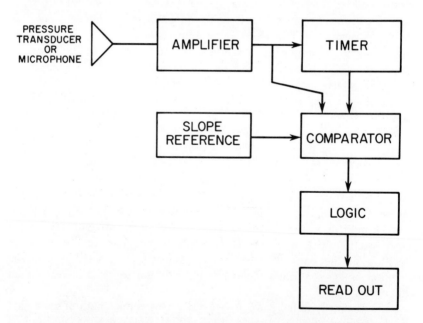

Figure 8. Speech comparator system. Various onset slope values of the leading edge of the envelope of the signal can be compared to an idealized slope value. F_1 and F_2 values of a syllable nuclei can be compared to predetermined F_1 and F_2 value within the comparator. The logic system gives various readout information. A stutterer with a programmed manual can practice easy onset skills.

tor, in his slope signal. A second comparator has two predetermined frequency values for the F pattern within the vowel of the syllable to be matched. These values are within the ranges of F_1 and F_2 of a given idealized vowel. For example, if a stutterer produces the syllable /pa/, he must match a specified onset slope at a selected time slot and F_1 and F_2 values at a preselected time slot within the comparator. A programmed text is used with this unit.

The merit of the system is that it gives a stutterer an idealized speech target to match. Easy onset can be defined by specific slope values. If excessive constriction in the vocal tract of the stutterer is predominant in his effort to produce a syllable, then he will not "hit" the idealized values within the comparator. The system also has automatic timing and amplitude features. These timing features may facilitate a sense of syntagma that is so vital for an ongoing speech. The system is currently being evaluated at the University of Cincinnati.

SUMMARY

A brief review has been given on the history of "visible speech." The concept of visible speech has developed into the current art of measurement in speech spectrography. Measurements (segmental durations and/or spectra) from spectrograms entail a great deal of foreknowledge of articulatory phonetics. The visible speech concept has further advanced the field of experimental phonetics to a procedure of speech analysis by synthesis. The application of a speech synthesizer and/or formant estimations and the application of consonant features are dependent upon the experimental phonetician's ability to establish an idealized model of phonemes as references. Variations (error) in these measurements have been noted to be inherent in the nature of the speech wave, and some error can be attributed to specific limitations of the spectrographic apparatus.

The process of segmentation is a method of parcelling out the spectrogram into discrete patterned events. These segments are measured for their temporal or spectral features. Consequently, the experimenter assigns specific articulatory gestures to these segments. Knowledge of these segments eventually may direct researchers to the processing mechanism of speech perception. Possibly, the central nervous system, with its various comparator mechanisms, is time locked to specific patterns of phrase-like units.

Data from experimental phonetics have led to the development of a computerized speech comparator system. This system is capable of comparing an input speech signal (syllable) to an idealized signal. For example, a stutterer can practice specific articulatory and laryngeal motor control patterns. The acoustic signal (electrical) of these patterns from the speaker are compared to an "idealized" pattern of the syllabic structure within the comparator. Timing features of this system allow for longer strings of utterances to be compared.

ACKNOWLEDGMENTS

The author is appreciative of editorial comments and technical help from Stephanie Bastin, Laura List, Tim Agnello, and especially from his wife, Norma. Of course, his teacher and friend, Professor John W. Black, was so instrumental in instigating it all.

REFERENCES

Agnello, J. G. 1963. A study of pause and its relationship to speech rate. Unpublished doctoral dissertation. Ohio State Unversity, Columbus.
Agnello, J. G. 1971. Transitional features of stutterers and non-stutterers. ASHA 12: (abstr.)
Agnello, J. G. 1973. Apparatus for Simultaneous Recording Speech Spectra and Physiological Data. United States Patent Office. 3: 743, 783.
Agnello, J. G. 1974. Rate and pause, instrumentally measured pause, perceived pause. In S. Duker (ed.), Time-Compressed Speech. Scarecrow Press, Metuchen, N.J.
Agnello, J. G., and R. E. McGlone. 1972. Distinguishing features of /p/ and /b/ from spectrographic intraoral airpressure comparison. J. Acoust. Soc. Amer. 48: 121.
Agnello, J. G., and P. Nohr. A speech comparator. In preparation.
Agnello, J. G., and M. E. Wingate. Transitional aspects of stuttering. In preparation.
Bell, A. M. 1900. Principles of Speech Sounds and Directions for Cure of Stammering. Volta Bureau, Washington, D.C.
Black, J. W. 1973. Introductory comments. In E. W. Scripture, The Elements of Experimental Phonetics. AMS Press, New York.
Borst, J. M. 1965. The use of spectrograms for the analysis and synthesis. J. Audiol. Eng. Soc. 4: 14–23.
Cooper, F. S., P. C. Delattre, A. M. Liberman, J. M. Borst, and L. J. Gerstman. 1952. Some experiments on the perception of synthetic speech sounds. J. Acoust. Soc. Amer. 24: 597–606.
Cooper, F. S., A. M. Liberman, and J. M. Borst. 1951. The interconversion of audible and visible patterns as a basis for research in the perception of speech. Proc. Nat. Acad. Sci. 37: 318–325.
Crandall, I. 1925. The sounds of speech. Bell System Tech. J. 4: 586–626.
Delattre, P. 1951. The physiological interpretation of sound spectrograms. Word 66: 864–875.
Delattre, P. C., A. M. Liberman, and F. S. Cooper. 1955. Acoustic loci and transitional cues for consonants. J. Acoust. Soc. Amer. 27: 769–773.
Eimes, P. D., E. R. Sigueland, P. Jusczyk, and J. Vigorito. 1971. Speech perception in infants. Science 171: 303–306.
Ellis, A. J. (trans.). 1954. In H. Helmholtz, Sensations of Tone. Dover, New York.
Fairbanks, G. 1954. A theory of the speech mechanism as a servosystem. J. Speech Hear. Disord. 19: 133–139.

Fant, C. G. 1956. On the predictability of formant levels and spectrum envelopes from formant frequencies. *In* M. Halle (comp.), For Roman Jakobson, pp. 109–120. Mouton, The Hague.

Fant, G. 1962a. Sound Spectrography. *In* A. Sovijarvi and P. Abato (eds.), Fourth International Congress of Phonetic Sciences, Helsinki. Mouton, The Hague.

Fant, C. G. 1962b. Descriptive analysis of the acoustic aspects of speech. Logas 5: 3–17.

Fant, G. 1968. Analysis and synthesis of speech process. *In* B. Malmberg (ed.), Manual of Phonetics, pp. 173–277. North Holland, Amsterdam.

Flanagan, J. L. 1972. Speech Analysis-Synthesis and Perception. Springer-Verlag, New York. p. 444.

Fletcher, H. 1929. Speech and Hearing. Van Nostrand, New York.

Helmholtz, H. von 1887. On the Sensation of Tone. Translated by A. J. Ellis, 1954. 2nd Ed. Dover, New York.

Hollbrook, A., and G. Fairbanks. 1962. Diphthong formants and their movements. J. Speech Hear. Res. 5: 38–58.

Koenig, W., H. K. Dunn, and L. Y. Lacy. 1946. The sound spectrograph. J. Acoust. Soc. Amer. 18: 19–49.

Kozhevnikov, V. A., and L. A. Chistovich. 1966. Speech: Articulation and Perception. 2nd printing. National Technical Information Services, Washington, D.C.

Ladefoged, P. 1972. Three Areas of Experimental Phonetics. Oxford University Press, Cambridge. p. 180.

Lehiste, I. 1967. Readings in Acoustic Phonetics. MIT Press, Cambridge, Mass. p. 358.

Lindblom, B. 1962. Accuracy and limitations of sonagraph measurements. *In* A. Sovijarvi and P. Abato (eds.), Fourth International Congress of Phonetic Sciences. Mouton, The Hague.

Lisker, L., and A. S. Abramson. 1964. A cross language study of voicing in initial stops: Acoustical measurements. Word 20: 384–422.

Lisker, L., and A. S. Abramson. 1967. Some effects of context on voice onset time in English stops. Lang. Speech 10: 1–28.

Lisker, L., and A. S. Abramson. 1971. Distinctive features and laryngeal control. Language 47: 767–785.

Öhman, S. E. G. 1965. Co-articulation in VCV utterances: Spectrographic measurements. J. Acoust. Soc. Amer. 39: 151–168.

Potter, R., G. Kopp, and H. Green. 1947. Visible Speech. Von Nostrand, New York. p. 439.

Robson, Ernest M. 1969. Transwhichics. Dufour Editions, Chester Springs, Pa. p. 108.

Smith, S. 1947. Analysis of vowel sounds by ear. Arch. Neerland. Phon. Exp. 20: 78–96.

Stevens, K. N., and A. S. House. 1961. An acoustical theory of vowel production and some of its implications. J. Speech Hear. Res. 4: 303–320.

Stevens, K. N., and D. H. Klatt. 1974. Role of formant transition in the voiced-voiceless distinction for stops. J. Acoust. Soc. Amer. 55: 653–659.

Wendell, M. V. 1973. Comparison of VOT and VTT of five and six year old stutterers and nonstutterers. Unpublished masters thesis. University of Cincinnati, Cincinnati.

Willis, R. 1829. On the vowel sounds and on reed organ pipes. Trans. Comp. Phil. Soc. 3.

The Problem of Speaker Identification and Elimination

Oscar I. Tosi, Ph.D.
Professor and Director
Speech and Hearing Research Laboratory
Michigan State University

CONTENTS

INTRODUCTION

Criminals use their voices as often as their weapons in the commission of their crimes. In this era of widespread usage of voice communication, the telephone also has become an instrument for commission of crimes, ranging from extortions and bomb threats to obscene calls. Tape recordings constitute an excellent means of collecting samples of both the questioned voice and the voices of suspected persons. Law enforcement agencies, in particular, and society, in general, are therefore extremely intcrested to have a reliable technique of voice identification or elimination that can be used either to convict or to acquit a defendant.

The subject of voice identification has become, during recent years, a controversial topic for the speech scientists. Some claim that it is possible presently to identify or eliminate reliably an unknown talker among several known ones, by using a combination of aural and visual examination of spectrograms. Others sustain that this method, as well as any other available method of voice identification, is unreliable and should not be used in a court of law. In many court cases where this type of evidence is presently submitted, it is a common experience to see experts who claim to be correct by supporting either one of the two opposite arguments of the issue.

Any method of identification or elimination has to be based on parameters that vary differently or less within the individual than among different persons. Although it is a common subjective experience to recognize an individual by his voice, if the listener is familiar with it, a complete quantitative description of relevant parameters to produce such identification is not presently available. Relevant parameters may differ according to the method used. Therefore, methods and experiments in this area are necessarily empirical, performed in the hope of determining reliable sets of parameters or features that can be used to produce with reasonable accuracy voice identification or voice elimination. The different methods of voice identification are not exclusive, of course, and can be used concurrently in practical cases of voice examination; for instance, the voice identification unit of the Michigan Department of State Police uses both the aural and visual method concurrently in all cases of voice identification or elimination.

The aural method of identification by itself is successfully used on a daily basis by everybody when dealing with familiar voices. Since remote antiquity people or even superior animals, like dogs, have experienced this phenomenon of identifying a familiar voice by listening. In modern times. the RCA Victor Company adopted as a trademark a picture of Caruso's dog recognizing his master's voice through a disc recording. Moreover, identification of individuals by their voices has long been an accepted court room practice (Kamine, 1969).

Until recently the only available technique for voice identification or elimination was based on aural examination, either using the long-term memory process or the short-term memory process. The long-term memory process is utilized when the voice to be identified is a familiar one to the listener. The short-term memory process is used when the unknown and known voices to be compared are available to the listeners through recordings.

Since the early 1940's, scientists have attempted to produce controlled experimentation and to devise new and more objective techniques for voice identification or elimination. One of these techniques was first described by

Gray and Kopp (1944), under the name "voice print," a term coined by these authors. Another approach in the search for a reliable method consists of analyzing different speech parameters through automatic or semiautomatic means, using the computer as a tool.

Up to the present a single, completely reliable technique of voice identification has not been found. Such a technique should yield correct speaker identification or eliminations in 100% of the cases, irrespective of the sample length, background noise, and recording system distortions; it should not be affected by the time elapsed between recordings from the same individual, by his physical or psychological condition, or by his effort to disguise his voice. Possibly such a single technique that possesses all these assets will be never found. However, scientific and field research could lead to the usage of a cluster of methods that might approach more or less closely these ideal requirements.

An operation related to voice identification and elimination is the Speaker Authentication, Recognition, or Validation Test, which consists of either accepting or rejecting a challenging speaker as a particular one within a limited library of voices stored in the memory bank of a computer. The challenging speaker is highly cooperative and pronounces the clue words with excellent articulation, and the transmission system possesses no significant distortions. This operation is essentially a discriminatory one: either accepting or rejecting the challenging speaker who claims to be a particular one within the library of voices. On the contrary, voice identification and elimination methods are not limited to discriminating a challenging speaker among a close, small library of known voices; there could be several suspected subjects involved. They may not be collaborative, and the transmission and recording system might be of poor quality. Nevertheless, as of today a completely practical and reliable system of speaker authentication does not exist.

Subjective and Objective Methods of Voice Identification and Elimination: Closed, Open, and Discrimination Tests

The methods of voice identification and elimination can be classified into two general groups: subjective methods and objective methods. Subjective methods are those operations performed by the human mind, and objective methods are those operations performed by mechanical or electronic means. Actually, there is a continuum of methods. The aural identification of "living" voices of speakers out of the sight of the listener is the most subjective end of this continuum, and the computer authentication of a speaker who claims to have his voice stored in the memory bank of the computer is the most objective end of this continuum.

Typically, all types of aural examination of voices and visual examination of speech spectrograms are considered subjective methods, although the latter is closer to the objective part of the spectrum of methods than the former.

Semiautomatic and automatic methods are considered objective, but the former is closer to the subjective part of the scale than the latter. Whether subjective or objective, voice examinations for legal purposes always require the intervention of an examiner, at least to prepare the samples and to interpret the results from the computer, and computers will perform only according to the instructions and programming produced by a human.

Tests of voice identification or elimination can be classified into three general groups, according to the composition of known and unknown samples: 1) discrimination tests, 2) open tests, and 3) closed tests.

In the discrimination tests the examiner is provided with a known sample and an unknown sample. He has to decide whether or not both samples belong to the same speaker. Two types of errors can be produced in this test: false identification, when the examiner decides both samples belong to the same subjects and this is not true, and false elimination, when the examiner decides both samples belong to different persons, but are actually from the same subject.

In the open tests the examiner is given several known samples and an unknown sample. He is told that the unknown may or may not be found among the known speakers. Here the test can yield three types of errors. First is the error of false elimination, when the unknown speaker is among the known speakers but the examiner is unable to find the unknown. The second and third types are errors of false identification, which can originate from two possibilities: 1) one of the known speakers is the same as the unknown, but the examiner selected a different one; and 2) none of the known is the same as the unknown speaker, but the examiner decided that one of them was the same as the unknown.

In the closed tests the examiner is told that the unknown speaker is one of the known speakers. Consequently, here only one type of error can be produced: error of false identification.

In the three types of tests discussed the examiner may include a confidence rating together with each decision, according to a scale, i.e., almost certain, fairly certain, fairly uncertain, almost uncertain. These confidence ratings allow the determination of the receiver operating characteristic, described in the next section.

The number of utterances refers to the repetitions of the same sample word taken from the same subject. Different utterances of the same word are useful for surveying the range of intraspeaker variation (see under Speech Production Theory and Speaker Variability).

Contemporary samples are defined as those utterances of the same words from a speaker obtained during the same recording session, and noncontemporary samples are those obtained during different recording sessions. In real life situations questioned voices and suspected voice samples are noncontemporary.

Receiver Operating Characteristic

The receiver operating characteristic is a plot of the probability that an examiner will decide "same" when this is true in a discrimination test involving a scale of confidence ratings, against the probability that he will decide "different" when this is not true. Each point of the receiver operating characteristic curve represents the cumulative percentage of the correct "same" responses versus the incorrect "same" responses, obtained for each grade of the confidence scale for a given number of tests. Cumulative refers to the summation of percentages of all superior levels of confidence to the one considered at each point of the curve, plus the percentages corresponding to that particular level.

In general, the larger the area subtended by the curve, the better is the discriminating ability the examiner possesses. Two different examiners may operate with different decision thresholds but possess the same discriminating ability. This situation would become apparent after determining the receiver operating characteristic of both examiners; their curves will coincide.

To determine the receiver operating characteristic of an examiner, it is necessary to submit him to a series of tests and to compute percentages as explained. The receiver operating characteristic of a computer is calculated a priori, according to the decision algorithm programmed.

Further information on receiver operating characteristics can be found in Egan, Schulman, and Greenberg (1959), Green and Swetts (1966), and in Hecker (1971).

SPEECH PRODUCTION THEORY AND SPEAKER VARIABILITY

In order to have a better understanding of the methods of voice identification, some basic ideas on speech production and speaker variability are necessary. These basic ideas are offered to the reader in this section.

Speech Production

The process of speech production, still not well understood and less quantified, can be generally divided into three levels, in which concatenated events occur successively with almost negligible delay (Figure 1). The first one could be labeled the *psycholinguistic level*. At this level the preparation of the talker message using words and syntactic rules takes place. This message is transduced into a correlated series of motor impulses within the speech centers (area of Brocca, thalamus, hypothalamus, etc.). Such first encoding of the message constitutes the *physiological level* of speech. This motor encoding activates, through the peripheral nervous system, the speech structures encountered along the vocal tract of the speaker. The stream of air produced

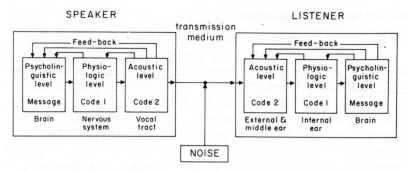

Figure 1. Block model of speech communication. The speaker's message is codified twice and consequently decodified by the listener. Noise in this model signifies any factor that deteriorates intelligibility.

by the lungs at a pressure above the atmospheric pressure, modulated by the vibration of the glottal folds or by turbulences at any articulatory constriction provides the basic source of sound for speech. The essentially unshaped spectra of these primary sources of sound are continuously modified by resonances in the cavities of the vocal tract, of which shapes and sizes are varied rapidly by the motor impulses. The variable speaker's output spectra constitute the second encoding of the message, being labeled the *acoustic level* of speech. The acoustic speech signal is transmitted through a medium (normally the atmosphere) to the listener, in whom this process is inverted, in order to decode, hopefully, the speaker original message.

In sum, from an acoustic point of view, to speak means to produce variable acoustic spectra correlated with a message through a particular phonetic code or language.

Speech Acoustic Spectra

The speaker output variable spectra carries not only semantic information, but also speaker-dependent features. Therefore, any method of speaker identification or elimination has to be based in some way on acoustic spectra. To arrive at the concept of speech spectrum, consider a very short segment of speech (about 50 msec) in which a phonetic utterance could be considered constant, i.e., the steady portion of a sustained vowel. In the time domain (amplitude versus time) (Figure 2) such a segment is correlated with a particular complex wave, which can be visualized on a readout device like the oscilloscope. Any complex wave is the summation of a series of simple or sinusoidal waves of different frequencies, amplitudes, and phases. The parameters of these components can be calculated by the Fourier analysis algorithm or obtained directly through a computer properly programmed or through an instrument called an acoustic spectrograph. Plotting of amplitude versus frequency of all simple waves components of a complex wave is called the *amplitude spectrum* of such a complex wave, or in the case discussed, the amplitude spectrum of the steady segment of speech analyzed (Figure 2). The plotting of phase versus frequency of these simple components is called the phase spectrum of that segment. In general, phase spectrum is disregarded in speech sciences. In ongoing speech the correlated complex wave is continuously changing in the time domain. Therefore, its spectrum in the frequency domain is also continuously changing. There is little doubt that one of the operations performed by the hearing structures of the listeners consists of analyzing the spectra of the variable acoustic signal produced by the speaker.

During very short intervals the speech waves can be quasiperiodic, i.e., the period of each wave within the interval is approximately constant; during other short intervals the speech waves can be aperiodic. Quasiperiodic waves, normally associated with vowel sounds, originate a type of spectrum called *discrete* or *line spectrum* (Figure 3) in which every sinusoidal component,

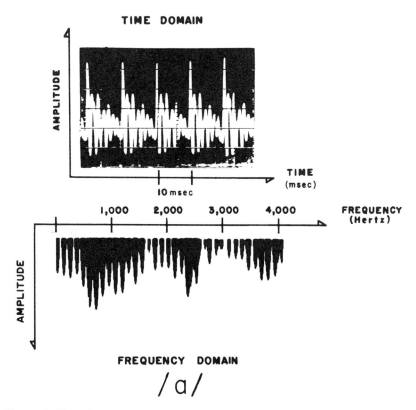

Figure 2. Time domain and frequency domain patterns from a quasiperiodic wave corresponding to the vowel /a/ uttered in isolation. The top graph was obtained from an oscilloscope. The bottom graph was obtained from a spectrograph with controls set at "section."

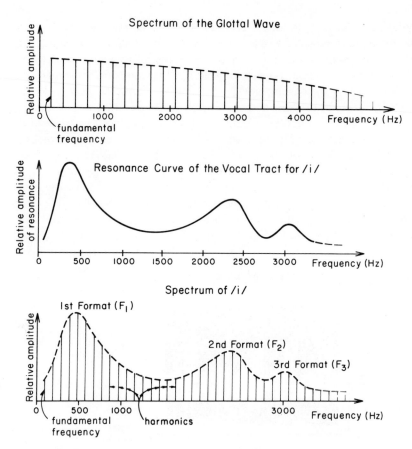

Figure 3. Model of resonances produced by the vocal tract to utter a quasiperiodic wave (i.e., a vowel) correlated with a discrete or line spectrum.

called harmonic, is clearly noticed through its frequency, integer of the fundamental frequency. This fundamental frequency coincides with the frequency of the first harmonic, with the frequency of the complex wave, and with the glottal frequency (frequency of vibration of the vocal folds) of the speaker in the short interval of time considered. Aperiodic waves, normally associated with unvoiced sounds (like /s/) originate a type of spectrum called *continuous spectrum* (Figure 4) in which acoustic power from the entire range of frequencies involved is present with no gaps. There also exists a mixed type of spectra correlated with voiced consonants (like /z/).

To produce all these types of varying-through-time spectra, the speaker utilizes the phenomenon of *resonance* (Figures 3 and 4). Resonance can exist with the interaction of at least two systems: an active system, the primary source of sound, and a resonance system that amplifies the amplitude of the primary source spectrum on some particular bands of frequencies and dampens the amplitude in other bands of frequencies. Each resonance system possesses a particular resonance curve according to the size, shape, and materials with which it is built. This resonance curve is a specification of the frequencies that are amplified and the frequencies that are dampened when the system is excited by a source containing these frequency bands.

As it was previously discussed, the speaker has available two primary sources of sound to produce speech, the glottal source and the frictional source, that can be used successively or simultaneously during ongoing speech, according to the instantaneous phonetic needs. The use of the glottal source originates the so-called voiced phonemes. The exclusive use of the frictional source originates the unvoiced phonemes. The spectra of these primary sources of sound is essentially flat and therefore not amenable to phonetic codification.

To establish a phonetic code, i.e., to speak, the spectra of the sources are modified at each instant by resonance in the vocal tract, conveniently shaped by the speaker through the articulatory movements. Each position of the articulators produces the desired phonetic spectrum that conveys a semantic meaning to the listener.

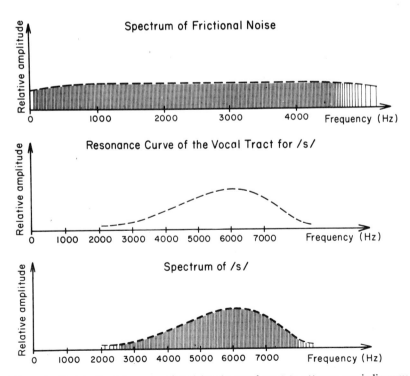

Figure 4. Model of resonance produced by the vocal tract to utter an aperiodic wave (i.e., a fricative) correlated with a continuous spectrum.

The frequency bands of relative higher amplitude of the variable output spectra are called formants in the case of vowels. There are also frequency bands of relative higher amplitude in the case of consonants. The relative position of the center frequency of these bands, their bandwidths, and relative amplitudes determine the different phonetic elements, as well as the speaker-dependent features, necessary for identification. However, these parameters are variable not only among different speakers, but also within the same speaker uttering the same phonetic elements. Coarticulation is one important factor responsible for these variations (Daniloff and Hammarberg, 1973; Stevens, House, and Paul, 1966).

Frequency range of speech comprises the glottal frequency up to about 7 kHz. However, most speech and speaker information is properly conveyed by a restricted range, up to about 4 kHz. Both the glottal spectrum and resonance curves of a vocal tract are dependent on anatomic and organic characteristics as well as on the functional or behavioral process experimented by each person during the learning stage of speaking.

Speech Acoustic Parameters and Speaker Variability

The most general acoustic parameters of speech are time, frequency, and intensity distribution within all bands of frequency simultaneously present in the instantaneous speaker output. Comparisons of these general spectral parameters or derived ones are the basis of all speaker recognition systems, both subjective and objective. Variation of these spectral parameters depends on phonetic content and speaker individuality. The phonetic source of variation can be minimized by limiting   comparisons only to similar sample sentences produced by the known and unknown speakers in voice identification tests. The problem is that even maintaining the text constant, values of the selected parameters will differ not only among different speakers, but also within the same speaker when different utterances of this same text are compared. The first type of variation is called *interspeaker variability;* the second type is referred as *intraspeaker variability.* Researchers of voice identification have searched for sets of efficient parameters, i.e., parameters that present the least intraspeaker variability and the most interspeaker variability in all conditions that may occur in normal or even in disguised speech. These efficient parameters are selected according to the particular method explored. Optimal selection for aural examination cannot be adequate for visual examination or for automatic recognition.

One recent study searching for efficient parameters in *automatic recognition* was conducted by Wolf (1972). He selected the following parameters: fundamental frequency at given locations of the sample sentences, amplitude of nasal consonants moment calculations with frequency band amplitudes of filtered vowels, mean frequencies of formants F_1 and F_2 in given locations of the sample sentences, spectrum slope at a given location of /u/, high frequency spectrum shape at the middle of /ʃ/, etc. Atal (1972) selected pitch contours for his method of automatic speaker recognition.

For *visual examination* of spectrograms the following parameters were considered (Tosi et al., 1972): mean frequencies and bandwidths of vowel formants, gaps and type of vertical striations, slopes of formants, duration of similar phonetic elements and plosive gaps, energy distribution of fricatives, plosives, and interformant spaces.

For *aural examination* perceptual parameters and voice-attribute rating tests like pitch, rate, intensity, and quality (Holmgren, 1967) have been used.

In sum, organic and learned differences are the sources of interspeaker variability. Time elapsed, psychological and physiological changes, circadian rhythm, and articulatory dynamics are the sources of intraspeaker variability. Additional variability is introduced by the effect of coarticulation when similar phonetic elements, extracted from different contexts, are compared. More variability is introduced by environmental reverberations, noise, and distortions of the transmission and recording systems. Considering all these sources of variability, there is little hope to develop a method, or rather a clustering of methods, that could provide a positive speaker identification in 100% of the cases examined, within a legally acceptable rate of error. In many cases, whatever the methods used, objective or subjective, the outcome of the examination has to be *no decision one way or the other* or *probability of identification or elimination,* if the examiner is unbiased and proceeding within strict rules of honesty.

SUBJECTIVE METHODS OF SPEAKER IDENTIFICATION AND ELIMINATION

Aural examinations and visual examinations of speech spectrograms are considered subjective methods of speaker identification, each within a different category of subjectivity. A summary of available experimental data is presented in this section.

Aural Examination of Voices

A listener may use the long-term memory process or the short-term memory process to identify or eliminate an unknown speaker as being the same as a particular known one. These two memory processes were defined at the start of the chapter.

The success of aural recognition based on long-term memory depends on the remembrance or the familiarity of the listener with the questioned voice, the time elapsed since last it was heard, the homogeneity of the "challenging" speaker's group, and the discriminating ability of the listener. The voice sample duration seems to be not critical after 1 sec of continuous speech. If a transmission or recording system is used to obtain challenging speakers' voice samples, distortions introduced by such a system may increase the percentage of errors. Filtering below 500 Hz and above 3,000 Hz seems to have no significant influence in the results of tests. Attempts of the challenging speaker to disguise his voice, or even to use whispered speech, may decrease greatly the correct identification percentages (Pollack, Pickett, and Sumby, 1954).

The first significant experiment done in the area of aural examination, using the long-term memory process, was performed by McGehee (1937). He used a total of 31 male and 18 female speakers, reading a paragraph of 56 words. Apparently, these speakers belonged to a phonetically homogeneous group, all graduate students. A total of 740 undergraduate students were employed as listeners in this experiment in which live voices were used exclusively. Listeners were divided into 15 panels, each panel participating in at least two sessions. During the first session they listened to a speaker behind a screen reading a paragraph. During the second session five speakers, including the one from the first session, read the same paragraph. Each listener had to indicate who, among these five speakers, was the one they had heard previously. The second listening session was spaced from 1 day to 5 months from the first one, according to the particular panel of listeners. The mean percentage of correct identifications varied from 83% to 13%. McGehee also investigated the effect of disguising the voice by changing the pitch, which drastically reduced the percentage of correct identifications. Other findings of this early study were that male and female voices are equally identifiable and that increasing the number of known speakers reduces the percentage of correct identifications. It is to be noted that all trials of identification were the closed type and that no recordings were used.

In a second study by McGehee (1944), sample voices were recorded on phonograph records at 78 rpm. Keeping the experimental design similar to that of the first study, he obtained approximately 7% fewer correct speaker identifications. In this study McGehee also attempted to produce an analysis of voice quality based on pitch, rate, and agreeableness scales. Speakers' voices were graded by three panels of judges: one panel trained in speech, one in music, and the third with no particular training to judge sound. McGehee found a close agreement from the three groups in most of the ratings.

Pollack, Pickett, and Sumby (1954) performed an experiment on aural recognition based on the long-term memory. All 16 speakers used in this experiment were familiar to the listeners, who performed the so-called "speaker-naming tests" for groups of from two to eight speakers. These authors investigated the effect of several variables on the percentage of correct identifications, namely, duration of the speech sample, filtering, and whispering. Their findings can be summarized as follows. Durations longer than 1 sec do not improve significantly the percentage of correct identifications, which reached a figure close to 95% after this interval of time. Whispered speech reduces approximately 30% the correct identifications, with other conditions constant. For low- and high-pass filtering, the authors concluded that "over a rather wide frequency range, identification performance is resistant to selective frequency of this type." The authors used monosyllabic words from the Harvard Psychoacoustic Laboratory PB (phonetically balanced) list as speech materials for this experiment.

Bricker and Pruzansky (1966) studied the effects of stimulus content and duration on aural talker identification. They used 16 listeners familiar with 10 speakers, who recorded all different materials through high fidelity equipment. The examiners listened to the tapes through a loudspeaker. The best examiner was able to obtain 100% correct identification when listening to sentences of mean duration of 2.4 sec containing about 15 phonemes. The worst examiner, for the same trials, obtained only 92% correct responses. These percentages dropped to 56% correct for samples of duration 0.12 sec containing only one phoneme. They found a significant interaction between particular phonemes and speakers for these brief excerpted phonetic materials. They also ran tests based on short-term memory, including two known subjects A and B, to be compared with one unknown X, using reversed excerpts. Listeners were not familiar with the speakers. Average results of correct identification in these closed tests reached the 75% level.

One of the rare studies in aural examination using open trials and short memory process was performed by Stevens et al. (1968). In this study the authors attempted to compare results obtained from aural examination and from visual examination of spectrograms, using the same materials and same examiners. They employed 24 highly homogeneous talkers from the point of view of perceptual attributes of speech. All of these speakers recorded twice, 1 week apart, repeating 10 times a reading list of nine words and two short sentences. These materials were dubbed into loops of 4.5-sec duration, each loop containing two utterances of the same word or one utterance of a short sentence. Spectrograms of these materials were also subsequently prepared. Six examiners performed open and closed tests of speaker identification and elimination with these materials, using separately aural and visual examinations. They did not receive training for either of the two methods; however, they were selected on the basis of their abilities to become aurally familiar with an ensemble of six previously unfamiliar voices. All tests included one unknown and eight known speakers. The examiners could listen to the nine loops representing these speakers, switching as necessary among the tape recorded channels.

In all cases the percentages of correct responses were significantly higher for aural examination than for visual examination. For the closed test types, mean errors yielded by aural examination ranged from 18 to 6%. Mean errors yielded by visual examination of spectrograms of the same materials ranged from 28 to 21%. The lower percentages correspond to later tests, when some learning effect had obviously interacted with the results. For the open test types results were as follows: aural method, 8 to 6% error of false identification and 12 to 8% error of false elimination; visual method, 47 to 31% error of false identification and 20% to 10% error of false elimination.

This writer feels that these percentages were biased, since the examiners had normal hearing and therefore were accustomed to discriminate voices aurally from the early stages of life, but they were not familiar with spectrograms, at least in that they had had no special training. Furthermore, the examiners in this study were selected on the basis of their aural ability, but their ability to match patterns was not tested. Also, the lengths of the samples used were inadequately short for spectrographic recognition. In a letter to prosecutor P. Lindhom (28 January 1971), Dr. Stevens acknowledged that these factors might be the reason for the high percentage of errors produced in his experiment.

Other conclusions of this study were that: 1) some speakers are more difficult to identify than others, even when the experimental speakers are homogeneous from the point of view of the perceptual attributes; 2) there are large differences in the ability of examiners to identify voices by either method; teams of visual examiners perform better than a single examiner; and 3) aurally, it is easier to identify a speaker listening to front vowels than to back vowels; longer utterances increase the probability of correct identifications using visual methods.

Other authors took a different approach to study aural identification, trying to determine significant perceptual attributes of speakers' voices, in order to create reliable classification scales. These scales might help an examiner to perform aural discriminations on a systematic and consistent basis. A classical study of this type was undertaken by Voiers (1964), who was able to isolate four significant perceptual scales—clarity, roughness, magnitude, and animation—as means to discriminate among speakers. Holmgren (1967) found that pitch, intensity, quality, and rate scales helped to classify better the uniqueness of each particular voice. However, in practical cases it was verified that the same set of numbers from the four scales might correspond to different voices. Therefore, perceptual scales should be considered only as a helping device for speaker identification or elimination.

In sum, aural examination of voices is the most familiar and natural system of speaker identification and elimination. It is accepted by any court of law for what it is worth. The expected percentage of error for open tests, using the short-term memory process (i.e., listening through recordings to the known and unknown voices) has not been accurately determined by experimentation. It might be as large as 20%, according to particular circumstances, especially if the examiner is forced to reach a positive decision in all tests, instead of selecting probabilities or choosing no decision one way or the other. Distortions and disguising of the voice can increase greatly the expected error percentages.

In spite of the modern trend to investigate automatic systems of speaker recognition, continued research on aural examination is worthwhile. Experimental designs should include open tests, low quality transmission, recording systems, and background noise to approach real life situations. Cartridge tape recorders, presently available, are ideal instruments for this type of research.

Visual Examination of Spectrograms

Spectrography The purpose of speech spectrography is to resolve the complex speech signal into its single components. This operation was first performed at the turn of the century for sustained vowels. The instrument used in these early studies was the mechanical Henrici analyzer. With such a machine, Black (1937) was able to produce tridimensional spectra of the same vowel as spoken by different speakers, plotting harmonic frequencies and corresponding intensities against time.

In 1941, a spectrograph project lead by Dr. Ralph Potter was started at the Bell Telephone Laboratories (Potter, Kopp, and Green, 1947). This machine was developed with the primary purpose of helping the military during time of war, and only when the war was over did the spectrograph become available to speech scientists. The input to the spectrograph is a recorded speech sample limited to segments 2.4 sec long. The output consists of a graphic display (spectrogram) of frequency intensity versus time for the sample analyzed. Frequencies are plotted on the vertical axis and time on the horizontal axis. Relative intensities are portrayed by the different degrees of darkness of the patterns produced. In the commercially available spectrographs, there are several options for setting the ranges of frequencies of analysis (60–4,000 Hz or 60–7,000 Hz, etc.) using logarithmic or lineal scales. The bandwidth of the scanning analyzing filter can be selected at 45 or 300 Hz. Also, it is possible to obtain bar or contour spectrograms with these machines.

The operation of the spectrograph consists essentially of performing a continuous Fourier analysis of the speech sample, at each instant of time. If the narrow-band filter (45 Hz) is selected, the actual Fourier harmonics of the input speech sample are displayed on the spectrograms. If the broad-band scanning filter (300 Hz) is utilized, the formants rather than the individual harmonics appear on the spectrogram (Figure 5). These two types of displays are called bar spectrograms. Since the relative intensity of each harmonic or each formant is portrayed by the different degrees of darkness of the patterns produced, and the intensity range of the speech harmonics or formants can be as large as 40 dB, a compressor circuit reduces the intensity of the input signal proportionally to the scanned range of frequencies. The reason for this procedure is to compensate for the reduced dynamic range of the Teledeltos paper (about 10 dB) where the spectrogram is printed, making it possible to

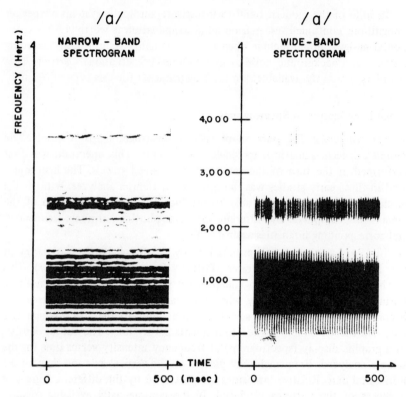

Figure 5. Narrow-band and broad-band spectrogram from the vowel /a/ of Figure 2.

record on the paper the weak, higher harmonics or formants of the speech signal.

Voiceprint Identification The original spectrograph design, marketed by Kay Elemetrics (Pine Brook, N.J.) was improved in 1966 by Anthony Presti, an engineer at the Bell Telephone Laboratories, who later joined the Voiceprint Laboratories, Inc. (N.J.), to market his new improved spectrograph with the brand name Voiceprint (Presti, 1966). He also introduced in the machine a display called "contour," where relative intensities are plotted by isobaric lines (contours) at 6-dB steps.

The sound spectrograph or sonograph can be considered a kind of universal instrument for researching and teaching the acoustics of speech or sound in general. In addition, it was used for practical applications such as improving the speech of deaf people. In 1944, Gray and Kopp found that spectrograms could be applied to identify speakers, since the spectrogram not only portrays the phonetic features of speech but speaker-dependent features as well. They wrote a report (Gray and Kopp, 1944) containing their experiences in this field and describing practical means to put this system into use, how to train examiners to identify questioned speakers, etc. They concluded their report with the following paragraph.

Voice print identification seems to offer possibility of a useful radio intercept feature and one that could be put into use without extensive training or elaborate equipment. As a study of combat conditions in the European and Pacific theaters indicates a need for such identification, it is suggested that a trial voice identification group be established to carry on work under actual or simulated field conditions to test the conclusions of this laboratory work.

To the best knowledge of this writer, such a test was not completed because of the end of the war and the problems of recordings. Tape recorders were not practically developed at that time.

Studies by Kersta During the early 1960's, Lawrence Kersta, a staff member of the Bell Telephone Laboratories, reexamined the Voiceprint method at the request of a law enforcement group.

He performed laboratory experiments using spectrograms from five clue words spoken in isolation by an unspecified population (Kersta, 1962). All the tests were of the closed type, using contemporary spectrograms, that is, spectrograms produced from each speaker sample obtained during the same recording session. The maximal number of known speakers in each trial of identification was 12. The examiners were requested to render a positive identification on all cases. These examiners were a group of high school girls trained by Kersta 1 week before the start of the experiment. They worked in pairs. The percentage of correct identifications in these experiments was better than 99%. Using only one cue word per speaker, this percentage diminished to approximately 97%. Kersta found also that the five clue words "a," "I," ' is," "on," and "you," produced slightly higher errors of identification than the words "to," "me," ' and," "the," and "that." In the Kersta papers there was no report of significant performance differences among examiners. Homogeneity and number of speakers were not discussed. Other experiments that Kersta performed, such as sorting spectrograms in order to form groups including the same speaker, also showed a high percentage of correct responses.

Kersta became absolutely convinced of the "infallibility" of spectrograms for identification purposes. He presented a paper to the November 1962 Meeting of the Acoustical Society of America, in which he compared the reliability of this method with that of the fingerprints.

In 1966, Kersta retired from Bell Telephone Laboratories and established his own company, Voiceprint Laboratories, Inc. with the goal of producing spectrographs on a commercial basis. He offered his professional services to identify persons through their voices, and to train police officers as speech spectrogram examiners.

The scientific community soon voiced its opposition to Kersta's claims. Some experiments which contradicted the extremely high success percentages reported by Kersta were produced. One of the most adamant opponents of Kersta at that time was Dr. Peter Ladefoged, who published a paper (Ladefoged and Vanderslice, 1967) contradicting the statements of Kersta.

Studies by Young and Campbell, Stevens et al., and Hazen Young and Campbell (1967) published a study dealing with closed tests of speaker identification by visual examination of spectrograms. Five talkers uttering two words were used as known speakers in each trial. Young and Campbell used 10 examiners, who received a maximum of 2.5 hr of training before the start of the experiment. During this training phase, using one word ("you" or "it") spoken in isolation, the identification success reached a mean of 78.4%. During the experimental tasks, spectrograms of the same two words (you, it) were used, but this time they were excerpted from a sentence rather than produced in isolation. The percentage of success decreased to a mean of 37.3%. Young and Campbell attribute these differences to the shorter stimulus represented by the excerpted words, as compared with the longer similar words uttered in isolation, and to the coarticulation factors. They recognized however, that the different experimental approach they took, as compared with that of Kersta, the difference in training of examiners, and possibly differences in population homogeneity could have accounted for the different score percentages obtained in both experiments.

Stevens et al. (1968) produced another experiment using separately aural and visual examination of spectrogram. Results from this experiment are presented earlier in this chapter in the section Aural Examination of Voices.

In a published thesis an experiment was reported on speaker recognition using five words physically excerpted from spectrograms obtained from spontaneous speech (Hazen, 1973). Hazen used seven panels of teams of two examiners who received a "few sessions" of training before the start of the experiment. There were different types of tasks to be performed, including absolute identification or elimination of one unknown speaker among 50 known speakers. Hazen forced the examiners to reach a positive decision in any of the 40 tests performed by each panel. The range of errors ran from 0.00 to 83.33% according to the type of task and the panel. The error was always larger when comparing words cut off from different speech contexts than for words taken from the same contexts. Considering the types of errors he obtained, Hazen concluded that identification using speech spectrograms should not be utilized "until sufficient and consistent data are gathered to establish accurately the limits of this technique" (p. 659).

Certainly, this would be a most reasonable conclusion if speech spectrograms of five physically excerpted words were used as sole means of identification by examiners with no experience, who are forced to render a positive decision in 100% of the cases examined. On the other hand, it should be pointed out that Hazen's idea of using words from spontaneous speech as opposed to words from readings was an excellent one, since in real life cases the questioned person indeed uses spontaneous speech. However, to section physically these words from ongoing speech spectrograms was not a commendable procedure since it is almost impossible to target the boundaries of a word in that condition. Furthermore, transient patterns are speaker-dependent features, and they became lost with this procedure. In addition, only 40 trials of absolute identification or elimination per panel (or 280 trials in total) do not constitute an impressive amount of statistical data to substantiate solidly any recommendation.

The merit of Hazen's study is in having reiterated what should not be done with spectrograms, namely, to segment physically spectrographic patterns of a given word from an ongoing text and to use random contexts for matching techniques.

Studies by Tosi et al. To date, the largest study on voice identification and elimination using speech spectrograms has been performed by Tosi et al. (1972) at Michigan State University. This study was possible through a large grant from the United States Department of Justice; it was carried from the beginning of 1968 to December 1970. This experiment included a total of 34,992 experimental trials of identification and elimination, according to different models, performed by 29 experimental examiners who were trained for 1 month.

Each trial involved up to 40 known voices, in various conditions: closed and open trials; contemporary and noncontemporary spectrograms; nine or six clue words spoken in isolation, in a fixed context, and in random context, etc. The 250 speakers used in this experiment were randomly selected from a homogeneous population of approximately 25,000 male students at Michigan State University.

The experimental examiners were forced to reach a positive decision (identification or elimination) in each test, taking an average time of 15 min. Their decisions were based solely on examination of spectrograms; listening to the voices was discarded from this experiment (Figure 6). The examiners graded their self-confidence in their judgments on a 4-point scale: 1 and 2, uncertain; 3 and 4, certain. Percentage error of false identifications obtained from the forensic models (open tests, noncontemporary spectrograms, ongoing speech texts) tested in this experiment was approximately 6.4%. Percentage error of false elimination from these models was approximately 12.7%. Kersta's models (closed tests, contemporary spectrograms, words spoken in isolation) were also tested in this experiment and yielded a percentage error less than 1%. Examiners' answers graded "uncertain" were computed in order to determine the possible percentages that would have been obtained if the examiners had not been forced to reach a positive conclusion in 100% of the tests. The computer analysis determined that in this case, percentage error of false identification for the forensic models would have been reduced approximately to 2.4%, percentage error of false eliminations approximately to 4.8%, and percentage of tests with "certain" answers to 74%.

Figure 6. Three speakers, A, B, and C, produced spectrograms from the same sentence. Spectrogram labeled 1 was obtained from a second utterance of this sentence by speaker B.

At the same time that the laboratory study was being conducted by Tosi, a field study was completed at the Crime Laboratory of the Michigan State Police, by Lt. Ernest Nash (Michigan Department of State Police, 1972), with the purpose of finding the difference between laboratory conditions and the actual situation a professional examiner encounters when handling forensic situations. This field study included 673 voices involved in actual criminal investigations.

After evaluation of laboratory conditions and field conditions, the following conclusions were reached. First, a *combined method of aural and visual examination* of spectrograms can be used in the investigation of a crime if the following standards are maintained.

1. The examiner must be a qualified professional trained in phonetics and speech sciences. A 2-year apprenticeship in field work should be required along with academic training before a voice examiner is qualified professionally.

2. The professional examiner must abstain from offering any positive conclusion when he has the least doubt on the exactness of such conclusion. Since this method is essentially subjective and relies heavily on the expertise of the examiner, prudence should be the cardinal principle that guides the examiner's decisions.

3. The examiner must be entitled to spend as much time and to demand as many voice samples of good quality as he deems necessary to reach a positive conclusion. Otherwise, he should select alternative decisions, such as probability of identification or elimination or simply no conclusion one way or the other.

Second, in keeping with these standards, the Michigan State Police decided to employ these *combined aural and visual methods* of speaker identification or elimination starting in December 1970.

In sum, subjective methods of voice identification or elimination can offer reasonable reliability if the listed standards are rigorously maintained.

Distortions caused by transmission and recording systems, background noise, or psychological or physiological alterations of the speakers will greatly decrease the percentage of cases in which a honest and well trained examiner could reach a positive identification using these subjective methods. However, the same statement could be applied to objective methods the day they will become sufficiently developed to be applied to forensic cases.

The crucial problem with subjective methods is testing the honesty and reliability of the examiner. Open discrimination tests, in which several voices in addition to the defendant voice are included, may serve to test the examiner as well as to obtain his receiver operating characteristic curve.

Bolt et al. (1973) have expressed their opposition to the use of speech spectrograms for legal purposes. Their conclusions are most reasonable, indeed, if they mean exclusion of aural examination and reaching positive decisions in 100% of the cases examined, irrespective of the conditions and frequency range of the voice samples, psychological, and physiological alterations of the speakers, distortions introduced by the recording and transmission systems, background noise, etc. These conditions, however, clearly contradict the standards specified by this writer and his colleagues (Black et al. 1973) for real life examinations.

OBJECTIVE METHODS OF SPEAKER RECOGNITION

Both automatic and semiautomatic methods of speaker recognition are considered objective, each according to a different degree of objectivity. These methods are presently in the early stages of development. To date, objective methods are more suitable for speaker authentication or verification than for speaker identification in legal cases. Automatic systems that include a limited library of voices (about 10), able to authenticate a collaborative speaker with an error of the order of 10% or even less, are presently available.

Further development of automatic methods is desirable because of the many assets these methods have, such as possibility of mathematical specification of the expected errors, the receiver operating characteristic, and the elimination or great reduction of human bias. Although a human operator is always necessary to prepare the samples and to interpret results from the computer, the necessary skill of such an operator could be reduced to minimal levels, compatible with the characteristics of each particular system. In addition, human fatigue, a factor that may contribute to errors in subjective methods, is almost eliminated.

Two functional steps are necessary in all automatic systems: 1) extraction of relevant parameters from the questioned and known speaker samples, and 2) consequent decision "same-different" (or no decision in some systems) according to rules based on a programmed algorithm. There are two general procedures to complete the first step in automatic or semiautomatic speaker

identification: 1) forming a matrix based on the spectra of the common
phonetic elements selected, or 2) extracting from these spectra a variety of
derived parameters that are considered relevant by each particular experimenter searching for an efficient speaker identification or elimination system
(Wolf, 1972).

To complete the second step, rules of decision are programmed. Generally, they consist of comparing statistically the data obtained from the first
step after introducing weighing factors, computing Euclidean distances, and
so forth (Li, Hughes, and House, 1969). An alternative   procedure consists
of forming hierarchical clustering groups with the data (Tosi, 1974). The
decision algorithm provides a choice of possible responses when comparing a
known speaker to the questioned one, such as "same-different-no decision,"
according to limits of decision arbitrarily set by the programmer.

One problem that plagues most objective systems is the automatic recognition and alignment of the common phonetic elements to the "known" and
"unknown" samples, which are the sources of the parameters on which to
base a decision. The risk consists of false targeting. In this case comparison
would be based on different phonetic elements, which may hinder greatly the
process. Several strategies have been devised to cope with this problem
(Hecker, 1971).

Semiautomatic Systems: Studies from the Stanford Research Institute and the Texas Instruments Company

Semiautomatic systems include recognition of the common phonetic elements from samples to be compared by a human operator. An excellent
development of a semiautomatic system was produced by scientists from the
Stanford Research Institute (Becker et al. 1972). In this system the operator
observes on a cathode ray tube the sample sentence waves and selects the
segments to be analyzed through a display window.

After this selection is made, amplitude and phase spectra of these segments (generally steady portions of a vowel) are obtained and compared with
similar ones obtained from other speech samples. Through a special algorithm
a decision among the following alternatives is reached: samples were produced by the same speaker, samples were produced by different speakers, or
no decision one way or the other.

By changing the decision algorithm, percentages of expected errors of
false identification, false elimination, and no decision consequently can be
changed in a known proportion. For instance, to have less than 1% chance of
error of false identification, the percentage of no decisions has to be as high
as 30%.

Companion to this study was the one conducted by Hair and Rekieta
(1972), in which they performed open tests by automatic means, including
32, 8, and 2 suspects, respectively. These authors claimed a 99% accuracy of
the system, provided some conditions are maintained. Also, according to

these experimenters, their semiautomatic system of voice identification could be easily implemented for use by law enforcement agencies.

Automatic Systems

Atal (1972) reported the use of pitch contours as an efficient parameter for automatic speaker recognition. Closed tests involving 10 speakers yielded 97% of correct identification using Atal's method.

Wolf (1972) described another automatic system using efficient parameters for voice identification (see under Speech Acoustic Parameters and Speaker Variability). Correct results from a population of 21 speakers, using such a set of parameters programmed in a computer, reached the 98% level in closed tests of speaker authentication.

Su and Fu (1973) published a study on automatic speaker identification. They based their method on statistical information derived from spectra of nasal consonants, spectra of words excerpted from ongoing speech, and spectra of continuous speech. Spectra of nasal consonants proved to be the best of the three clues for speaker identification, and spectra from excerpted words was the least favorable. Using readings from 10 speakers, three female and seven male, in closed tests of voice identification, they obtained percentages of correct responses from 100 to 10%, according to the materials and decision algorithms used. In their report, they included a complete review of the available literature on automatic speaker identification up to 1973.

In 1973, during a sabbatical leave spent at the Galileo Ferraris Institute of Torino, Italy, this writer experimented with choral speech spectra applied to voice identification (Bordone et al., 1974). This study attempted to eliminate the problem of temporal alignment of common phonetic elements from the unknown and known voices to be compared, as well as to eliminate the requirement demanded by many systems of voice identification of having "known" and "unknown" samples of similar texts. Choral spectra are defined as the spectra of mixed temporal segments of different speech produced by the same talker (Tarnóczy, 1958).

In this Torino study choral spectra of different texts recorded by 20 speakers were compared through a special computer algorithm. The purpose was to test whether or not it is possible to produce reliable discriminations based on relative individual invariances of such spectra, irrespective of text or language used by the speakers.

The speakers, 14 male and six female, all had education beyond high school, had no noticeable speech defects, and spoke fluent Piamontes, Italian, and French. All were natives of Piedmont and therefore had a high degree of phonetic homogeneity. They recorded three times, within 1-week intervals, a 10-min text in Piamontes, Italian, and French, respectively. Texts consisted of items from two newspapers and a book. Recordings were obtained within a sound-isolated room and using a high quality system.

Recordings of each language were temporarily segmented into 14 parts

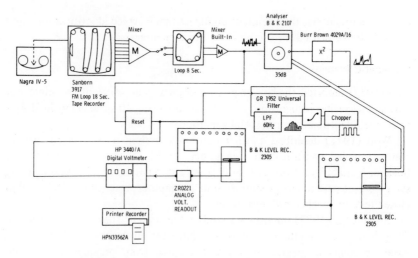

Figure 7. Block instrumentation to obtain choral spectra.

and dubbed into loops each approximately 20 sec long, utilizing a Sanborn 3917 FM tape recorder. The mixed output from these loops, played back simultaneously, were re-recorded into an 8-sec long single loop, obtaining a total of nine of these choral speech loops per speaker. Each loop therefore was defined by speaker, language, and recording session, respectively. These loops were analyzed through a special spectrographic system (Figure 7). Intensity of all loops was adjusted to a common peak value of 25 dB re an arbitrary zero.

Output from this system consisted of 180 choral speech spectra, each representing a speaker, language, and recording session. Range of spectra was from 63 to 6,300 Hz, processed through a 1/3 octave filter. Spectra were digitally sampled every 4/100 octave, obtaining 156 readings of relative decibels versus frequency for each spectrum (Figure 8).

These digital data were transferred into IBM cards and processed through a hierarchical clustering algorithm, implemented on the CDC 6500 computer at Michigan State University.

Hierarchical clustering algorithms provide one way of investigating the following question.
1. Are the spectra for a particular speaker more similar to one another than to the spectra for other speakers?
2. Are the spectra from one language more similar to one another than to those from other languages?
3. Do the answers to the first two questions remain consistent in time?

Similarity matrices of spectra were computed in this study by two different methods: 1) sum of absolute differences between energies of corresponding frequencies on all pairs of spectra, and 2) squared root of the sum of the squared differences between these energies. The hierarchical clustering algorithm translates these similarity matrices into a dendrogram or tree. Cutting the dendrogram at various levels clusters the spectra into groups that enclose the most similar components.

The various methods to cluster these spectra, as described earlier, were explored. In all cases spectra clustered very well according to subject rather than to language or recording session. Errors of clustering or "identifying" speakers ran from 30 to 5% according to the methods used for cluster and for computing percentages. This find suggests that each speaker possesses relative invariances in his/her choral spectra, irrespective of the text or language used.

Recently, Li and Hughes (1974) published a study dealing with speaker differences as they appear in correlation matrices of cintinous speech spectra. They measured the differences between any combination of two matrices from a population of 30 speakers. They defined intraspeaker difference as the difference bewteen matrices obtained from spectra of different texts read by the same speaker. Interspeaker difference was defined by matrices of spectra from the same text read by different speakers. The results indicated that there is only a 1% overlap distribution of these differences to confound absolute identification of a given speaker.

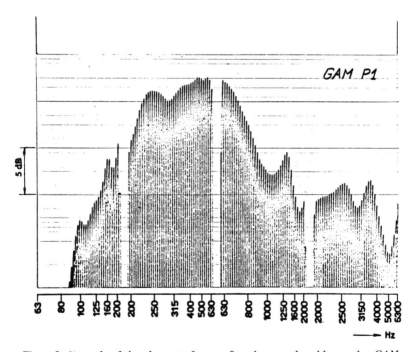

Figure 8. Example of choral spectra from an 8-sec loop produced by speaker GAM.

Conclusions

As a conclusion to this section of objective methods of speaker recognition, the writer should state that, while highly desirable, these methods could not be used independently of a human examiner for legal purposes, even if in the future they could be greatly improved. On the other hand, objective methods should not preclude simultaneous usage of subjective methods in legal examinations. Rather, a clustering of objective and subjective methods used to conduct a legal voice examination will strengthen the conclusion in case no contradiction is founded.

LEGAL SITUATION OF SPEAKER IDENTIFICATION AND ELIMINATION IN THE UNITED STATES

Court Cases before 1970

Legal evidence on voice identification or elimination presented before 1970 was based, in most cases, on aural examination. Witnesses testified simply that they recognized or did not recognize the voice of the defendant as being the same as the questioned voice. Since tape recorders were not available before or immediately after World War II, aural recognitions depended on the long-term memory process; phonographic recording was impractical for obtaining voice samples. Usually the weight given to these testimonies was not too significant. A historic case using this type of evidence was *People v. Hauptmann* (1935).

In most recent cases tape recordings of the questioned voice were available, and therefore witnesses could use the short-term memory process for their aural examinations. For instance, in the case *New Jersey v. DiGiglio* (1970), Tosi used exclusively aural examination and the short-term memory to eliminate Mr. DiGiglio as being the same person as the one whose voice was recorded through the telephone. The expert witness in this case was able to demonstrate the different quality and pitch of the two voices examined, as well as the existence of a permanent hoarseness in the voice of Mr. Digiglio, due to a chronic monochorditis, that did not appear in the questioned voice.

After 1965, L. Kersta presented legal evidence using the method called Voiceprint (Gray and Kopp, 1944) in several cases. The first case using exclusively visual examination of spectrograms was *People v. Straehle* (Westchester County Court, New York, 1966). One of the last cases in which Kersta acted as an expert witness presenting Voiceprint evidence was *California v. King* (1968). Expert witness for the defense was Dr. Peter Ladefoged, professor of phonetics at the University of California, Los Angeles, who challenged very successfully the credentials of Kersta, as well as the reliability of Voiceprints to identify persons. The defendant was acquitted by the appellate court. In the *New Jersey v. Cary* (1968) case, Kersta testified before the Superior Court of New Jersey in favor of exclusive usage of speech spectrograms for voice identification. Tosi stated that more scientific experimentation was necessary. The court ruled that this was the case; thus, evidence was not accepted. After this case, Kersta did not appear anymore as an expert witness, on the grounds of poor health.

In total, Kersta and his employees at the Voiceprint Laboratories presented evidence in approximately 15 cases, until 1973, the year that this corporation went into bankruptcy. A list of these cases was not available to this writer. In addition, personnel of the Voiceprint Laboratories performed voice examination for approximately 200 clients including civil, commercial, and criminal cases (Kersta, 1974, unpublished data).

Voice Identification Unit of Michigan Department of State Police

During the last part of 1966 and the beginning of 1967, the commanding officers of the Crime Laboratory of the Michigan Department of State Police became interested in investigating the possibility of using speech spectrograms to identify criminals through their voices. Since the Voiceprint Laboratories were offering a training course for police officers at that time, two fingerprint technicians from the Michigan State Police, detectives Ernest Nash and Louis Wilson, were selected to participate in such a course. In addition, this author was requested to evaluate the Voiceprint method as a consultant to the Michigan State Police. After spending approximately 10 days at the Voiceprint Laboratories, observing the training Nash and Wilson received, discussing with Kersta his experiments, and collecting data from Kersta's trainees, this author wrote a report (Tosi, 1967) expressing essentially that: "the method of identifying persons by speech spectrograms shows promise, but before it could be endorsed or rejected for investigation of crimes, it is necessary to perform a comprehensive and independent study, including forensic models and variables not tested by Kersta."

Such a study (Tosi et al., 1972) was performed from 1968 to December 1970 at the Department of Audiology and Speech Sciences, Michigan State University, with funds granted by the United States Department of Justice. At the same time, a voice identification unit, headed by Nash, was created within the Michigan State Police, to study real life cases, in order to compare conditions and spectrograms obtained within these conditions with those obtained at the Tosi laboratory. It was agreed that no material from the Voice Identification Unit would be used as legal evidence during the period of experimentation.

In December 1970, results from the experiment were available. Error of false identifications within forensic models, forcing relatively naive examiners to reach a positive conclusion in all cases, was approximately 6.3%. Errors of false elimination within the same models was approximately 12.7% (as reported under studies by Tosi et al.). The Michigan State Police decided that these percentages, together with the experience gained by Nash in field cases during the last 3 years, granted the application of speech spectrograms to investigation of crimes. However, sine qua non conditions for forensic usage were that: 1) police examiners had to conduct aural examinations in addition to visual examinations in each case investigated; 2) they must be free to choose within five alternative answers after completing each examination (positive identification, positive elimination, probability of identification, probability of elimination, and no decision one way or the other); and 3) police examiners must use extreme caution, selecting the "no decision" alternative in all cases where they had the slightest doubt that the defendant was the same as the questioned person.

With these guidelines, the Voice Identification Unit of the Michigan State Police started offering voice identification evidence based on this combined aural and visual method throughout the United States and Canada. The first case in which this type of evidence was presented by the Crime Laboratory of Michigan State Police was *Minnesota v. Trimble* (December 1970). In this case Nash was able to eliminate 12 suspected persons, finally identifying Ms. Trimble as the person who made the telephone call instrumental in this murder case. The expert for the defense, Dr. Ladefoged, finally agreed with this identification, and Ms. Trimble confessed during the trial that she actually did make the call.

As a consequence of this case, his personal experiences, and the Tosi study, Dr. Ladefoged agreed that in some cases it is possible to identify persons by using the combined aural and visual examination of spectrograms (*U.S. v. Raymond*, 1971). Other recognized speech scientists like Drs. Henry Truby and John Black also agreed with these statements. This initial success and the success of other examinations that followed, including confessions from suspected persons identified by Nash, confirmed to the commanding officers of the Michigan State Police the usefulness of the Voice Identification Unit.

In 1971, Detective Wilson was transferred at his request from the Voice Identification Unit to his original fingerprint job. The Voice Identification Unit of the Michigan State Police Department was expanded with the incorporation of two new examiners, Detective Lonnie Smrkovski in 1971, and Detective Malcolm Hall in 1972. These two examiners were trained by Kersta and by Nash, and both, as Nash did, took courses of audiology and speech sciences at Michigan State University in order to improve their expertise in this area.

The Voice Identification Unit completed approximately 4,000 voice examination cases from December 1970 to May 1974. In approximately 65 cases, voice identification evidence was presented in court by Nash. Approximately 1,900 suspected voices were eliminated; for 1,500 voices no opinions or probabilities of identification or elimination were given after completing the examination (Nash, personal communication).

In June 1974, Nash was granted a leave of absence from the Michigan Department of State Police and was replaced by Detective Smrkovski as head of the Voice Identification Unit.

International Association of Voice Identification

After the creation of the Voice Identification Unit of the Michigan State Police, many law enforcement agencies felt the urge to create similar units. Since the Voiceprint Laboratories offered a 10-day training course in Voiceprint and spectrographs, available to anyone who could afford tuition, there began to be concern about the possibility that examiners with little experience would start offering legal evidence.

In order to establish qualifications of examiners, to avoid misuse of voice identification by untrained personnel, and to encourage research on this area, a nonprofit International Association of Voice Identification was incorporated in Michigan on 14 May 1971. Officers of this association for the period May 1971–May 1974 were: president, Lt. Ernest Nash; vice president, Dr. Oscar Tosi; and secretary-treasurer, detective Lonnie Smrkovski. Mr. Lawrence Kersta was elected president of the board and the lawyer for the Association was the Honorable Fred Stackable. However, Dr. Tosi resigned as director of the board and vice president on 16 May 1974 because of disagreement with procedures of the board and the president.

This association has three categories of associates: members, trainees, and friends. Members are those persons who qualify through a 2-year apprenticeship in real life cases under the supervision of a member, and who pass a theoretical-practical examination. Persons with an advanced degree in audiology and speech sciences are exempted from the theoretical examination. There was also a grandfather clause for the members Kersta, Nash, Tosi, and Ladefoged. Trainees are those associates completing their 2-year practical apprenticeship. There are no requirements to become a friend of the association.

The association has also appointed as honorary members some speech scientists who have produced outstanding contributions to the field of audiology and speech sciences. As of May 1974, the Association listed three honorary members, eight members, 12 trainees, and 14 friends.

In 1971, the House of Representatives and the Senate of Michigan issued a resolution commemorating the incorporation of the International Association of Voice Identification and commending the goals set by its bylaws.

Court Cases after 1970

Since the first case in which voice identification evidence based on aural and visual examination of spectrograms was presented by Nash in December 1970 (*Minnesota v. Trimble*), the Voice Identification Unit of the Michigan Department of State Police continued successfully to offer this type of evidence, with no major opposition or significant expert witnessing presented by the defense, until 1972.

In *California v. Hodo* (1972), the evidence presented by Nash was challenged by several scientists, who, besides expressing an adverse opinion on the reliability of the spectrograms in general, indicated that the samples utilized by Nash were too distorted to be of any practical value. The same situation occurred in the case *California v. Jackson* (1972). Also due to strong defense expert team, the prosecution opted to dismiss the case *U.S. v. O'Hara* in Orlando, Florida (1972). One of the points brought by the defense was that the FBI was not using speech spectrograms as evidence, meaning that the FBI considered them to be unreliable.

According to the opinions of some speech scientists, the absolute statements of Nash during some of the trials, as well as the poor samples used by this officer in some cases, produced such strong opposition from many of the persons employed by the defense as expert witness. Drs. Papcun and Ladefoged (1973) presented a paper at the 86th Meeting of the Acoustical Society reviewing two cases presented by Nash, criticizing samples used by this officer and discussing the court rulings. Poza (1974) published a paper including similar criticisms. Jones (1973, 1974), a professor of law, was also highly critical of using spectrograms in court cases; however, he did not have enough expertise on voice identification, as Drs. Ladefoged, Papcun and Poza did have, to produce solid criticism in this matter.

In August 1973, in *California v. Chapter,* the Court ruled that Nash had produced several errors in the evidence he presented. This was the first case where the evidence presented by Nash was not admitted by the Court. In March 1974, in the case of *Michigan v. Chaisson,* the court ordered Tosi to analyze the samples presented by Nash as evidence against the defendant. Tosi expressed that he was unable to use such samples to attempt any kind of examination. However, he was able to offer a probability of identification on the basis of new samples obtained from the defendant, ordered by the court. The prosecution then dismissed the case.

There was a kind of consensus among some persons that all these circumstances have jeopardized the position of the Voice Identification Unit and that a different approach than the one previously imparted should be taken in the future.

FUTURE OF VOICE IDENTIFICATION

Possibly, no combination of methods may ever produce absolutely positive identification or eliminations in 100% of the cases submitted. Reasonably, it could be stated that the better the quality and extension of available samples, the better the qualifications of the examiner, and the more comprehensive the cluster of methods used, the better the chance of obtaining reliable decisions in a large percentage of cases. Continuing research in this area, using both subjective and objective methods, is most desirable.

Criticism from several scientists against voiceprints, i.e. identification of speakers *exclusively* through speech spectrograms, is most reasonable if these critics mean rendering positive decision in 100% of the cases examined. As Bolt et al. (1973) have pointed out, there are distortions attributable to the speaker himself, the system of transmission and recording, environmental noise, and resonances that could interact very strongly against the ability of spectrograms to convey speaker-dependent features. It should be absolutely clear that this writer has never endorsed the reliability of speech spectrograms in 100% of the cases analyzed. From the very beginning (*Minnesota v. Trimble*, 1970) he carefully has circumscribed in court the restrictions and standards that must be maintained to use subjective methods of voice identification, namely, combination of aural and visual examinations, five alternative decisions after each examination, including "no decision" one way or the other, extension and quality samples, training, and professional honesty of the examiner (Black et al. 1973; Tosi et al., 1972).

These restrictions and standards simply mean that any sample distorted by the psychological or physical condition of the subject, or by the transmission and recording systems, must automatically yield a "no decision" or probabilities, but never a positive identification. On the other hand, both combined methods, the aural and the visual ones, are subjective, and therefore their reliability depends heavily on the examiner. If the examiner fails to maintain the high standards and thresholds required for a minimal reliability, subjective methods are prone to fail completely.

Practical forensic experience will dictate whether aural and visual examinations in actual life cases should be complemented with semiautomatic methods and whether the examiner should be periodically tested to determine his receiver operating characteristic, in order to satisfy the critical requirements for voice identification reliability.

REFERENCES

Atal, B. 1972. Automatic speaker recognition based on pitch contours. J. Acoust. Soc. Amer. 52: 1687–1697.

Becker, R. W., F. R. Clark, F. Poza, and R. J. Young. 1972. A semiautomatic speaker recognition system. Stanford Research Institute Report 1363, Stanford, Cal.

Black, J. W. 1937. The quality of a spoken vowel. Arch. Speech. 2: 7–27.

Black, J. W., W. Lashbrook, E. Nash, H. Oyer, C. Pedrey, O. Tosi, and H. Truby. Reply to speaker identification by speech spectrograms: some further observations. J. Acoust. Soc. Amer. 54: 535–537.

Bolt, R., F. Cooper, E. David, P. Denes, J. Pickett, and K. Stevens. Speaker identification by speech spectrograms: some further observations. J. Acoust. Soc. Amer. 54: 531–534.

Bordone, C., R. Dubes, R. Pisani, G. Sacerdote, and O. Tosi. 1974. Invariances of talkers' choral spectra. Presented at 87th Meeting of the Acoustical Society of America, April 23–26, New York.

Bricker, P., and S. Prozansky. 1966. Effect of stimulus content and duration on talker identification. J. Acoust. Soc. Amer. 40: 1441–1449.

Daniloff, R. G., and R. E. Hammarberg. 1973. On definition of coarticulation. J. Phonet. 1: 185–194.

Egan, J., A. Schulman, and G. Greenberg. 1959. Operating characteristics determined by binary decisions and by ratings. J. Acoust. Soc. Amer. 31: 768–773.

Gray, C. H., and G. A. Kopp. 1944. Voiceprint identification. Bell Telephone Laboratories Report, pp. 13–14, New Jersey.

Green, D., and J. Swetts. 1966. Signal Detection and Psychophysics, pp. 404–408. John Wiley & Sons, New York.

Hair, G., and T. Rekieta. 1972. Speaker identification final report. Stanford Research Institute Report 1363. Stanford, Cal.

Hazen, B. 1973. Effects of different phonetic contexts on spectrographic speaker identification. J. Acoust. Soc. Amer. 54: 650–660.

Hecker, M. 1971. Speaker recognition: An interpretative survey of the literature. ASHA Monogr. 16: 82–86.

Holmgren, G. 1967. Physical and psychological correlates of speaker recognition. J. Speech Hear. Res. 10: 57–66.

Jones W. 1973. Danger–Voiceprints ahead. Amer. Crim. Law Rev. 11: 549–573.

Jones, W. 1974. Evidence vel non. The non sense of Voiceprint identification. Kentucky Law J. 62: 301–326.

Kamine, B. S. 1969. The voiceprint technique: Its structure and reliability. San Diego Law Rev. 6: 213–241.

Kersta, L. G. 1962. Voiceprint identification. Nature 196: 1253–1257.

Ladefoged, P., and R. Vanderslice. 1967. The voiceprint mystique. Working Papers in Phonetics. Vol. 7. University of California, Los Angeles.

Li, K., and G. Hughes, 1974. Talker differences as they appear in correlation matrices of continuous speech spectra. J. Acoust. Soc. Amer. 55: 883–837.

Li, K., G. Hughes, and A. House. 1969. Correlation characteristics and dimensionality of speech spectra. J. Acoust. Soc. Amer. 46: 1019–1025.

McGehee, F. 1937. The reliability of the identification of the human voice. J. Gen. Psychol. 17: 249–271.

McGehee, F. 1944. An experimental study of voice recognition. J. Gen. Psychol. 31: 53–65.

Papcun, G., and P. Ladefoged. 1973. Two voiceprint cases. Presented at the 85th Meeting of the Acoustical Society of America, November 10–15, Los Angeles.

Pollack, I., J. Pickett, and W. Sumby. 1954. On the identification of speakers by voice. J. Acoust. Soc. Amer. 26: 403–406.

Potter, R., G. Kopp, and H. Green. 1947. Visible Speech. Van Nostrand, New York. Reprinted (1966) by Dover, New York.

Poza, F. 1974. Voice Print Identification: Its Forensic Application. Proceedings of the Carnahan Crime Countermeasures Conference, University of Kentucky, Lexington.

Presti, A. J. 1966. High-speed sound spectrograph. J. Acoust. Soc. Amer. 40: 628–634.

Stevens, K., A. S. House, and A. P. Paul. 1966. Acoustical description of syllabic nuclei: An interpretation in terms of a dynamic model of articulation. J. Acoust. Soc. Amer. 40: 123–132.

Stevens, K. N., C. E. Williams, J. R. Carbonell, and B. Woods. 1968. Speaker authentication and identification: A comparison of spectrographic and auditory presentation of speech material. J. Acoust. Soc. Amer. 44: 1596–1607.

Su, L., and K. Fu. 1973. Automatic speaker identification using nasal spectra and nasal coarticulation as acoustic clues. Report from the Purdue University School of Electrical Engineering. TR-EE 73-33. Air Force Office of Scientific Research Grant 69-1776. Lafayette, Ind.

Tarnóczy, T. 1958. Détermination du spectre de la parile avec une méthode nouvelle. Acustica 8: 392–395.

Tosi, O. 1967. Report to Michigan department of state police. Also presented at 1968 International Congress of Logopedics and Phoniatrics, Paris, France.

Tosi, O., H. Oyer, W. Lashbrook, C. Pedrey, J. Nicol, and E. Nash. 1972. Experiment on voice identification. J. Acoust. Soc. Amer. 51: 2030–2043.

Voiers, W. 1964. Perceptual bases of speaker identity. J. Acoust. Soc. Amer. 36: 1065–1073.

Wolf, J. 1972. Efficient acoustic parameters for speaker recognition. J. Acoust. Soc. Amer. 51: 2044–2056.

Young, M., and R. Campbell. 1967. Effects of contexts on talker identification. J. Acoust. Soc. Amer. 42: 1250–1254.

The Measurement of Parameters of Speech Underwater: A Unique Application of Speech Science

Russell L. Sergeant, Ph.D. [1]
Associate Professor
Communication Sciences Program
School of Health Science
Hunter College of the City University of New York

CONTENTS

INTRODUCTION

Speech science applies to the study of vocal communications in many different situations. Those related to disordered speech are probably the most familiar to speech pathologists and audiologists. To speech scientists, the ability of swimmers and deep sea divers to communicate effectively by voice is a unique area for study. With recent emphasis upon underwater work in general, there has been a tremendous growth in research activity related to underwater communication by voice. Although not nearly so publicized as

[1] Formerly with Naval Submarine Medical Research Laboratory, Groton, Connecticut.

433

the lunar voyages of the past 2 decades, recent undersea ventures have been extremely difficult and hazardous encounters with an unfamiliar environment. Vocal communication is important to these types of operations.

Missions Under the Sea

The oceans attract man for a variety of reasons. With energy crises and dismal forecasts of oil depletions in the foreseeable future, there is a vigorous search for new sources of fuel from beneath the oceans. The diver is an important member of teams that set up and maintain large, complex oil-drilling structures such as those seen in the Gulf of Mexico off the Texas and Florida coasts. It is natural that oceanologists also have utilized the capabilities of divers and swimmers to study the oceans. With the convenience of scuba (self-contained underwater breathing apparatus), many people follow hobbies which lead them to the water to fish, collect rocks, or whatever. In other more economic adventures, divers and swimmers conduct underwater salvage and repair tasks, not to mention the routine performance of military operations.

Because of the added interests in underwater activities, continuing investigations have been made of man's ability to exist and work within the sea. Underwater life support systems are studied by physiologists, psychologists, medical researchers, and others interested specifically in how man functions in the abnormal, stressful, hazardous, and exotic environments typical of the world under the sea. This work is being done by scientists whose special programs of research are aimed at gathering basic information about all aspects of human performance, including that of underwater communication.

Man Underwater

There are six basic ways that man gets into the water. First, he can simply go swimming. In this case, he relies on what Mother Nature has given him. He is restricted, with rare exception, to shallow depths for short periods of time, and in fact spends most of his time splashing around on top of the water. For this, speech occurs above water.

In the second method, man wears scuba gear which enables him to submerge for much longer periods of time to depths of 100 feet or so. Some equipment permits communication, but often there is no communication at all. For the third way, man dons a special diving hard hat attached to a deep sea diver's suit and is lowered on a tethered line to depths from the surface to 1,600 feet. Specially regulated breathing mixtures are supplied through the tethered line, which also carries a hard wire communication link. Speech deteriorates progressively for the deep sea diver at greater depths and with the introduction of exotic gas mixtures.

Vehicles for underwater use can transport divers from one location to another at far greater speeds than those of normal swimming. In addition, these vehicles can carry other devices such as cameras, communication equipment, and so forth. This fourth way of being underwater is specially useful to television crews, military groups, explorers, or anyone interested in traveling long distances underwater.

Undersea habitats make up a fifth category. A habitat is a large steel container which is lowered to the bottom of the sea, and the pressure inside is equal to that on the outside. Convenient access hatches allow swimmers to go easily from the hyperbaric gas environment inside to the pressurized water outside. Figure 1 is an artist's conception of a habitat on the floor of the ocean. Hyperbaric pressure chambers located at various diving installations have basically the same characteristics as undersea habitats except that the chamber is not lowered into the water and the pressure outside is normal. This category illustrates two different speaking situations; one within a hyperbaric gaseous atmosphere and the other submersed in pressurized water.

The sixth way man is able to stay underwater is to ride in a submarine or diving bell. However, because the atmosphere inside is highly regulated to be identical with normal atmospheric conditions, the resultant speech is normal and thus has little bearing on undersea speech and its resultant complications.

Once again, the purpose of this chapter is to present a unique application of the field of speech science to problems associated with talking in under-

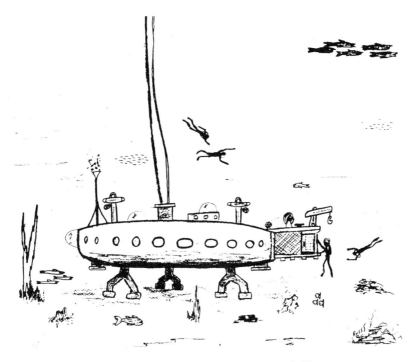

Figure 1. Artist's conception of an undersea habitat.

water environments. Conditions are described under which deep sea divers, swimmers, and scuba divers communicate by voice. The major effects on production and perception of speech are considered, and current methods used to counteract undesirable effects are reviewed.

SOURCES OF SPEECH DISTORTION

The causes of distortion to the speech of swimmers and divers depends to a large extent on the diving situation in which the talker finds himself. These causes can be organized according to the following categories: psychological, interference by noise, increased pressure effects, breathing gas mixture, intermittent back pressures, and equipment. In any single diving situation several different categories usually combine to reduce communicability.

The effects of psychological factors are difficult to describe and more difficult to place in their proper perspective. Apprehension and experience are of paramount importance to individual differences among divers, including their ability to talk well. Operations underwater can be dangerous and loaded with mental and physical strains. Good communications during such times can be vital. For example, in the emergency where the diver's life line is accidentally cut, he must be either raised to the surface immediately or provided with an alternative source of breathing gas. Communication could ensure his recovery.

Nevertheless, it is well known that the speech of deep sea divers all but disappears as he is lowered below about 100 feet into the water. The cause of this absence of any practical communication is the difficulty in implementing a reliable and effective voice communication system. Protocols that the deep sea diver must follow during his time of submergence are typically written so that there is little or no need for verbal activity, not so much because speech would not help, but because acceptable communication by voice either does not exist or is unreliable. Although the presence of tension, stress, and apprehension is recognized, psychological factors are much less debilitating to either the talker or listener than are other direct causes of distortion to speech underwater.

High levels of unwanted noise are characteristic of hyperbaric chambers and interfere with speech perception. During periods when the atmosphere within the chamber is compressed or decompressed rapidly, there is intense noise caused by gas moving through valves and pipe openings. The noise, similar to white noise, can be so loud that hearing conservation measures must be followed. Luckily the periods of intense noise are short. Although some communication by voice is possible with microphones and earphones specifically designed for use under noisy conditions, most talking can and does wait for the much longer periods of relative quiet.

Another example of interference by high levels of noise exists inside the deep sea diver's helmet. Much lower in intensity than the noise of pressure chambers, the breathing gas produces a loud hissing as it enters the helmet. When combined with the diver's speech and picked up by the microphone inside the helmet, there is a very poor speech-to-noise (S/N) ratio, and intelligibility suffers. A simple method for improving the situation is to instruct the diver to talk more loudly and clearly, therby improving the S/N ratio of the signal that reaches the listener at the surface. However, the noise still interferes with reception within the helmet by the diver. Other examples of external noise, such as from ships passing overhead, waves and surf, underwater tools and equipment, etc., rarely pose serious difficulty to underwater voice communications.

The two major determinants of serious deterioration to speech in hyperbaric environments are the increase in ambient pressure and the mixture of gas breathed by the diver. Both pressure and gas mixture alter the ability of the talker to generate normal speech. When the deep sea diver descends to depths below approximately 100 feet, breathing air causes an elated feeling accompanied by disorganized behavior similar to that of a drunk person. This nitrogen narcosis has been called "rapture of the deep" and leads to the "rule of the martini," which states that every increase of 1 atmospheric pressure absolute (equivalent to increasing depth by 33 feet) is equivalent to imbibing one martini.

Diving physiologists interested in eliminating the consequent dangerous behavior associated with breathing compressed air discovered that replacement of the nitrogen in air with helium stops narcosis. However, helium introduces drastic changes to the voice such that men sound like little boys. This speech has been popularly called "Donald Duck" speech. In addition to a change in the voice quality of helium speech, there is an accompanying degradation in intelligibility that is exacerbated by conditions of increased pressure. A more detailed account of the effects of pressure and gas mixture is presented later.

Have you ever tried yelling when you were swimming underwater? Results are poor! Among other things there are very rapid alterations in the amount of pressure into which you shout. A similar situation exists when the scuba swimmer speaks into his facemask. Various degrees of back pressures build up and quickly fade away inside the hoses just outside his mouth. The demand valve which regulates the breathing gas to the diver effects the pressure. Little is known about the specific damage to speech that these intermittent back pressures cause, but there is no question that they interfere with the normal outflow of voice from the vocal tract, and thereby interfere with the ability of the scuba diver to generate clear and distinct speech.

Most of the distortions to speech discussed thus far concern the talker's ability to produce speech. Another type of distortion is equipment oriented. Electronic components of underwater voice communication systems suffer from the same kinds of malfunction as do other communication systems. However, they additionally must be able to withstand the unusual disturbances of pressure and humidity. The microphones designed for pressure chambers do not need special waterproofing, but they must function properly at pressures ranging from normal to over 30 times normal atmospheric pressures. Microphones carried by scuba divers must be waterproofed, rugged, and matched to the acoustic characteristics of the facemask enclosure. When helium speech must be processed, the microphone must respond to frequencies higher than usual and under hyperbaric conditions. Otherwise, necessary information for processing words like "thank" and "sank" or "fix" and "six" is missing. Often the failure to select a proper microphone has rendered unscramblers ineffectual.

Earphones used by swimmers and divers have not been a major source of difficulty to voice communications since the primary change in output of receivers under hyperbaric conditions is one of intensity. This is easily controlled with a volume knob. Of course waterproofing techniques must be applied to receivers for them to function properly. In general, the problems of communicating by voice in underwater environments are more closely associated with the talker's inadequate generation of speech and the capability of the microphone to properly pick up that speech, rather than the adequacy of the receiver.

The above sources of speech distortion can act independently or in combination with each other, depending on the dive. For   example, the speech of a scuba diver swimming around a habitat located several hundred feet below the surface would be affected by the psychological aspects of the task, pressure and gas mixture, possible distortion from back pressures in his facemask, and very likely some unpredictable equipment inadequacies. Nevertheless, with proper selection and use of equipment, including a good helium speech unscrambler, the diver's speech can be understood by others in spite of the usual difficulties associated with the unusual environment and the generation of abnormal speech.

SHALLOW WATER PROBLEMS

Communication problems among bathers do not exist. During the brief periods that they swim beneath the surface they do not speak because they have no need to. When floating or swimming on top of the water, or just standing with their heads above water, they can and do talk. Scuba swimmers, on the other hand, spend more time completely submerged, and the need to communicate may be great. Without means to communicate vocally, standard hand signals and gestures may help, but poor visibility at increased depths, muddy water, or darkness can easily preclude the possibility of communicating visually. Of course, the diver could shout directly into the water, but this technique produces severely distorted and unintelligible speech, and furthermore, is limited to distances of several feet.

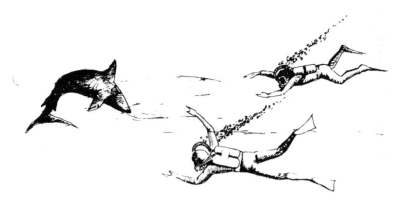

Figure 2. Scuba divers.

Small enclosures with a mouth opening on one end and a diaphragm on the other have been designed for divers. They operate on the principle of minimizing the acoustic mismatch of impedance for signals which pass from air into the water. However, the improvement afforded by these units over directly shouting into the water is questionable. Serious communication by shouting either directly or through a special device into water is impractical.

The advent of scuba equipment has enabled free-swimming divers, such as the two shown in Figure 2, to spend longer periods of time underwater. With early versions the diver held a bit located at the end of the air hose between his gums. Needless to say, the scuba mouthpiece precludes talking. Full facemasks and later oral-nasal masks were improvements which allowed installation of small microphones and more free movement of the human speaking mechanism, but very special requirements for diver microphones were not immediately recognized. By 1957, the United States Navy had designed its first underwater voice communication system for fleetwide use. It was basically a redesign of different components typically found in other communication systems. Elkins (1972) described this initial system as "a masterpiece of packaging for this era but (it) provided an intelligibility of less than 14 percent."

By the mid 1960's commercial companies foresaw future marketing possibilities for an effective means for divers and swimmers to speak to one another. Consequently, new systems began to appear in diving equipment catalogs. Aquasonics[2] was probably the first company to design a scuba mouthpiece specifically for purposes of voice communication. Speech produced in their Nautilus mask was 70% intelligible according to evaluations by the Navy (see Elkins, 1972), but physiologically the diver was exposed to hazards of carbon dioxide build-up in his breathing mixture.

[2] Now affiliated with Hydro Products, San Diego, California.

During the past decade further improvements to shallow water voice communication systems were developed, but the major emphasis was less toward improving the intelligibility of speech as counteracting problems in wiring, waterproofing, increased distance of aquatic transmission, reliability, size, costs, etc. Today, communication systems can be purchased which can provide understandable speech to and from divers, but transmissions through the water, unless via wire, are limited to distances of several hundred yards.

DEEP WATER PROBLEMS

Deep water diving refers to dives at depths from 200 feet to depths near 1,500 feet. Problems encountered are more abundant and severe than those for swimmers and shallow water divers, and include distortions to speech caused by very high ambient pressures as well as different mixtures of breathing gas.

Hard Hat Diving

In 1869, the familiar deep sea diver's helmet shown in Figure 3 was designed. A voice communication capability was added in 1925. It consisted of a transceiver located inside the helmet and connected by wire to an amplifier unit with its loudspeaker or earphones located at the diving control station. Except for this important addition, there has been almost no change in the initially designed hard hat.

At depths less than 100 feet, the deep sea diver can be understood fairly well on the surface receiver using the old 1925-style communication system. However, to maintain reliable and secure communications at greater depths, the diver usually reverts to standard diving signals similar to the sign language of deaf persons when he is working with another diver, or to pulls on a rope to signal people at the surface. As noted, tasks for deep sea divers were typically organized to minimize communication of any kind. Experience, training, and intensive preplanning were the alternatives to the preferred luxury of control through use of highly dependable voice communication capabilities.

After the long history of minimal changes to the hard hat designed in 1869, new models having significant improvements and looking quite different are now appearing from different companies. In addition to the lightweight characteristics of fiberglass and the all around visibility provided by plexiglass, more recent advances in microphones and unscramblers of helium speech are being incorporated into the latest voice communication systems. Although many needs for improved underwater capability to communicate continue, major advances in the state-of-the-art have changed the overall picture during the last decade. For example, a diver submerged to a depth of 600 feet on helium and oxygen could not be understood in 1968 even by

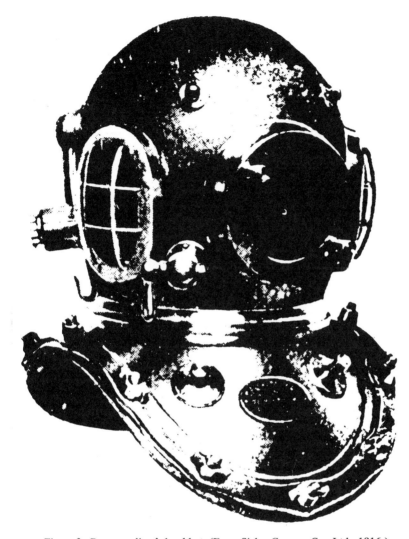

Figure 3. Deep sea diver's hard hat. (From Siebe, Gorman Co., Ltd., 1916.)

other experienced divers. Intelligibility tests of such speech produced mean scores below 20%. Today, test results of 95% for speech recorded from depths to 1,500 feet are possible.

Hyperbaric Pressure Chambers

Rooms that can be pressurized from one to many times normal atmospheric pressures are used to medically treat gangrene and decompression sickness. People are taught techniques of diving inside these rooms, and scientists conduct research in various aspects of diving operations in them. Called hyperbaric pressure chambers, these rooms are located at diving installations and in some well equipped hospitals. Figure 4 is a view looking into one of these chambers. Communications inside are influenced by the noise level of incoming or escaping gases, reverberations from the inner steel walls, the ambient pressure, introduction of helium-rich breathing mixtures, and the choice of the individual components comprising the communication system.

In most underwater communication situations, the receiver poses little or no difficulty. The diver's ability to generate normal and acceptable speech does change, and that is a primary source of difficulty in communicating by voice in deep sea diving operations and within hyperbaric pressure chambers. The selection of a microphone must be consistent with these changes of diver's speech. In addition, it must function properly under the extreme ambient pressure. Although noise-cancelling microphones should eliminate the effects of loud noise, the high levels produced by air-venting noises during compression and decompression inside the chamber usually preclude adequate communicaton with divers inside. Even face-to-face communicating during these intense levels of noise is visual, not acoustic.

As previously mentioned, deterioration of speech under conditions of high ambient pressure occurs during the generation of speech. The difficulty is not in the transmission of good speech through the gas medium or reception by the listener, but in the actual formulation of speech sounds by

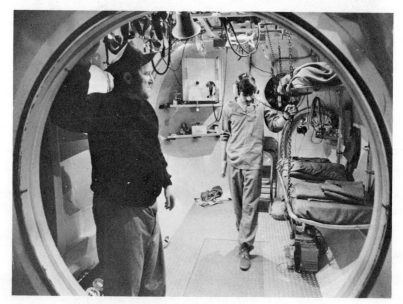

Figure 4. View looking into a hyperbaric pressure chamber.

the talker. Some people believe that special microphones, for instance a throat microphone, can eliminate the difficulty. This is as absurd as trying to correct a lisper's faulty "s" the same way. A more favorable S/N ratio is obtained with a noise-cancelling microphone, and consequently the more easily heard speech is more intelligible. However, the basic alteration of the diver's speech, which occurs in the generating of it, is caused by increase in pressure and the presence of helium. These alterations are not influenced by the selection of the microphone.

There continues to be a need to change the diver's speech back to something which not only sounds more normal but is also more intelligible. This suggests that training to speak more normally under these conditions of distortion would be appropriate. However, training and experience produce very minor improvement. A better approach is to develop a means to unscramble divers' gibberish. Devices designed to do just that are considered later under the section on correcting helium speech.

Undersea Habitats

Along with exotic explorations to the very depths of the oceans, the concept naturally arose to inhabit that exotic world and build cities under the sea. Man could build houses and buildings where he could eat, sleep, work, and play, all within the confines of artificial atmospheres, swimming out periodically to harvest the wonders of the sea. If he lived in one of these hyperbaric dwellings, the problem of decompression after forays into the water would be solved. Dreams of this sort became a possibility after pioneers such as Cousteau and Bond conducted experiments in which man stayed for days, weeks, and longer inside pressure chambers placed upon the ocean's floor.

For the speech scientist there was the challenge produced by the need for effective communication by voice inside and around these habitats. In fact, the problems were not unlike those already being investigated for the deep sea diver or people working within pressure chambers located on land. An umbilical cord provides life support, breathing gas, power, and communication links to the undersea chambers. Microphones do not need to be as waterproof as the ones for the deep sea diver or swimmer, but they must have extended frequency response and be immune to effects of high ambient pressure. In addition, an unscrambling device is required when helium is part of the breathing atmosphere.

MEASUREMENT OBSTACLES

The speech scientist's standards for accuracy in the study of the acoustics of speech are very high. Noise levels, frequency response of earphones and microphones, spectrum analyses of the voice, and other measurements demand highly calibrated instruments, and the collection of information or data must follow precisely controlled procedures. Very often, a secondary calibration can be used to evaluate one instrument with another that has previously undergone precise calibration. For example, it is not unusual to compare a microphone scheduled to collect experimental data with another which has been accurately calibrated at the factory where it was manufactured. However, when measurements are to be made under hyperbaric conditions during the experiment, then secondary calibration techniques such as this are unacceptable. The response of the typical laboratory microphone is usually based on performance under normal atmospheric pressures; this is inappropriate to the underwater situation. Further difficulties arise because the special procedures for performing primary calibrations are difficult to implement.

Because of the difficult problems in measurement, Sergeant and Murry (1971) and Thomas, Preslar, and Farmer (1972) devoted substantial time and effort first determining and later following techniques which would yield accurate information about the performance of microphones under hyperbaric atmospheres typical of deep sea environments. They did that work not because of an interest in the techniques of calibration per se, but to pursue accurately their more basic research interests in underwater speech and hearing.

One has to be constantly alert to the uniqueness of underwater operations whenever equipment is considered. Components must be protected from wetness and increased ambient pressure. Many preliminary problems must be solved in order to conduct meaningful research. At the University of Florida (Gainesville, Fla.), Hollien (Hollien and Tolhurst, 1969) developed a divers communication research system (DICORS), which incorporated precision instrumentation in an underwater apparatus to allow experimental control of subject position, stimulus presentation, and subject response. Figure 5 shows DICORS assembled on land for later submersion into water for an experiment. A monitoring TV camera allows the experimenter to observe the submerged subject from a dry control room. In addition to studies of divers' speech performance, DICORS has been utilized to evaluate different commercially available underwater voice communication systems.

Several points must be considered in order to collect adequate samples of speech from submerged divers during research projects. The transmission of instructions to the subject is difficult, especially if movement is to be limited and the head held at a particular axis. Simple methods of presenting instructions and stimuli to the subject have to be devised. In one technique typewritten material is sealed between two plexiglass sheets. Special subject response switches that are unaffected by moisture or pressure are valuable. For acceptable research to be conducted in the area of underwater voice communications, specific techniques associated with diving operations and familiarity with associated equipment must be fully and carefully melded with required procedures and basic knowledge of speech science.

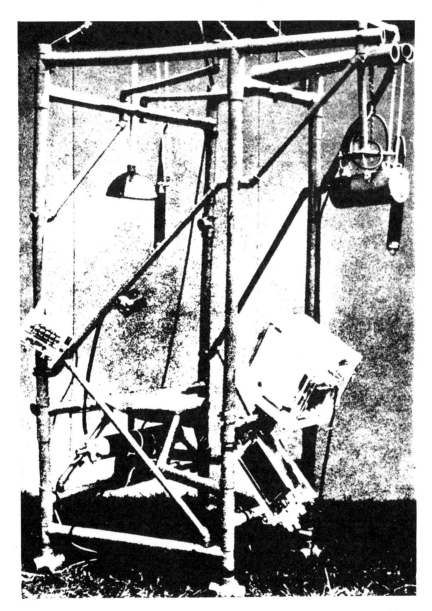

Figur 5. Diver Communications Research System (DICORS) developed at the University of Florida. (From Hollien, Rothman and Feinstein, 1973.)

SPEECH DISTORTIONS CAUSED BY THE SPEAKING MEDIUM

The two major causes of distortion to the deep sea diver's speech are oriented to the medium within which he talks. Undesirable changes in his speech occur when the atmosphere is at very high levels of ambient pressure and when it is made up of exotic breathing mixtures, typically rich in helium. Both factors interfere with the talker's ability to generate proper speech.

Effects of High Pressure

Effects of pressure can be heard in the diver's speech as he descends to depths of about 100 feet or greater. The quality of his voice becomes nasal and crisp. In contrast to the transposition of acoustic spectrum caused by helium, Fant (Fant and Sonesson, 1964; Fant et al., 1971) theorized that the lower limit of the natural frequency of resonance for the human vocal tract is drastically raised as ambient pressure increases. There is a shunting of acoustic energy through the walls of the vocal tract such that the location of the first formant is restricted to the upper part of its normal range.

Using Fant's formula, Sergeant (unpublished data) determined the lower limiting frequency, F_m, for the average adult male. He then compared these values first with predictions based on the hypothesis that formants remain the same for increased pressure provided that the gas mixture is the same, and also with measurements of the formant centers of speech produced by divers who breathed air at normal atmospheric pressure and under pressures equivalent to 300 feet underwater. Figure 6 shows the results. The broken diagonal line represents no change in formant position from the surface to 300 feet. The plotted data show that formants, low and high, had a minor shift upward of about 175 Hz when pressure increased to the 300-foot level. Note how the line of fit for the data points bends upward at the lower ends of the frequency scales, so that if the line were continued it would pass over the point of the calculated F_m. None of the data points is lower than that calculated point.

Fant et al. (1971) presents a similar figure using data from a diver who was breathing a mixture of helium, nitrogen, and oxygen inside a pressurized chamber. It shows the same upward shift at the lower frequencies, further supporting his theory of the minimal possible frequency of resonance in the human vocal tract. Sergeant (unpublished data) evaluated spectrograms of specific vowels produced by divers as they breathed air, first on the surface and later within a chamber pressurized to 300 feet. As the pressure increased from normal to the hyperbaric condition, measurements of the locations of the first formants of vowels that normally have low ones, [i] and [u], revealed a marked upward shift to positions just above the calculated lower limits. On the other hand, vowels such as [ae] and [a], whose first formants usually lie well above the lower limit, did not have a similar upward shift. Instead they only shifted about the same amount as all other formants, i.e., 175 Hz. Apparently, the lower limiting frequency acted to shift just the lowest formants of speech.

The acoustic changes noted above interfere with the intelligibility of speech. Transitions between vowels and consonants are affected, as is the perception of specific phonemes. When a talker descends from surface pres-

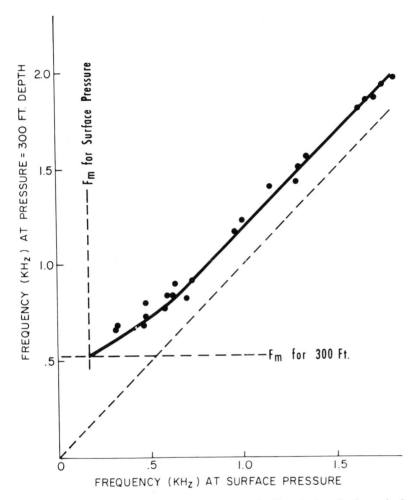

Figure 6. Measurements of the formants of speech. The abscissa is the scale for measurements obtained at normal atmospheric pressure, and the ordinate is for speech at pressures equivalent to 300-foot submersion in water. Each plotted point represents two measurements, one at each ambient pressure. The broken horizontal line indicates the lower limiting frequency (F_m) of natural resonance of the vocal tract at 300 feet. The broken vertical line indicates F_m at the surface. The broken diagonal line theorizes no shift in the speech formants for increase in ambient pressure.

sures to pressures found 250 feet below the surface, and he continues to breathe air, intelligibility scores drop from 95% to slightly below 75%. If the breathing mixture also changes, as is usual for deep sea conditions, deterioration to speech becomes even more severe. Interestingly, the semivowels [r], [l], and [w] are not significantly affected by increases in pressure alone. By contrast, a significant loss in intelligibility occurs for [b] and [tʃ], with responses dropping below 50% for compressed air at 250 feet. Sounds which are relatively difficult to discriminate at normal atmospheric pressures do not change appreciably as pressure increases. They just continue to rank low in relative phonemic intelligibility.

When considering the above type of information, theoretical implications for constructing special vocabularies for use in deep submergence diving must be made with caution because helium is usually added to breathing mixtures for deeper diving. In fact, one rarely encounters situations in which divers breathe pure mixtures of air at depths greater than approximately 100 feet. Consequently, the effect of hyperbaric conditions upon the perception of speech usually is confounded with breathing gas.

Effects of Breathing Mixtures

To counteract the unsatisfactory use of air, inert helium is added to the diver's breathing mix. Physiologically, narcosis and other problems are solved. Unfortunately, the helium causes a deterioration to the diver's speech by raising the spectrum of his voice about an octave, the so-called "Donald Duck" speech.

Acoustic analysis of helium speech shows that fundamental periodicity does not change. The rate of vocal fold vibration is approximately the same. Figure 7 contains two spectrographs of speech, one generated while the talker breathed air, the other while he breathed helium and oxygen. The formants

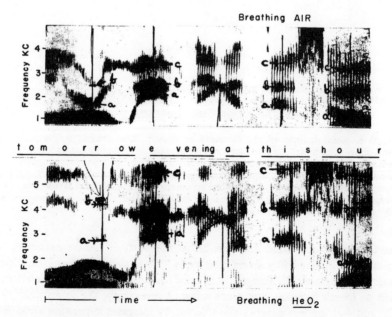

Figure 7. Spectrograms of speech in air and in a mixture of helium and oxygen. (From Sergeant, 1963.)

for the helium speech are approximately one half octave above those for air. Because the cavities of the vocal tract determine the natural resonance frequencies which make up the acoustic spectrum of vowels, it is possible to determine what physical changes in the speaking mechanism pertinent to vocal output will take place as the diver's breathing mixture changes from air to helium. If he remains at normal atmospheric pressure, the size, shape, and other dimensions of the cavities are identical. In fact, the only significant change is in the gases within the vocal tract. This change from exhaled air to helium increases the velocity of sound within the resonating cavities, and consequently, the natural frequencies of resonance in the voice spectrum shift upward. It is possible to calculate that shift in frequency of the formants by determining the two velocities of sound from basic information about the two exhaled gases. The following formula determines the velocity, c, of sound in a gaseous medium:

$$c = \sqrt{\frac{\Upsilon P_o}{d}}$$

where Υ is the ratio of specific heats for a gas, P_o is ambient pressure, and d is the density of the gas. Then the shift in formant frequency can be calculated from the two velocities with the following formula:

$$\frac{c_x}{c_{\text{air}}} = \frac{F_x}{F_{\text{air}}}$$

where c is the velocity of sound in a gaseous medium, F is the formant frequency, and the subscripts x and air refer to a breathing mixture of the gas under study and of air. Simply, the ratio of velocities of sound in any gas to air equals the ratio of formants of speech produced in that gas to formants in air. Remembering that we are interested here in the expired gas mixtures contained within the vocal tract, it is possible to calculate the shift in formant frequencies from two pieces of information. One is a precise knowledge of the composition of the two expired gases, and the other is information about certain basic properties of those gases.

To test the above theories of shift in formant frequencies, evaluations were made of the speech of divers breathing air, helium and oxygen (Heliox), nitrogen and oxygen (Nitrox), and hydrogen and oxygen (Hydrox). Table 1 summarizes the data according to measurements of formant centers, calculated velocity ratios, and tests of intelligibility. Through the use of breath-by-breath analyses during talking, the theory of upward shift in formants is supported. It is presumed that deterioration in speech is a direct result of these acoustic changes.

At normal atmospheric pressures, helium speech sounds very different from normal speech, and the ability to recognize different talkers disappears.

Table 1. Relations among gas mixture, velocity of sound, formants of speech, and intelligibility of speech[a]

Gas mixture and depth	Calculated velocity ratio (gas to air)	Measured formant ratio (gas to air)	Speech intelligibility (%)
Air, surface	1.00	1.00	70
Heliox, 200 feet	2.44	2.40	32
Hydrox, 200 feet	2.44[b]	2.40	36
Nitrox, 200 feet	1.00	1.07	59

[a]From Sergeant (1973).
[b]Assumes 4.5% nitrogen contamination.

However, the intelligibility is excellent if high fidelity microphones are used or if the communication is face to face. Cooke and Beard (1965) noted that speech intelligibility did not depreciate with helium mixtures at altitudes as high as 35,000 feet. However, with the increases in ambient pressure to which divers are exposed, there is progressively more marked deterioration, to the point that beyond depths of 600 feet perception is completely obliterated without the aid of a helium-speech processor.

Noise can affect speech perception in two ways. It can be present at the listener's ear producing a poor S/N ratio there, or it can be at the talker's ear, where it interferes with his internal auditory feedback mechanism as he monitors the production of his speech. McKay and Sergeant (1968) studied the effects of noise at the listener's ear and found no difference in intelligibility scores for speech in air and helium, provided that the noise level was relatively soft (S/N > +5 dB) or loud (S/N < −15 dB). The speech was either highly intelligible or unintelligible. With moderate levels of noise, the intelligibility of the helium speech deteriorated more rapidly than did the speech in air. At an S/N of −5 dB, the helium speech was 10 percentage points less intelligible. Although the difference is small, the point is demonstrated that helium speech is more susceptible to interference by noise than is normal speech.

The effects of helium and masked auditory feedback upon speech perception were studied by Willott and Sergeant (1968). Subjects visually monitored their voice levels with a VU meter to determine a comfortable speaking level in a quiet room. Later they used the VU meter to speak at that same level while their ears were exposed via earphones to random noise at a 95-dB sound pressure level re 0.0002 dyne/cm^2. Care was taken to ensure that the noise inside the phones did not reach the talker's microphone. Talkers' speech was recorded when they read aloud material from intelligibility tests first with 95-dB noise in their earphones, and later with that noise turned off. This was done when they breathed air and when they breathed an 80:20 mixture of helium and oxygen. The recorded materials were combined electronically with random noise for presentation to listening panels in order to eliminate ceiling effects.

Results showed that for both the air and helium conditions, masking noise at the talkers' ears improved their intelligibility scores by 10 percentage points. Camp (1956) also found an increase in talker intelligibility when loud masking noise was introduced at the ears. Apparently, loud noise triggers a mechanism which makes people speak more precisely.

The upward shift of energy in the spectrum of helium speech suggests the possibility of selectively filtering out unwanted noise with a resultant improvement to perception. However, Sergeant (1966) found that no condition of filtering increases intelligibility above that resulting from the use of a high quality system with no filtering. Helium speech, like speech in air, is quite distortion-resistant to effects of filtering.

The acoustic spectrum of divers' speech is affected by increased pressure during deep dives as well as by the introduction of helium into the breathing mixture. Considering the importance of the acoustic nature of speech to perception, Murry, Sergeant, and Angermeier (1970) conducted comparative sutides of the nature and severity of phonemic confusions in diving environments. Their purpose was to determine the appropriate steps for improving diver communicability. The data from four studies are given in Table 2 to indicate rank orders of phonemic intelligibility of speech in air and in helium at normal and hyperbaric pressures. The rankings can be used to generalize about the effectiveness of phonemes with regard to their usefulness in special

Table 2. Specific phonemic intelligibility (%) and its rank order (R) for each of four environmental conditions (specific phonemic intelligibility is the percentage correct for each phoneme (Stim) based on the number of presentations)[a]

Air breathing mixture						Helium and oxygen breathing mixture					
Surface			250-foot depth			Surface			200-foot depth		
R	Stim	%	R	Stim	%	R	Stim	%	R	Stim	%
1	ʃ[b]	97	1	ð	98	1	1	90	1	h[b]	87
2	m[b]	97	2	w	96	2	m	78	2	r[b]	87
3	n	95	3	tʃ	95	3	b	75	3	g	81
4	3	92	4	ʃ	94	4	g	73	4	j	80
5	θ	86	5	r	91	5	n	61	5	s[b]	79
6	t	79	6	g[b]	89	6	p	59	6	n[b]	79
7	d[b]	76	7	v[b]	89	7.5	r	55	7	z	78
8	f[b]	76	8	θ	88	7.5	d	55	8	t[b]	75
9	b[b]	75	9	s	83	9.5	k	49	9	k[b]	75
10	v[b]	75	10	g[b]	82	9.5	t	49	10	l	71
11	s[b]	75	11	d[b]	82	11.5	f	48	11	p[b]	68
12.5	g	60	12	l	79	11.5	w	48	12	b[b]	68
12.5	z	60	13	f	78	13	s	28	13	d_3	66

[a]From Murry et al. (1970).
[b]Rank order determined before rounding off to the nearest percentage correct.

diving vocabularies. However, caution must be applied because different values of phonemic intelligibility probably exist among the various possible combinations of phonemes, especially in those words having consonantal blends.

CORRECTION OF HELIUM SPEECH

There has always been a need for divers to communicate. Before the introduction of a transceiver into the helmet of the hard hat diver, hand signals and jerks upon the diver's tether were used. At depths greater than about 200 feet, helium speech interferes with communicability. Since the basic need for communication remains, there arose the new requirement for a processor which would be able to unscramble the diver's unintelligible helium speech. Until a means of converting helium speech into an acceptable signal was developed, diving protocols for underwater operations continued to be written, knowing the severe limitations of vocal communication.

Elkins (1972) reviewed the basic requirements of the ideal speech communications system. He listed the following points important to such a system.

The divers' training and experience
The input or fidelity of the microphone
The conversion of helium speech
The output characteristics of the system
A small size, enabling easy portability by divers
Controls that are easy to manipulate under water
A minimal requirement for power

Of these, the characteristics of the microphone and the success of conversion determine whether or not intelligible speech is possible. The microphone must respond accurately to the higher frequencies of the upward shifted voice spectrum caused by the helium, and the conversion must be in real time to be of practical use.

All early attempts to unscramble helium speech were doomed to failure from an improper microphone. One approach used existing shallow water microphones which were appropriate to speech in air but not in helium. Consequently, most of the input information required for conversion was lost before getting to the converter. The other typical approach was to use a laboratory quality microphone. However, that was unsuccessful because the frequency response characteristics changed drastically either from the extreme ambient pressures or whenever the microphone was installed within the confines of facemasks. It would be interesting to reevaluate, with a good microphone, unscrambling equipment designed during the 1960's and considered at that time to be unacceptable.

Morrow and Brouns (1971) recently designed a successful gradient microphone for use within diving masks or within hyperbaric chambers. The unit is insensitive to mask cavity acoustics, withstands pressurization and decompression, performs to 10,000 Hz in helium environments, and is amenable to the wet marine environment. This microphone represents a breakthrough in the accurate pick-up of speech within hyperbaric environments.

Probably the first attempts to unscramble helium speech were simply to slow down a taped recording of it. Provided a fairly good quality microphone was part of the recording set-up, the improvement in intelligibility is remarkable. In fact, even the poorer transceivers typically installed inside pressure chambers enable a signal to be understood at depths to 200 feet or more. Three difficulties of the "slow down" technique are: 1) that the conversion is not in real time, 2) the technique ceases to work at those very deep depths where there is the more severe combined effect of pressure and gas mixture, and 3) the much slower speech, although actually more intelligible, still sounds unusual enough to preclude talker recognition.

In 1966, Copel (1966) utilized a heterodyning technique to convert the abnormal helium speech spectrum back to a more normal one. Minor improvement to intelligibility was achieved. However, the technique theoretically was incorrect because it lowered frequencies within several bandwidths by a constant number of cycles. Instead, the spectrum should be lowered by multiplying it by a constant factor, such as 0.58, for an 80:20% mixture of helium and oxygen.

Shortly after Copel's unscrambler was developed, Golden (1966) treated recordings of helium speech obtained inside a habitat located at a depth of 200 feet. He applied formant-restoring vocoder techniques developed at the Bell Telephone Laboratories (Murray Hill, N. J.). Although the equipment was large and expensive (he made use of existing complex computers at the Bell Telephone Laboratories), Golden demonstrated the possibility of appropriate changes that can improve the intelligibility of helium speech as well as make it sound more natural.

During the late 1960's a number of different unscramblers were designed. A brief history of this progress is presented by Tolhurst (1972). After evaluating the improvement to intelligibility of commercially available unscramblers, Rothman and Hollien (1972) concluded that until 1970 "none of the unscramblers provided substantial enough speech improvement to allow for adequate diver-to-diver or diver-to-surface communication."

A milestone in the development of helium speech unscramblers occurred with the development by Gill, Morris, and Edwards (1970; British patent application 29400/70, 1970) of the Admiralty Research Laboratory Processor of Helium Speech. Evaluations of that unit by Murry (1971) revealed excellent intelligibility for the speech of divers talking inside a hyperbaric chamber during a record-breaking dive to 1,500 feet. The breathing atmo-

454 Russell L. Sergeant

sphere contained more than 99% pure helium. Of special interest was the fact that the voices of the divers not only sounded normal, but talker recognition became possible for the first time. The transducer of that processor was a hydrophone which functioned similarly to Morrow's gradient microphone and also produced an accurate high frequency response.

SUMMARY

The world beneath the sea offers a unique application of the field of speech science. The voice becomes distorted by the unusual conditions of the different environments in which the diver must work as well as by tensions and apprehension associated with being under water. Shallow water problems of the scuba diver primarily relate to compatibility of components which comprise the voice communication system with other equipment, enabling the diver to breathe. For operations in deep water or within hyperbaric pressure chambers, there are three considerations. Once the unique problems of measurement are solved, effects of ambient pressures and exotic breathing mixtures must be considered. After an active decade of research by various organizations to design a device which would unscramble hyperbaric helium speech, Gill, Morris, and Edwards (1970) developed a highly successful processor which not only returns intelligibility to the helium speech of deep sea divers but also restores the capability for listeners to recognize which individual diver is doing the talking.

Research in the development of future underwater communication systems will improve existing equipment by making components lighter, smaller, more reliable, cheaper, and easier for the swimmer to carry. Perceptual tests of speech performance will continue to be important as a metric to evaluate future systems designed to improve the ability of man to communicate vocally underwater.

REFERENCES

Camp, R. T. 1956. The effect of noise environment upon speaker intelligibility. Joint project, Ohio State University Research Foundation and U.S. Navy School of Aviation Medicine. Joint project report 63. 12 p.

Cooke, J. P., and S. E. Beard. 1965. Verbal communication intelligibility in oxygen-helium, and other breathing mixtures, at low atmospheric pressures. Aerosp. Med. 36: 1167–1172.

Copel, M. 1966. Helium voice unscrambling. IEEE Trans. Audio. Electroacoust. 14: 122–126.

Elkins, J. H. 1972. Requirements of the ideal helium-speech communications system: General and specific. *In* R. L. Sergeant and T. Murry (eds.), Processing Helium-Speech: Proceedings of a Navy-Sponsored Workshop— August 1971, pp. 39–52. Naval Submarine Medical Research Laboratory Report 708, Groton, Conn.

Fant, G. M., J. Lindqvist, B. Sonesson, and H. Hollien. 1971. Speech distortion at high pressures. *In*: C. J. Lambertson (ed.), Underwater Physiology. Academic Press, New York.

Fant, G., and B. Sonesson. 1964. Speech at high ambient air-pressure. Speech Transmission Lab. Q. Prog. Status Rep. 2: 9—21.

Gill, J. S., R. Morris, and M. G. Edwards. 1970. A time-domain processor for helium speech. I.E.R.E. Conf. Proc. 19: 523—528.

Golden, R. M. 1966. Improving naturalness and intelligibility of helium-oxygen speech using vocoder techniques. J. Acoust. Soc. Amer. 40: 621—624.

Hollien, H. H., B. Rothman, and S. H. Feinstein. 1973. The auditory sensitivity of divers at high pressures, CSL/ONR Tech Rep. 50. Communication Sciences Laboratory, University of Florida, Gainesville. 17 p.

Hollien, H., and G. Tolhurst. 1969. A research program in diver communication. Naval Res. Reviews 22: 1—13.

McKay, C. L., and R. L. Sergeant. 1968. The intelligibility of helium-speech as a function of speech-to-noise ratio. Naval Submarine Medical Research Laboratory Report 555, Groton, Conn. 5 p.

Morrow, C. T., and A. J. Brouns. 1971. Speech communication in diving masks. I. Acoustics of microphones and mask cavities. J. Acoust. Soc. Amer. 50: 1—22.

Murry, T. 1971. The intelligibility of processed helium speech at depths greater than 1000 feet. Naval Submarine Medical Research Laboratory Report 697, Groton, Conn. 6 p.

Murry, T., R. L. Sergeant, and C. Angermeier. 1970. Navy diver/swimmer vocabularies: Phonemic intelligibility in hyperbaric environments. Naval Submarine Medical Research Laboratory Report 648, Groton, Conn. 16 p.

Rothman, H. B., and H. Hollien. 1972. An investigation of helium-speech unscramblers under controlled conditions. *In* R. L. Sergeant and T. Murry (eds.), Processing Helium-Speech: Proceedings of a Navy-Sponsored Workshop—August, 1971, pp. 39—52. Naval Submarine Medical Research Laboratory Report 708, Groton, Conn.

Sergeant, R. L. 1963. Speech during respiration a mixture of helium and oxygen. Aerosp. Med. 34: 826—829.

Sergeant, R. L. 1966. The effect of frequency passband upon the intelligibility of helium-speech in noise. Naval Submarine Medical Research Laboratory Report 480, Groton, Conn. 5 p.

Sergeant, R. L. 1973. The intelligibility of hydrogen speech. J. Acoust. Soc. Amer. 54: 300(A).

Sergeant, R. L., and T. Murry. 1971. Reciprocity calibration of microphones under high ambient pressures. Naval Submarine Medical Research Laboratory Report 671, Groton, Conn.

Siebe, Gorman and Co., Ltd. 19 April 1916. Advertisement in The Syren and Shipping Illustrated, London.

Thomas, W. G., M. J. Preslar, and J. C. Farmer. 1972. Calibration of condenser microphones under increased atmospheric pressures. J. Acoust. Soc. Amer. 51: 6—14.

Tolhurst, G. 1972. A history of helium-speech processing instrumentation. *In* R. L. Sergeant and T. Murry (eds.), Processing Helium-Speech: Proceedings of a Navy-Sponsored Workshop—August, 1971, pp. 4—10. Naval Medical Research Laboratory Report 708, Groton, Conn.

Willott, J. F., and R. L. Sergeant. 1968. Auditory feedback and helium-speech. Naval Submarine Medical Research Laboratory Report 544, Groton, Conn. 5 p.

Author Index

Subject Index